INTRODUCTION TO
HUMAN BIOCHEMICAL
AND
MOLECULAR GENETICS

INTRODUCTION TO

HUMAN
BIOCHEMICAL
AND
MOLECULAR
GENETICS

Arthur L. Beaudet, M.D.
Charles R. Scriver, M.D.C.M.
William S. Sly, M.D.
David Valle, M.D.
Victor A. McKusick, M.D.
John B. Stanbury, M.D.
James B. Wyngaarden, M.D.
Donald S. Fredrickson, M.D.
Joseph L. Goldstein, M.D.
Michael S. Brown, M.D.

McGRAW-HILL, INC.
HEALTH PROFESSIONS DIVISION
New York   St Louis   San Francisco   Colorado Springs   Auckland
Bogotá   Caracas   Hamburg   Lisbon   London   Madrid   Mexico   Milan   Montreal
New Delhi   Panama   Paris   San Juan   São Paulo   Singapore   Sydney   Tokyo   Toronto

1234567890   MALMAL   9876543210

ISBN 0-07-004262-4

The editor was Gail Gavert.
The production supervisor was Annette Mayeski.
The cover was designed by MN'O Production Services, Inc.
Malloy Lithographers, Inc., was printer and binder.

Library of Congress Cataloging-in-Publication Data

Introduction to human biochemical and molecular genetics / Arthur L.
    Beaudet . . . [et al.].
      p.   cm
      Includes bibliographical references.
      ISBN 0-07-004262-4 :
      1. Genetic disorders. 2. Molecular genetics. 3. Biochemical
genetics. I. Beaudet, Arthur L.
      [DNLM: 1. Genetics, Biochemical. 2. Genetics, Medical.
3. Hereditary Diseases.   QH 431 I613]
RB155.5.I57   1990
616'.042--dc20
DNLM/DLC
for Library of Congress   90-5414
                                                                        CIP

CONTENTS

AUTHORS' AFFILIATIONS

Arthur L. Beaudet, M.D.
Investigator, Howard Hughes Medical Institute; Professor, Institute for Molecular Genetics and Departments of Pediatrics and Cell Biology, Baylor College of Medicine, Houston, Texas

Michael S. Brown, M.D.
Paul J. Thomas Professor of Medicine and Genetics, University of Texas Southwestern Medical Center, Dallas, Texas

Donald S. Fredrickson, M.D.
Researcher, Molecular Disease Branch, National Heart, Lung and Blood Institute; Scholar, National Library of Medicine, National Institutes of Health, Bethesda, Maryland

Joseph L. Goldstein, M.D.
Paul J. Thomas Professor of Genetics and Chairman, Department of Molecular Genetics, University of Texas Southwestern Medical Center, Dallas, Texas

Victor A. McKusick, M.D.
University Professor of Medical Genetics, The Johns Hopkins University School of Medicine; Physician, The Johns Hopkins Hospital, Baltimore, Maryland

Charles R. Scriver, M.D.C.M.
Professor of Biology, Human Genetics and Pediatrics, Departments of Biology and Pediatrics and Center for Human Genetics, McGill University, Montreal, Canada

William S. Sly, M.D.
Alice A. Doisy Professor of Biochemistry and Professor of Pediatrics; Chairman, Edward A. Doisy Department of Biochemistry and Molecular Biology, St. Louis University School of Medicine, St. Louis, Missouri

John B. Stanbury, M.D.
Honorary Physician, Massachusetts General Hospital; Division of Health Science and Technology, Massachusetts Institute of Technology, Boston, Massachusetts

David Valle, M.D.
Investigator, Howard Hughes Medical Institute; Professor of Pediatrics, Medicine, and Molecular Biology & Genetics, The Johns Hopkins University School of Medicine, Baltimore, Maryland

James B. Wyngaarden, M.D.
Associate Director for Life Sciences, Office of Science and Technology Policy, Executive Office of The President, Washington, D.C.

When we were preparing the sixth edition of *The Metabolic Basis of Inherited Disease* (MBID), we surmised that the first chapter of that text could serve as a useful, brief introduction to the principles of biochemical, molecular, and human genetics. This material is an overview, distilled and refined through six editions and 30 years of scientific effort.

Undergraduate and graduate students in biomedical science, medical students, and faculty members can use this little book as an ancillary to their courses and in conjunction with the parent text, MBID. To that end, we kept all the cross references to specific chapters within this version; interested readers will find detailed discussion of particular problems in the larger text. The complete bibliography is retained to give readers a broad introduction to the literature. The Summary Table, which lists the Mendelian disorders and other genetic diseases covered in MBID, is also reproduced here to indicate the present breadth of knowledge about these disorders.

The parent text and its offspring differ in significant ways, including the following:

• Dr. Victor McKusick has provided the most current (January 1990) version available of the human gene and morbid anatomy gene map, located in Appendix 1, "Genetic Map of the Human Genome Autosomes, and X, Y, and Mitochondrial Chromosomes." We also explain how to use the material in this appendix. The gene map used in the first printing of the parent book, dated March 25, 1988, and the present version differ significantly!
• An alphabetized list by disorder in Appendix 2 indicates location on the human genome map of mapped mutations.
• We have compiled a new Selected Readings list. It features books and journals we have found useful, entertaining, or both.
• "Analysis and Diagnosis of Human Inherited Disease by Recombinant DNA Methods," an appendix in the parent text, does not appear here.

THE RATIONALE FOR PARENT AND OFFSPRING

The Metabolic Basis of Inherited Disease, sixth edition, reflects a wealth of knowledge. The fruits of molecular genetics now appear in one chapter after another. If MBID has had an abiding rationale, it was that the causes of all diseases listed in the text were Mendelian and the diseases (so-called inborn errors of metabolism) were exceptions to be treated for their illumination of human biology and for the insight they gave into pathogenesis of disease. But always there was the feeling that one did not understand cause as well as one should because not enough was known about the genes. That situation is changing rapidly. Every week there are new data about loci and structure of numerous normal genes affecting the phenotype (those identifiable or observable characteristics of an organism) encoded by them.

Basic principles and lessons of human genetics, exemplified in disease after disease, include: the biochemical basis of Mendelian inheritance; dominance and recessivity; gene, gene product, and phenotype relationships; allelic and nonallelic heterogeneity; molecular analysis of mutations; monogenic, multifactorial, and environmental interactions; linkage disequilibrium; haplotype analysis; selective advantage; biochemical and molecular diagnosis; heterozygote and newborn screening methods; and pathogenesis. What the present little book offers is a concise, historical perspective and summation of what we know about them as they relate to a well-known set of phenotypes reflecting human genetic variation.

WHAT THE PARENT TEXT CAN TELL YOU—AND WHY YOU WANT TO KNOW

Some topics in the current edition of MBID are particularly well suited for additional reading, for example:

Phenylketonuria, the prototypic amino acid disorder, illustrates a complex enzymology, demonstrates allelic and nonallelic heterogeneity, shows how dietary therapy relaxes selection, and provides examples of the genetic and molecular aspects of mutation.

Disorders of propionate and methylmalonate metabolism are typical illustrations of organic acidemia and how vitamins interact with metabolic pathways.

Familial hypercholesterolemia is the modern day example of how intense study of patients with a single inherited disease can lead to broad new insights into biology and medicine. It illustrates extensive molecular heterogeneity and the biochemical basis for a dominantly inherited disorder. It also reveals how individual genes may interact and how they and nongenetic factors precipitate disease (e.g., atherosclerosis) in the predisposed patient.

The mucopolysaccharidoses provide prototypic examples of lysosomal storage diseases. There are examples of multiple phenotypes due to different mutations at a single locus and of indistinguishable phenotypes due to mutations at different loci.

I-cell disease exemplifies how a defect in posttranslational processing can lead to secondary abnormalities in many different enzymes.

The G_{M2} gangliosidoses embody principles and practices for heterozygote screening in populations at risk for prevention of genetic disease.

Synthesis of hormones require enzymes, and there are inborn errors of hormone synthesis. *Congenital adrenal hyperplasia* is the classic disease in this category and now there are recognizable diseases of hormonal end-organ unresponsiveness, for example, the *androgen resistance syndromes*.

Coagulation factor VIII deficiency (hemophilia A) illustrates many themes of classical genetics and modern mutation analysis. The triumphs and failures of replacement therapy for hemophilia provide other important lessons.

Hemoglobinopathies, Duchenne muscular dystrophy, and cystic fibrosis are common, important human genetic disorders that teach us many lessons. A major development, in fact, since the publication of MBID 6/e has been the cloning and characterization of the cystic fibrosis gene (*Science* 245;1059, 1066,1073:1989).

Disorders of collagen synthesis and function demonstrate how complex, specialized, posttranslational processing and intricate macromolecular structures can be disturbed by mutations affecting the parent molecule and its processing machinery. Different mutations in the same gene can give rise to mild or severe phenotypes, or even to dominant or recessive alleles.

The past editors of MBID—John B. Stanbury, James B. Wyngaarden, Donald S. Fredrickson, Joseph L. Goldstein, and Michael S. Brown—in their turn wrote the introductory chapter to successive editions of the parent text. This text therefore reflects those strata; the former editors are our co-authors now. In addition, Victor A. McKusick and his assistant, Joanna M. Strayer, kindly provided the material in Appendixes 1 and 2. As with the parent text, many people contributed to the preparation of this volume, notably Gail Gavert and J. Dereck Jeffers at McGraw-Hill; Loy Denis; and our own assistants: Grace Watson (AB), Lynne Prevost and Hugette Rizziero (CRS), Elizabeth Torno (WS), and Sandy Muscelli (DV).

Arthur L. Beaudet
Charles R. Scriver
William S. Sly
David Valle

INTRODUCTION TO

HUMAN BIOCHEMICAL
AND
MOLECULAR GENETICS

INTRODUCTION TO HUMAN BIOCHEMICAL AND MOLECULAR GENETICS

The medical model of disease holds that *manifestations* are the result of a *process* which has a *cause*. The manifestations of disease are assembled in *diagnosis* and they constitute a *taxonomy*. The process which underlies them is the *pathogenesis* of disease. The cause of disease is either an event that overwhelms homeostatic mechanisms (an *extrinsic* cause) or one that undermines them (an *intrinsic* cause). Most diseases involve a combination of both (a multifactorial cause).

This text has three unifying themes, the first and central one being that the causes of the diseases described are mutations (intrinsic). Because these mutations are usually expressed as *disadaptive phenotypes* (i.e., clinical manifestations) in the universal environment, they are simply inherited and classified as *Mendelian disorders*. Some chapters describe more complex causes with non-Mendelian inheritance as in the case of Down syndrome (Chap. 7,* a chromosomal disease) and diabetes mellitus (Chap. 10, a multifactorial disease). The discussion of LDL receptor deficiency (Chap. 48) and other lipoprotein disorders illustrates how a disease of heterogeneous etiology (coronary artery disease) is being broken down into its component causes, some cases being caused by single gene defects and some cases being of multifactorial etiology. This edition, when compared with earlier editions, reveals an enormous increase in our knowledge about genetic cause at the molecular level. This knowledge is applied increasingly through the use of recombinant DNA methods in clinical counseling.

This text's second unifying theme deals with pathogenesis in great detail. Knowledge of the pathophysiology of a disease explains its manifestations, is necessary for rational treatment, and may even suggest that treatment is not feasible.[1] It can be taken for granted that at least partial knowledge of pathogenesis is important for the treatment of most inborn errors of metabolism. Successive editions document the expansion of knowledge about cause and pathogenesis of inherited diseases. In due course, this text, or one like it, should become a fundamental textbook for the theory and practice of medicine, since most diseases in developed societies have a genetic determinant. Every individual is a deviant in terms of biochemical individuality,[2] meaning that every person has an inherited predisposition to disease (diathesis) in a particular circumstance. This is no new idea; Garrod expounded it thoroughly and

clearly in his second book.[3] The difference between then and now is simply that molecular methods have made it possible to see in our DNA our inherited predispositions. We can either avoid the occurrence of serious disease genotypes through genetic counseling procedures or ameliorate symptoms through treatment. Therapy of inherited diseases constitutes the third unifying theme of this text.

The power of current cellular, molecular, and metabolic techniques is that they provide a vast amount of new information. There is the astounding prospect of identifying the biochemical defects for a large proportion of the thousands of disease phenotypes catalogued by McKusick in *Mendelian Inheritance in Man*.[4] At the Human Gene Mapping conference held in 1987, the chromosomal location of more than 1300 genes and 2000 anonymous DNA segments had been identified.[5] A detailed map of the human genome is becoming a reality (see Appendix 1 below and Chap. 6), and there are serious proposals to sequence the entire human genome.[6]

This avalanche of new information brings with it important new perspectives and goals. Metabolic, molecular, and genetic details are now available for hemoglobinopathies, phenylketonuria, Tay-Sachs disease, and many other disorders included in the chapters of this volume. Diseases such as cystic fibrosis, Duchenne muscular dystrophy, Huntington disease, adult polycystic kidney disease, and hereditary retinoblastoma, which have long resisted definition of the biochemical defect, are now yielding to investigation. Several gaps in current knowledge are likely to be the focus of future endeavors. Studies of inherited disorders of morphogenesis (which are often autosomal dominant) and of the function of the central nervous system (for which, it is said, a third of our genes are dedicated) will facilitate the understanding of these complex biologic processes. Elucidation of the biochemial basis of phenotypes caused by interaction between nongenetic factors and genetic variation at multiple loci will become increasingly feasible. We can hope to achieve an increased understanding of the homeostatic disturbances which underlie the clinical phenotypes of disorders whose molecular and biochemical lesions are already known. Challenges are posed to our understanding of pathogenesis both by classic questions such as what mechanism causes mental retardation in phenylketonuria and when

---

*Chapter numbers refer to *The Metabolic Basis of Inherited Disease*, sixth edition.

3

new genes are cloned before we comprehend their biochemistry, as in the case of hereditary retinoblastoma (Chap. 9). Efforts to understand the molecular and biochemical bases underlying human genetic variation are more vigorous than ever. New techniques allow for the study of unique individuals in great detail. Garrod[7] quoted a letter written by William Harvey in 1657 to emphasize the value of studying human variants:

Nature is nowhere accustomed more openly to display her secret mysteries than in cases where she shows traces of her workings apart from the beaten path; nor is there any better way to advance the proper practice of medicine than to give our minds to the discovery of the usual law of Nature by careful investigation of cases of rarer forms of disease. For it has been found, in almost all things, that what they contain of useful or applicable is hardly perceived unless we are deprived of them, or they become deranged in some way.

This thesis has many modern proponents. Basic scientists are attracted to the study of human genetic diseases in increasing numbers, and the most prestigious scientific journals vie to report the latest accomplishments. Reports such as the identification of the human gene determining sex[8] and of the product of the Duchenne muscular dystrophy gene[9] are prominently reported in leading newspapers. This is a golden era for the study of inherited metabolic disease.

DEVELOPMENT OF THE CONCEPT OF INHERITED METABOLIC DISEASE

Inborn Error Concept (Garrod)

The history of human biochemical genetics began at the turn of the twentieth century, when Sir Archibald Garrod initiated the brilliant studies of alkaptonuria that were to culminate in his Croonian Lectures in 1908[10] and in his monograph, *Inborn Errors of Metabolism*, which appeared in 1909 and in modified form in 1923.[11]

Garrod had observed that patients with alkaptonuria excreted large, rather constant quantities of homogentisic acid throughout their lifetimes, whereas other persons excreted none at all.[12] He observed that this condition had a familial distribution and that, while frequently one or more sibs were involved, parents and more distant relatives were normal. There was a high incidence of consanguineous marriages in the parents of his patients, as well as in the parents of similar patients studied elsewhere. On conferring with Bateson, one of the earliest of the great school of British geneticists, Garrod learned that these observations could readily be explained if the defect were inherited as a recessive condition in terms of the recently rediscovered laws of Mendel.[13,14]

From his observations of patients with alkaptonuria, albinism, cystinuria, and pentosuria, Garrod developed the concept that certain diseases of lifelong duration arise because an enzyme governing a single metabolic step is reduced in activity or missing altogether.[15] Garrod viewed the accumulation of homogentisic acid in alkaptonuria as evidence that this substance is a normal metabolite in the dissimilation of tyrosine, and he correctly attributed its accumulation to a failure of oxidation of homogentisic acid. A half-century later, Garrod's hypothesis was proved by the demonstration of deficient activity of homogentisic acid oxidase in the liver of a patient with alkaptonuria.[16]

Similarly, the failure of pigment formation in the skin in albinism, the excretion of large amounts of cystine in the urine in cystinuria, and the appearance of pentose in the urine in essential pentosuria were viewed by Garrod as the results of blocks in normal metabolic pathways. He attributed the first instance to failure of melanin formation and the other two to excretion of metabolites accumulating proximal to a metabolic block.

One Gene–One Enzyme Concept (Beadle and Tatum)

The term *gene* was first applied to the hereditary determinant of a unit characteristic by Johannsen in 1911.[17] The relation between gene and enzyme attained clear definition in the one gene–one enzyme principle, first succinctly stated by Beadle in 1945.[18] This formulation, now a biologic precept, emerged gradually from studies of eye color in the fruit fly, *Drosophila*, by Beadle and Tatum[19,20] and Ephrussi.[21] It received extensive support from the classic studies of Beadle and Tatum on induced mutants of *Neurospora crassa*, in which acquisitions of requirements for specific metabolites in the culture medium were traced to losses of single chemical transformations, each dependent on a different enzyme.[22,23]

The one gene–one enzyme concept that developed from these experiments has been well expressed by Tatum[23] as follows:

1. All biochemical processes in all organisms are under genetic control.
2. These biochemical processes are resolvable into series of individual stepwise reactions.
3. Each biochemical reaction is under the ultimate control of a different single gene.
4. Mutation of a single gene results only in an alteration in the ability of the cell to carry out a single primary chemical reaction.

The one gene–one enzyme hypothesis has since been refined[24] and extended to cover proteins that are not enzymes, as well as complex proteins composed of nonidentical polypeptide chains linked in various ways. The functional unit of DNA which controls the structure of a single polypeptide chain is frequently called a *cistron*.[25] The one gene–one enzyme principle has been redefined as the one cistron–one polypeptide concept. Posttranslational cleavage to generate multiple peptides, alternative splicing, and alternative promoter sequences contribute to complexities of the concept. Some examples of the complexity and variations involved in the one gene–one enzyme concept are presented in Table 1-1.

The one gene–one enzyme concept had immediate explanatory potential for the inborn errors of metabolism that Garrod had described. It appeared that inherited diseases such as alkaptonuria were produced by mutations in genes encoding enzymes in the same way that vitamin-dependent mutants of *Neurospora* lacked single enzymes required for vitamin synthesis. It was not until 1948 that the first enzyme defect in a human genetic disease was demonstrated by Gibson. This was the deficiency of the NADH-dependent enzyme required for

Table 1-1 Complexity and Variations in the One Gene–One Enzyme Concept

Concept	Examples	Chapter or (Reference)
One gene–one enzyme	Phenylalanine hydroxylase	15
	Hypoxanthine-guanine phosphoribosyl-transferase	38
One gene–nonenzymatic protein	Collagens	115
	Spectrin	95
One gene–RNA product	Transfer RNA, ribosomal RNA	1,2
One enzyme activity requires multiple subunits from separate genes	Propionyl CoA carboxylase	29
	Hexosaminidase A	72
One subunit functions in multiple enzymes	Hexosaminidases A and B	72
	E_3 subunit of dehydrogenases	22,32
One polypeptide chain with multiple enzyme activities	Orotate phosphoribosyl transferase and orotidine-5′-phosphate decarboxylase	43
	CAD tri-enzyme protein	(Ref. 26)
Deficiency of one enzyme causes multiple secondary enzyme deficiencies	Cobalamin C and D	82
	UDP-N-acetylglucosamine (GlcNAc): glycoprotein GlcNAc 1-phosphotransferase	62
Posttranslational cleavage of a peptide	ACTH (adrenocorticotrophic hormone), endorphins	(Ref. 27,28)
Alternative promoters for transcription	Amylase	(Ref. 29)
Alternative splicing of pre-mRNA	Calcitonin	(Ref. 30)
	Muscle proteins	(Ref. 31,32)
DNA rearrangements prior to transcription	Immunoglobulins	109
	T-cell receptors	110
Posttranscriptional modification of mRNA	Apolipoproteins B-100 and B-48	44B
Overlapping reading frames in DNA and RNA, suppression, frameshifting	Bacterial release factor	(Ref. 33)
	Retroviruses	(Ref. 34)

the reduction of methemoglobin in recessive methemoglobinemia.[35] This was soon followed by the description in 1952 by Cori and Cori of glucose-6-phosphatase deficiency in von Gierke disease (glycogen storage disease, type I)[36] and in 1953 by Jervis of phenylalanine hydroxylase deficiency in phenylketonuria.[37]

Molecular Disease Concept (Pauling and Ingram)

Direct evidence that human mutations actually produce an alteration in the primary structure of proteins was first obtained in 1949 by Pauling and his associates.[38] Studying hemoglobin extracted from erythrocytes of patients with sickle-cell anemia, Pauling showed that sickle hemoglobin migrated differently in an electric field than did normal hemoglobin. Heterozygotes for the sickle-cell trait produced both normal and abnormal hemoglobin molecules. The subsequent studies of Ingram established that the electrophoretic abnormality arose because sickle-cell hemoglobin had a valine substituted for a glutamic acid residue at a particular point in the amino acid sequence.[39] This finding closed one era of discovery in human biochemical genetics: Inborn errors of metabolism were caused by mutant genes that produced abnormal proteins whose functional activities were altered.

Reverse Genetics

With the identification of a restriction fragment length polymorphism (RFLP) at the β-globin locus by Kan and Dozy,[40] the concept of a new and virtually inexhaustible source of genetic markers for the exploration of inherited human disease

became a reality. Quickly thereafter, Botstein et al.[41] proposed the feasibility of creating a linkage map of the human genome using RFLPs. Following these strategies, it became possible using genetic linkage analysis to identify DNA markers close to human disease loci.

"Reverse genetics" has been used to describe a variety of investigative approaches but is used here to describe the strategy of mapping and cloning genes prior to the identification of their products[42] (Chap. 2). For the great majority of disorders described in this volume, the gene product and its general function were identified long before the molecular characterization of the gene as exemplified for hemoglobin and phenylalanine hydroxylase. The reverse genetic strategy utilizes genetic information to clone a gene prior to the identification of the product. This approach was developed in bacterial genetics and has been extended in recent years to the study of Drosophila as exemplified by the characterization of homeotic genes which are involved in development.[43] The construction of a genomic map of the location of RFLPs is allowing for the extension of this approach to human diseases. Information gained from rare patients with visible cytogenetic abnormalities in association with single gene disorders, so-called contiguous gene syndromes, also has played a major role in early successes using reverse genetics (Chap. 9). The genes for chronic granulomatous disease[44] (Chap. 114), Duchenne muscular dystrophy[45] (Chap. 118), and hereditary retinoblastoma[46] (Chap. 9) were cloned by these approaches. The genes for Huntington disease,[47] adult polycystic kidney disease,[48] neurofibromatosis,[49] Von Hippel-Lindau disease,[50] polyposis of the colon,[51] and others have been mapped to specific sites in the human genome and are likely to be cloned in the foreseeable future. The continuing value of individual patients as experiments of nature was exemplified by the identification of a single patient with a deletion of chromosome 5 in association with polyposis of the colon leading to the mapping of the polyposis locus using RFLPs.[51,52]

The practice and performance of investigation of inherited disease are changing with this explosion of techniques. While the role of the individual laboratory remains prominent, often multiple laboratories, each with particular areas of expertise, contribute to the investigation of a disorder. As part of efforts to map the human genome, a massive international collaboration has been organized under the auspices of Centre d'Étude du Polymorphisme Humain (CEPH) (Chap. 6).[53] DNA samples on over 500 individuals from 40 large sibships have been prepared and are being analyzed for RFLPs by laboratories around the world. The data are returned to a computerized data base for collaborative analysis to construct a human gene map.

Recent molecular studies of cystic fibrosis represent another example of international collaboration and interaction (Chap. 108). Laboratories around the world collected samples from cystic fibrosis families for the purposes of linkage analysis. The first linkage to a protein polymorphism was reported from Copenhagen,[54] while the first DNA linkage which allowed chromosomal assignment was discovered in Toronto using a DNA probe isolated by a laboratory in Boston.[55] With the assignment of the cystic fibrosis locus to chromosome 7, more closely linked DNA markers were identified in Salt Lake City[56] and London.[57] A collaboration of nine laboratories provided detailed linkage data for 211 families in a short time.[58] The expansion of collaborative efforts has been accompanied by an increasing role of commercial laboratories in the investigation of inherited disease, which was once the almost exclusive purview of academic investigators.

With international proposals to map and sequence the human genome, it is possible that most human genes will be identified before any relationship to product or phenotype is established. This rather anonymous genetics has been experienced to some extent with the availability of the entire sequence for human mitochondrial DNA and the identification of open reading frames (coding segments) prior to information regarding the products or phenotypes which might be associated with these genes. While "anonymous" genetics may not seem attractive as an intellectual pursuit, its impact on the study of inherited disease is certain to be great.

MOLECULAR BASIS OF GENE EXPRESSION

The human genome is estimated to contain about 50,000 to 100,000 genes, each of which is composed of a linear polymer of DNA. The genes are assembled into lengthy linear arrays that together with certain proteins form rod-shaped bodies called *chromosomes*. All normal nucleated human cells other than sperm or ova contain 46 chromosomes, arrayed in 23 pairs, one of each pair derived from each of the individual's parents. The striking discovery that genes are not continuous sequences of DNA but consist of coding sequences (exons) interrupted by intervening sequences (introns) led to a new and more complex view of gene expression.

Some approximations regarding the magnitude and organization of the human genome are presented in Fig. 1-1. The estimated 50,000 to 100,000 genes are distributed within the 3 billion base pairs of DNA which constitute a haploid genome.

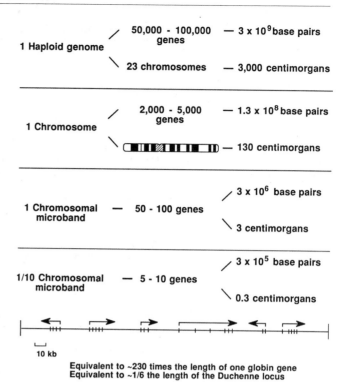

Fig. 1-1 Perspectives on the amount of DNA, number of genes, and genetic distance in the human genome. The arrows in the lowest panel indicate hypothetical transcripts with vertical lines indicating exons within genes.

Linkage studies indicate that the human genome comprises approximately 3000 centimorgans (cM) in recombination distance. A centimorgan (1/100 of a Morgan) is a measure of genetic distance reflecting the probability of a crossover between two loci during meiosis. One centimorgan approximately equals a recombination fraction of 0.01 or a 1 percent chance of a crossover during meiosis. Thus an average chromosome would contain 2000 to 5000 genes within 130 million base pairs of DNA and would be equivalent to about 130 cM of genetic material. A typical microband on a stained chromosome contains 3 to 5 million base pairs and 50 to 100 genes. This representation oversimplifies many issues. Estimates of the total number of genes are imprecise. Although the average recombination distance is estimated to be approximately 1 cM per million base pairs of DNA, there is wide variation in this rate over shorter distances, as well as differences in recombination distance according to sex (Chap. 6). Genes range in size from very small (1.5 kb for a globin gene) to very large (perhaps 2000 kb for the Duchenne muscular dystrophy locus). Cis-acting regulatory elements (i.e., on the contiguous DNA strand) may occur at a considerable distance from the coding region, e.g., 50 kb 5' and 20 kb 3' to the β-globin gene,[59] thus extending the functional domains of genes and complicating the definition of boundaries.

The human genome also includes numerous nonfunctional sequences and highly reiterated sequences.[60] There are 300,000 to 500,000 copies of the *Alu* repeat sequence (the most reiterated sequence which derives its name from the frequency with which it is cut by the restriction enzyme *Alu*I) in the human genome. Many other reiterated sequences occur with lesser frequency. Many genes have additional nonfunctional copies (pseudogenes), and the sequence distribution of human DNA is not uniform. For example, HTF (*Hpa*I tiny fragment) islands are G-plus-C-rich regions which occur near the 5' end of constitutive genes and are thought to have some relationship to regulation of gene expression.[61] The functional significance of the majority of DNA which occurs outside coding regions remains to be determined.

The Molecular Flow of Information

Much is known about how living organisms store, transmit, and utilize their genetic information. The picture is most detailed for prokaryotic organisms, but information is being acquired rapidly for the more complex eukaryotic organisms. Two excellent textbooks[62,63] provide a more systematic and comprehensive treatment of cellular and molecular biology than is included here. The fourth edition of *Molecular Biology of the Gene* by Watson and colleagues[64] provides a detailed view of the molecular flow of information in prokaryotic and eukaryotic organisms.

The genetic information carried on chromosomes is transmitted to daughter cells under two different sets of circumstances. One of these occurs whenever a somatic cell (i.e., a nongerm cell) divides. This process, called *mitosis*, functions to transmit two identical copies of each gene to each daughter cell, thus maintaining a uniform genetic makeup in all cells of a single organism. The other set of circumstances prevails when genetic information is to be transmitted from one individual to an offspring. This process, called *meiosis*, functions to produce germ cells (i.e., ova or spermatozoa) that possess only one copy of each parental chromosome, thus allowing for new combinations of chromosomes to occur when the ovum and sperm cell fuse during fertilization and restoring the *diploid* state.

During the process of meiosis, the 46 chromosomes of an immature germ cell arrange themselves in 23 pairs at the center of the nucleus, each pair being composed of one chromosome derived from the mother and its homologous chromosome derived from the father. At a specified point in the meiotic process, the two partner chromosomes separate, only one of each pair going into each daughter cell, or gamete. Thus, meiosis produces gametes with a reduction in the number of chromosomes from 46 to 23, each gamete having received one chromosome from each of the 23 pairs. The assortment of the chromosomes within each pair is random, so that each germ cell receives a different combination of maternal and paternal chromosomes. During the process of fertilization the fusion of ovum and sperm cell, each of which has 23 chromosomes, results ultimately in an individual with 46 chromosomes.

The independent assortment of chromosomes into gametes during meiosis produces an enormous diversity among the possible genotypes of the progeny. For each 23 pairs of chromosomes, there are 2^{23} different combinations of chromosomes that could occur in a gamete, and the likelihood that one set of parents will produce two offspring with the identical complement of chromosomes is one in 2^{23} or one in 8.4 million (assuming no monozygotic twins). Adding even further to the enormous genetic diversity in humans is the phenomenon of *genetic recombination* (see "Genetic Linkage and the Human Gene Map," below, and Chap. 6).

The Structure of DNA

Most organisms store their genetic information in *deoxyribonucleic acid (DNA)*. DNA is a linear polymer of four different monomeric units, collectively called *deoxyribonucleotides* or simply *nucleotides*, that are linked together in a chain by phosphodiester bonds (Fig. 1-2). A typical DNA molecule consists of two interwound polynucleotide chains, each containing several thousand to several million monomers (Fig. 1-3). Each nucleotide in one chain is specifically linked by hydrogen bonds to a nucleotide in the other chain. Only two nucleotide pairings are found in DNA: deoxyadenosine monophosphate with thymidine monophosphate (or A-T) and deoxyguanosine monophosphate with deoxycytidine monophosphate (or G-C). Thus, the sequence of nucleotides of one chain fixes the sequence of the other, and the two chains are therefore said to be *complementary* to each other.

The sequence of the four nucleotides along a polynucleotide chain varies among the DNAs of unrelated organisms and in-

Fig. 1-2 A polynucleotide chain. One of each of the four different monomeric units of DNA is present in this tetranucleotide. The monomers of DNA are, from top to bottom, deoxyguanosine monophosphate (or G), deoxycytidine monophosphate (or C), deoxyadenosine monophosphate (or A), and thymidine monophosphate (or T). Each nucleotide consists of a phosphate group, a deoxyribose moiety, and a heterocyclic base. G and A have purine bases, and C and T have pyrimidine bases. The phosphodiester bonds that link adjacent nucleotides extend from the 3' position of one deoxyribose moiety to the 5' position of the next; this gives the chain a chemical polarity. An abbreviated way of writing the same sequence is shown at the top right. In RNA (see text) ribose, which contains a 2'-hydroxyl group, replaces deoxyribose, and uridine monophosphate (or U) replaces T. U differs from T in the substitution of ribose for deoxyribose and in the loss of the 5-methyl group.

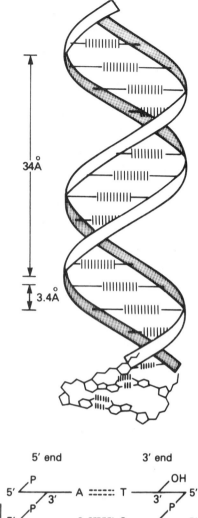

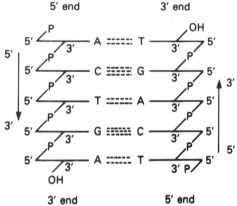

Fig. 1-3 The structure of DNA. *Top.* The two interwound hydrogen-bonded polynucleotide chains of DNA are shown. The hydrogen bonds are indicated by vertical hatches. The distance between adjacent nucleotide pairs is 3.4 Å. The distance between adjacent turns of the double helix is 34 Å or about 10 nucleotide pairs. *Bottom.* An alternative representation in which the opposite chemical polarities of the two chains can be clearly seen. (*From Kornberg.*[65] *Used by permission.*)

deed is the molecular basis of their genetic diversity. Because most genetic characteristics are stably transmitted from parent to progeny, the sequence of nucleotides in DNA must be faithfully copied or replicated as the organism reproduces itself. This occurs by unwinding of the two chains and polymerization of two daughter chains along the separated parental strands. The nucleotide sequence and hence the genetic information is conserved during this process because each nucleotide in the daughter chains is paired specifically with its

complement in the parental or template chains before polymerization occurs.

The DNA of higher organisms, separated from the great bulk of cellular components by a nuclear membrane, is wound into a tightly and regularly packed chromosomal structure consisting of nucleoprotein elements called *nucleosomes.* Each of these nucleosomal elements is in turn composed of four (sometimes five) protein subunits, *histones,* that form a core structure about which are wound approximately 140 nucleotide pairs of genomic DNA. Histone structure is remarkably well conserved throughout the eukaryotic kingdom. Such conservation argues strongly that strict functional requirements, presumably related to the detailed architecture of the nucleosome, impede divergent evolution. The nucleosomes, arranged as "beads on a string," become further organized into more highly ordered structures consisting of coils of many closely packed nucleosomes that in turn must form fundamental organization units of the eukaryotic chromosome.

Nucleosomal structure may serve a variety of purposes, for example, in simply compacting the enormous amount of DNA (about 6×10^9 base pairs) comprising the human diploid genome. Aside from such a packing function, this ubiquitous structure must also be reconciled with a train of enzymes that acts upon DNA to permit its orderly replication and transcription. Undoubtedly, these functions are subserved and modulated by other proteins that little resemble the monotonous structure of the histones and that recognize specific structural features of a DNA sequence. A fundamental question in eukaryotic molecular biology is how this nucleoprotein structure permits access to specific proteins and is differentially made available in the course of cellular growth and development.

The double-helical model of DNA immediately suggested the manner in which genes could be replicated for transmission to offspring. The actual replication process is mechanically complex but conceptually simple. The two strands of DNA separate, and each is copied by a series of enzymes that inserts a complementary base opposite each base on the original strand of DNA. Thus, two identical double helices are generated from one.[64-66] Details of the mechanisms of DNA replication in *Escherichia coli* are becoming known.[65,67-69]

The Genetic Code

DNA makes RNA (transcription) makes protein (translation) in the accepted paradigm (Fig. 1-4). The sequence of bases in a specific gene ultimately dictates the sequence of amino acids in a specific protein. This collinearity between the DNA molecule and the protein sequence is achieved by means of the *genetic code.*[64] The four types of bases in DNA are arranged in groups of three, each triplet forming a code word or *codon* that signifies a single amino acid.

In this manner, triplet codons exist for each of the 20 amino acids which occur in proteins (Fig. 1-5). Inasmuch as 64 different triplets can be generated from the four bases and only 20 amino acids exist, the genetic code is said to be *degenerate.* That is, most amino acids are specified by more than one codon. Each codon, however, is completely specific. Thus, the double-stranded sequence adenine-adenine-adenine (or AAA) in the transcribed (antisense) strand and thymine-thymine-thymine (or TTT) in the nontranscribed (sense) strand of DNA codes for uridine-uridine-uridine (or UUU) in mRNA, which is translated to phenylalanine in protein (Fig. 1-4).

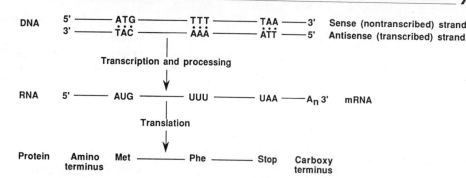

Fig. 1-4 DNA is transcribed and processed to yield mRNA which is translated to yield protein.

DNA-RNA Protein

To translate its genetic information into a protein, a segment of DNA is first transcribed into messenger ribonucleic acid (messenger RNA). The messenger RNA contains a sequence of purine and pyrimidine bases that is complementary to the bases of the transcribed (antisense) strand of the DNA. By this mechanism each adenine of DNA becomes a uridine of RNA, each cytosine of DNA becomes a guanine of RNA, each thymine of DNA becomes an adenine of RNA, and each guanine of DNA becomes a cytosine of RNA. Thus, each DNA triplet codon is translated into a corresponding RNA triplet codon.

The messenger RNA for each gene is processed extensively by modifying enzymes within the cell nucleus. It then crosses the nuclear membrane and enters the cytoplasm, where it serves as a template for the synthesis of a specific protein.[64] To translate the messenger RNA code into a protein, the messenger RNA binds to a complex structure called a *ribosome*, which is composed of a different type of RNA (ribosomal RNA) and a large number of proteins. In order to be inserted into its proper place in the protein sequence, each of the 20 amino acids is attached in the cytoplasm to an additional type of RNA (transfer RNA). Each amino acid is attached to a specific set of transfer RNAs (Fig. 1-6). Each transfer RNA contains an "anticodon loop," which includes a sequence of three bases that is complementary to a specific codon in the corresponding messenger RNA. For example, phenylalanine is attached specifically to a transfer RNA whose anticodon loop contains the sequence AAA, which is complimentary to the messenger RNA codon UUU, which codes for phenylalanine.

Under the influence of a host of cytoplasmic factors (initiation factors, elongation factors, and termination factors), peptide bonds are formed between the various amino acids that are aligned along the messenger RNA chain (Fig. 1-7). Eventually, a terminator codon is reached and the completed polypeptide is released from the ribosome. Inasmuch as the primary sequence of bases in the coding regions of the DNA determines the corresponding primary sequence of amino acids in the protein, the gene and its protein are said to be *collinear*. This means that any alteration of the sequence of bases in the gene will result in an alteration of the protein at a specific point in its sequence.

Control of Gene Expression

The proper rate and timing for transcription and translation are subject to complex controls. Cis-acting sequences are DNA regions at a distance but on the same duplex DNA molecule, and trans-acting factors (usually proteins) are encoded by other genes (usually unlinked). The trans-acting factors interact with the cis sequences to control the process of transcription. Many of the cis-acting transcriptional control elements occur short distances upstream from the initiation site for transcription (see Chap. 2), but some have been described at greater distances upstream and downstream from the initiation site for transcription (e.g., 5 to 50 kb). Regulation of gene expression also occurs posttranscriptionally involving RNA processing, translational control, and posttranslational control.

Some of our understanding about interactions between trans-acting factors and cis-acting sequences in mammalian cells comes from prokaryotes, especially studies of the *lac* and lambda repressors.[71] The mammalian cis-acting sequences include the TATA consensus, the CAAT consensus, Sp1 binding sites, enhancers, upstream activating sequences (UAS), hormone responsive elements, and others.[72–75] The TATA and CAAT consensus sequences occur upstream of the start site for transcription in many genes and bind transcription factors. There is evidence for multiple types of DNA binding proteins. Some DNA binding proteins, such as the λ repressor and the tryptophan repressor,[76] contain a "helix-turn-helix" motif, while others have a "zinc finger" motif which binds to DNA.[75] More recently, a third DNA binding motif, the "leucine zipper," has been suggested.[77] The DNA binding finger proteins contain Zn^{2+} molecules bound to amino acid residues. Proteins suggested to represent DNA binding proteins with Zn^{2+} fingers include transcription factor Sp1, transcription factor TFIIIA, numerous *Drosophila* proteins (e.g., the *Kruppel* gene product), and yeast transcription factor ADR1.[74,75] In addition mammalian and avian proteins suggested to have DNA binding Zn^{2+} finger motifs include the glucocorticoid receptor, the estrogen receptor, the progesterone receptor, the c-*erb*-A protein, the vitamin D receptor, the mineralocorticoid receptor, and the product of the sex determining gene.[8,74,75] A strategy for cloning DNA binding proteins by screening expression DNA libraries with oligonucleotides has been described.[78] Studies of the control of mammalian gene expression are progressing rapidly, and human mutations already are identified in the cis regulatory sequences (e.g., globin genes, Chap. 93) and are likely to be identified in trans-acting factors.

MUTATION AS THE ORIGIN OF NORMAL VARIATION AND GENETIC DISEASE

Broadly defined, a *mutation* is a stable, heritable alteration in DNA which can be passed from cell to progeny. Some mutations are genetically lethal and cannot be passed from one gen-

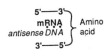

Second RNA nucleotide

	U	**C**	**A**	**G**	
U	UUU / AAA ⎱ Phe, UUC / AAG; UUA / AAT ⎱ Leu, UUG / AAC	UCU / AGA, UCC / AGG, UCA / AGT, UCG / AGC ⎱ Ser	UAU / ATA ⎱ Tyr, UAC / ATG; UAA / ATT ⎱ Stop, UAG / ATC	UGU / ACA ⎱ Cys, UGC / ACG; UGA / ACT Stop; UGG / ACC Trp	U C A G
C	CUU / GAA, CUC / GAG, CUA / GAT, CUG / GAC ⎱ Leu	CCU / GGA, CCC / GGG, CCA / GGT, CCG / GGC ⎱ Pro	CAU / GTA ⎱ His, CAC / GTG; CAA / GTT ⎱ Gln, CAG / GTC	CGU / GCA, CGC / GCG, CGA / GCT, CGG / GCC ⎱ Arg	U C A G
A	AUU / TAA, AUC / TAG ⎱ Ile, AUA / TAT; AUG / TAC Met	ACU / TGA, ACC / TGG, ACA / TGT, ACG / TGC ⎱ Thr	AAU / TTA ⎱ Asn, AAC / TTG; AAA / TTT ⎱ Lys, AAG / TTC	AGU / TCA ⎱ Ser, AGC / TCG; AGA / TCT ⎱ Arg, AGG / TCC	U C A G
G	GUU / CAA, GUC / CAG, GUA / CAT, GUG / CAC ⎱ Val	GCU / CGA, GCC / CGG, GCA / CGT, GCG / CGC ⎱ Ala	GAU / CTA ⎱ Asp, GAC / CTG; GAA / CTT ⎱ Glu, GAG / CTC	GGU / CCA, GGC / CCG, GGA / CCT, GGG / CCC ⎱ Gly	U C A G

First RNA nucleotide (left axis)   *Third RNA nucleotide* (right axis)

Fig. 1-5 The genetic code. The RNA codons appear in boldface type; the complementary DNA codons are in italics. A = adenine; C = cytosine; G = guanine; T = thymine; U = uridine (replaces thymine in RNA). In RNA, adenine is complementary to thymine of DNA; uridine is complementary to adenine of DNA; cytosine is complementary to guanine and vice versa. "Stop" = punctuation. The three-letter and single-letter abbreviations for the amino acids are as follows: Ala (A) = alanine; Arg (R) = arginine; Asn (N) = asparagine; Asp (D) = aspartic acid; Cys (C) = cysteine; Gln (Q) = glutamine; Glu (E) = glutamic acid; Gly (G) = glycine; His (H) = histidine; Ile (I) = isoleucine; Leu (L) = leucine; Lys (K) = lysine; Met (M) = methionine; Phe (F) = phenylalanine; Pro (P) = proline; Ser (S) = serine; Thr (T) = threonine; Trp (W) = tryptophan; Tyr (Y) = tyrosine; Val (V) = valine.

eration to the next, while others are less deleterious and are tolerated in the descendants under permissive conditions. From the viewpoint of evolution, mutations are essential for the generation of sufficient genetic diversity to permit species to adapt to their environment through the mechanism of natural selection.

Mutations involving gross alterations (millions of base pairs) in the structure of a chromosome include duplications, deletions, and translocations of a portion of one chromosome to another. Mutations can involve even the entire genome (3 bil-

lion base pairs) as in triploidy where there is a third copy of the whole chromosome constitution. On the other hand, mutations can be minute, involving a deletion, insertion, or replacement of a single base. Single-base or very small mutations are called *point mutations*. If deletions or insertions of a single base occur in a coding region, they give rise to *frameshift mutations* because they alter the reading frame of the genetic code such that every triplet distal to the mutation in the same gene is altered. Frameshift mutations grossly alter the protein sequence and frequently result in termination of the peptide chain shortly beyond the mutation site because of the occurrence of a termination codon in the altered reading frame. Small deletions or insertions can also affect transcription, splicing, or RNA processing, depending on their location.

When one base is replaced by another in the coding region, the point mutations may be of three types: (1) a *synonymous mutation* (constituting about 23 percent of random base substitutions in coding regions), in which the base replacement does not lead to a change in the amino acid but only to the substitution of a different codon for the same amino acid (e.g., a replacement of a single base pair in the DNA so that an RNA codon for phenylalanine will be transcribed into RNA not as UUU but as UUC, which still codes for phenylalanine); (2) a *missense mutation* (about 73 percent of base substitutions in coding regions), in which the base replacement changes the codon for one amino acid to another (e.g., the replacement of a base pair in DNA in the codon for phenylalanine such that it will be transcribed into RNA not as UUU but as UUA, which would change the codon to leucine); and (3) a *nonsense mutation* (about 4 percent of base substitutions in coding regions), in which the base replacement changes the codon to one of the termination codons (e.g., the replacement of a base pair in the codon for tyrosine such that it is transcribed into RNA not as UAU but as the stop codon UAA).[79]

In addition to these point mutations, there are larger deletions which may affect a portion of a gene, an entire gene, or

Fig. 1-6 A diagrammatic representation of a tRNA molecule. Each base in the tRNA is represented by a box. The structure is shown with interacting complementary sequences indicated by a row of dots. Each conserved loop is shown (DHU = dehydrouridylic acid loop; TψC = thymidylic acid-pseudouridylic acid-cytidylic acid loop). The anticodon position is indicated. All tRNAs end with a CCA sequence at their 3′ terminus that serves as the amino acid acceptor portion of the molecule. (After L. Stryer.[70])

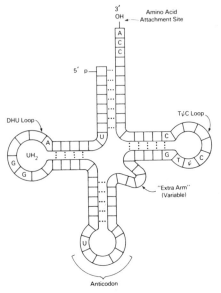

Fig. 1-7 The elongation reactions in protein synthesis. The figure diagrammatically represents the ribosome (60 S and 40 S subunits), the tRNA moieties (hairpinlike structures), and the associated mRNAs. The first elongation intermediate (*upper left*) shows a peptidyl tRNA, the peptide portion of which is represented by leucine and three dots, at the donor site on the ribosome interacting with a leucine codon, AUU. In the presence of GTP and elongation factor 1 (EF-1), tyr-tRNA binds to the next available codon at the receptor site. The peptide is transferred to the oncoming tyr-tRNA by an enzymatic activity associated with the 60 S subunit of the ribosome. The next step involves release of the deacylated tRNA (leucine) and the translocation of the mRNA and the newly elongated peptidyl tRNA to the donor site, exposing the next available codon, CAU, for recognition. The later reaction requires elongation factor 2 (EF-2) and consumes GTP. The entire process is repeated until a termination codon is encountered, and the finished peptide is released in the presence of appropriate termination factors.

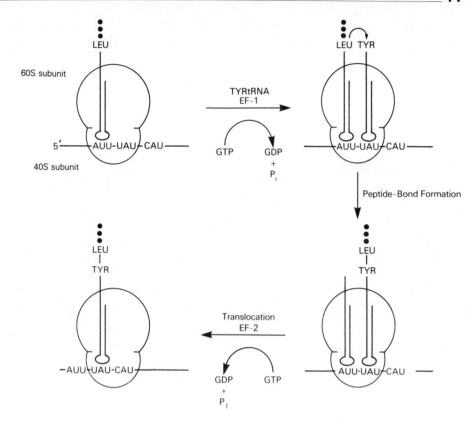

a set of contiguous genes. Such deletion mutations may interrupt or remove the coding region of a gene causing the absence of its protein product. Alternatively, a deletion can bridge between the coding regions of two genes and produce a fusion resulting in the production of a hybrid protein containing the initial sequence of one protein followed by the terminal sequence of another protein. This latter type of mutation may occur particularly by unequal crossing over between tandemly repeated homologous genes such as the globin genes (Chap. 93). The range of mutations seen at the human β-globin locus provides a good perspective on the extent of heterogeneity of mutations that can occur (Chap. 93). Over 200 missense mutations causing amino acid substitutions with various phenotypes are known at the β-globin locus.[4] Various δ-β and β-δ fusions are known. Numerous transcriptional, splicing, and RNA processing mutations cause β thalassemia[80] as depicted in Fig. 1-8.

The type and frequency of human mutations is a very complex topic. Mutations causing chromosomal aneuploidy occur

at increasing frequency with advancing age of the mother. Smaller mutations occur with increased frequency with advancing age of the father, although the molecular nature of the mutations seen with advanced paternal age is just becoming known. Some loci, such as those for Duchenne muscular dystrophy and achondroplasia, are subject to very high rates of new mutation. In the instance of Duchenne dystrophy, this may be related in part to the unusually large size of the gene. The structure of the gene, its position within the genome, and the constraints on the gene product may contribute along with other factors to the frequency of new mutations causing phenotypic effects at a locus. The occurrence of 5-methylcytosine, particularly at the sites of CpG base pairs, provides sites of increased mutational frequency, apparently due to spontaneous deamination of 5-methylcytosine yielding a thymine base. An enzymatic mechanism exists for selective methylation of cytosine residues after replication. The propensity for deamination of 5-methylcytosine leads to increased frequency of RFLPs for at least some restriction enzymes, which include CpG pairs in the recognition site,[81] and accounts for certain mutational hot spots causing hemophilia A (Chap. 86) and other human disorders. The availability of recombinant DNA techniques is leading to an increasing definition of the exact

Fig. 1-8 Location of 30 mutations causing β thalassemia. Symbols are △ = frameshift and nonsense mutations; ◇ = RNA splicing mutants; ● = transcription mutants; ○ = RNA cleavage mutant. (From S. E. Antonarakis et al.[80] Used by permission.)

β - Globin Gene

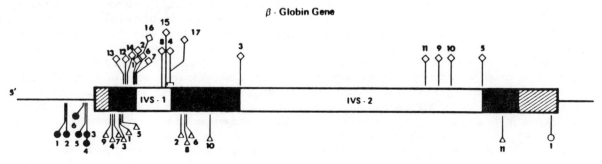

nature of new mutations, determination of whether they arose from a maternal gamete or from a paternal gamete, and identification of whether the mutation is of recent or ancient origin. Mutations which are widespread in the population but are descended from a single event can be recognized by the occurrence of specific haplotypes of RFLPs surrounding the mutations (see discussions of thalassemia, phenylalanine hydroxylase, and cystic fibrosis in various chapters). A haplotype is a group of genetic markers linked together on a single chromosome such as a group of close RFLP markers[80] or a group of HLA alleles (see Chap. 4).

When mutations occur in germ cells, the altered expression of the mutant gene does not affect the phenotype of the individual in whom the mutation occurs but is manifest only in subsequent generations. Usually such *new mutations* are recognized as sporadic events in human populations. On the other hand, when a mutation occurs in somatic cells at an early development stage, it may affect the individual harboring the mutation, but is not passed to subsequent generations. The individual harboring such a somatic cell mutation is said to be a *mosaic* because two populations of cells are present: normal cells and cells harboring the mutant gene. Mutations occurring in an early germ line cell can give rise to gonadal mosaicism so that numerous mutant gametes may be descended from a single event.

GENETIC DIVERSITY IN HUMANS: GARROD'S CHEMICAL INDIVIDUALITY AND THE CONCEPT OF POLYMORPHISM

Garrod recognized that the aberrant metabolism seen in a condition such as alkaptonuria might imply far more extensive chemical individuality, and he wrote[13]:

> If it be, indeed, the case that in alkaptonuria and the other conditions mentioned we are dealing with individualities of metabolism and not with the results of morbid processes the thought naturally presents itself that these are merely extreme examples of variations of chemical behaviour which are probably everywhere present in minor degrees and that just as no two individuals of a species are absolutely identical in bodily structure neither are their chemical processes carried out on exactly the same lines.

Garrod further said that "diathesis is nothing else but *chemical individuality*" which he described as follows[3]:

> . . . the factors which confer upon us our predispositions to and immunities from the various mishaps which are spoken of as diseases, are inherent in our very chemical structure; and even in the molecular groupings which confer upon us our individualities, and which went to the making of the chromosomes from which we sprang.

It becomes increasingly apparent that individuals have a molecular and biochemical individuality which is extraordinary. While there is often a tendency in medicine to regard patient populations as a homogeneous group of "wild-type individuals" or normal humans with "normal values" for all determinants, this is an erroneous conception. The aggregate of our genes determines who dies of myocardial infarction on a high fat diet, who develops cancer upon smoking, who only carries *Meningococcus* in the nasopharynx while another develops meningitis, who develops postoperative thromboembolism, and, perhaps, who is susceptible to alcoholism. These are risks that are substantially influenced by the genotype of the individual. Williams[2] emphasized the hypothesis that "everyone is a deviate" as follows:

> The existence in every human being of a vast array of attributes which are potentially measurable (whether by present methods or not), and probably often uncorrelated mathematically, makes quite tenable the hypothesis that *practically every human being is a deviate in some respects.*

Garrod's concept of chemical individuality has found its explanation over the past two decades with the realization that the gene for a given protein frequently exists in different forms in different normal individuals. Subsequently it was recognized that even more extensive variation exists in the DNA sequence of genomes between individuals. The widespread nature of this genetic diversity first became apparent when it became possible to study enzymes by electrophoresis of crude cell extracts and thereby to detect structurally variant forms of enzymes without the necessity of purification. With the use of this technique, studies by Harris in humans[82] and by Lewontin and Hubby in *Drosophila*[83] demonstrated that many proteins existed in two or more forms in the population. These multiple forms are due to the existence in the population of multiple genes (called *alleles*) at the same genetic locus coding for the same protein. At each genetic locus, each individual possesses two alleles, one derived from each parent. If the two alleles are identical, the individual is said to be *homozygous;* if they differ, the individual is *heterozygous.* The various alleles have been derived from a single precursor allele by mutations that have occurred during the evolution of the species; in general, they differ from each other only in the substitution of one base for another (missense mutations). In the vast majority of cases, the proteins produced by both alleles at a given locus are equally functional, i.e., the amino acid difference is "neutral" or nearly so from the standpoint of natural selection.

Based on population studies of 71 enzymes and other proteins that lend themselves to analysis by electrophoresis or other techniques, Harris has found that 28 percent of genetic loci show multiple alleles in the population.[79] Moreover, the average individual is detectably heterozygous at 7 percent of his or her loci. Since most detection methods require a change in the charge of the protein, they can detect only about one-third of the actual base changes that are possible, since only one-third result in a substitution of an amino acid with a different charge. Thus, all individuals may actually be heterozygous at as many as 20 percent of their loci.

At most genetic loci (such as that for the β chain of hemoglobin), there is one standard allele that accounts for the vast majority of the alleles in the population, whereas the alternate alleles are rare. At other genetic loci (such as that for the α chain of haptoglobin, a plasma protein), no single allele occurs with sufficient frequency to be designated as standard or normal. This latter situation represents an extreme example of genetic polymorphism. In strict terms, *polymorphism* is said to exist in a given population when the most common allele at a given locus accounts for fewer than 99 percent of the alleles in the population. By definition, when a polymorphism exists at a genetic locus, at least 2 percent of the population must be heterozygous at that locus.[79] Table 1-2 lists some plasma proteins and cellular enzymes for which electrophoretically determined polymorphisms have been demonstrated.

Harris' estimate that at least 28 percent of the genes for soluble blood proteins in humans show polymorphism is dis-

Table 1-2 Plasma Proteins and Cellular Enzymes that Exhibit Electrophoretically Detectable Polymorphisms

Protein	Locus symbol
Plasma proteins	
Haptoglobin (α chain)	HP
Transferrin	TF
Vitamin D-binding protein	GC (for group-specific component)
Ceruloplasmin	CP
α₁-Antitrypsin	PI (for protease inhibitor)
α₁-Acid glycoprotein	ORM (for orosomucoid)
β₂-Glycoprotein I	BG
Properdin factor B	BF
Complement	
Second component	C2
Third component	C3
Fourth component	C4
Sixth component	C6
Enzymes	
Pancreatic amylase	AMY2
Cholinesterase	CHE2
Red blood cell enzymes	
Acid phosphatase 1	ACP1
Adenosine deaminase	ADA
Adenylate kinase	AK1
Carbonic anhydrase 2	CA2
Diaphorase (NADPH-dependent)	DIA2
Esterase D	ESD
Galactose-1-uridyl transferase	GALT
Glucose-6-phosphate dehydrogenase	G6PD
Glutamic-pyruvic transaminase	GPT
Glutathione peroxidase	GPX1
Glutathione reductase	GSR
Glyoxalase I	GLO
Peptidase A	PEPA
Peptidase C	PEPC
Peptidase D	PEPD
Phosphoglucomutase 1	PGM1
Phosphoglucomutase 2	PGM2
Phosphogluconate dehydrogenase	PGD
Uridine monophosphate kinase	UMPK
White blood cell enzymes	
Aconitase (soluble)	ACO1
Cytidine deaminase	CDA
α-L-Fucosidase	FUCA2
α-Glucosidase	GAA
Glutamic-oxaloacetic transaminase (mitochondrial)	GOT2
Hexokinase 3	HK3
Malic enzyme (mitochondrial)	ME2
Phosphoglucomutase 3	PGM3

SOURCE: Data from Giblett[84] with updated gene symbols.

crepant with estimates for total cellular (fibroblast) proteins[85,86] where the variation is less for several possible reasons. Despite these differences, the frequency of protein polymorphism is high. The appreciation of polymorphism has been extended by the discovery of extraordinary variation at the DNA sequence level. Attention was focused on DNA polymorphism by the discovery of RFLPs by Kan and Dozy.[40] Extensive subsequent data suggest that approximately 1 in 100 to 1 in 200 bp in the human genome is polymorphic; this is consistent with heterozygosity at 1 in 250 to 1 in 500 bp.[87] A site is defined as polymorphic when at least 1 percent of the chromosomes have a sequence different from the majority. Although perhaps not an ideal usage, the term *allele* is now often extended to describe any nucleotide variation such as DNA fragment size differences detected as RFLPs even

when these are not associated with an expressed gene locus. It is possible to detect single base DNA polymorphisms that represent synonymous differences or amino acid polymorphisms in coding regions, but polymorphism at a DNA level occurs with even greater frequency outside coding regions in parts of the genome which may have little or no effect on gene expression. The polymorphism within the genome extends beyond single base differences to include insertions, deletions, and variation in numbers of short tandemly repeated sequences. The latter types of variation provide highly polymorphic sites due to the variable number of tandem repeats (VNTR) as discussed in Chap. 6.

With the recognition of the extensive amount of polymorphism in DNA (millions of nucleotide differences between two random haploid genomes), including variation in nonexpressed sequences, it becomes obvious that the majority of DNA polymorphism is not associated with phenotypic effects. Presumably a modest fraction of genomic polymorphism is associated with effects on the phenotype that account for variation such as racial differences and human individuality without a significant effect on health or disease. Another proportion of polymorphism would be associated with phenotypic variation that might have relatively subtle and complex effects on susceptibility to disease. These variations would include genes affecting susceptibility to hypertension, atherosclerosis, malignancy, psychiatric illness, and infection. These genetic differences would provide the basis for polygenic and multifactorial disorders to be discussed below. Finally, a few genetic variations have such profound effects on the phenotype that they give rise to a disease condition in a relatively consistent manner (i.e., in the universal environment with minimal modifying effect from the remainder of the genome). These few genetic variations are referred to as *single gene* or *monogenic* disorders, and they constitute the basis for most of the diseases discussed in this volume. However, even the phenotype caused by these single gene disorders is often subject to modification by the genotype at other loci and by environmental factors. As knowledge increases, this becomes clearer and is exemplified by the effect of the number of α-globin loci on the phenotype when the β-globin locus is mutant in sickle-cell anemia.[88,89] Other examples can be found in the disorders of apolipoproteins where the phenotype is affected by the genotype at other loci and by environmental factors (Chaps. 44 to 51); the determinants of Hartnup disease versus Hartnup disorder are another illustration (Chap. 101).

GENETIC LINKAGE AND THE HUMAN GENE MAP

The most recent update of McKusick's catalog of *Mendelian Inheritance in Man*[4] lists 4344 loci, of which about 75 percent are associated with a disease phenotype,[90] indicating that over 3000 single-gene-determined human diseases are known to exist. This implies that at least 3000 of the 50,000 or so human genes have undergone mutation so as to cause human disease. The chromosomal location of more than 1300 of these genes is now known (Fig. 1-9).

The ability to locate genes relative to each other on the human chromosomes grew out of the pioneering studies of Morgan and his school in the first two decades of this century.[91] Using the fruit fly *D. melanogaster*, Morgan demonstrated that genes are aligned in a linear manner on the chromosomes and

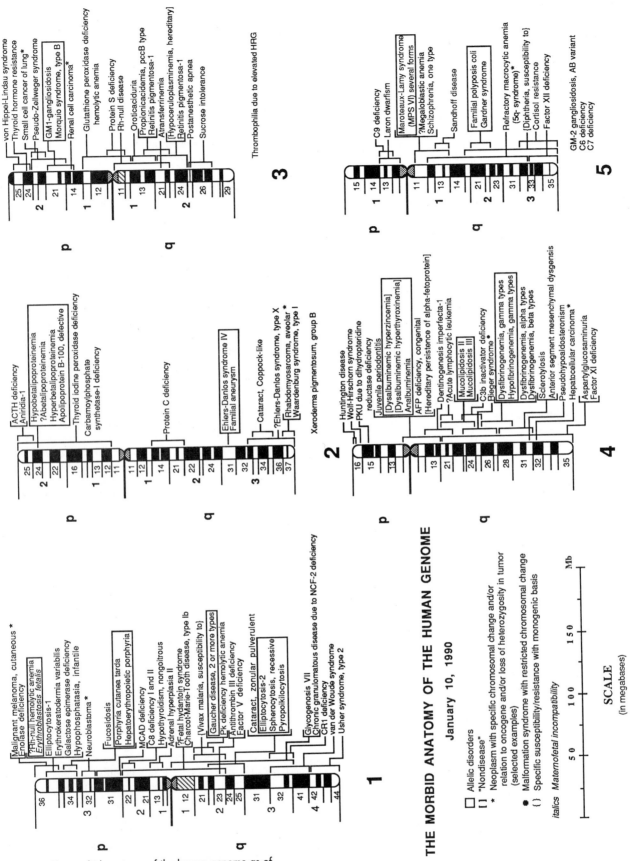

THE MORBID ANATOMY OF THE HUMAN GENOME
January 10, 1990

☐ Allelic disorders
[ ] "Nondisease"
* Neoplasm with specific chromosomal change and/or relation to oncogene and/or loss of heterozygosity in tumor (selected examples)
● Malformation syndrome with restricted chromosomal change
( ) Specific susceptibility/resistance with monogenic basis

italics Maternofetal incompatibility

SCALE
(in megabases)

Fig. 1-9 The morbid anatomy of the human genome as of January 10, 1990. See Appendix 1 for details by individual chromosomes, disease and adjacent normal loci, location by banding pattern, gene symbol, McKusick number, and corresponding locus in mouse genome.

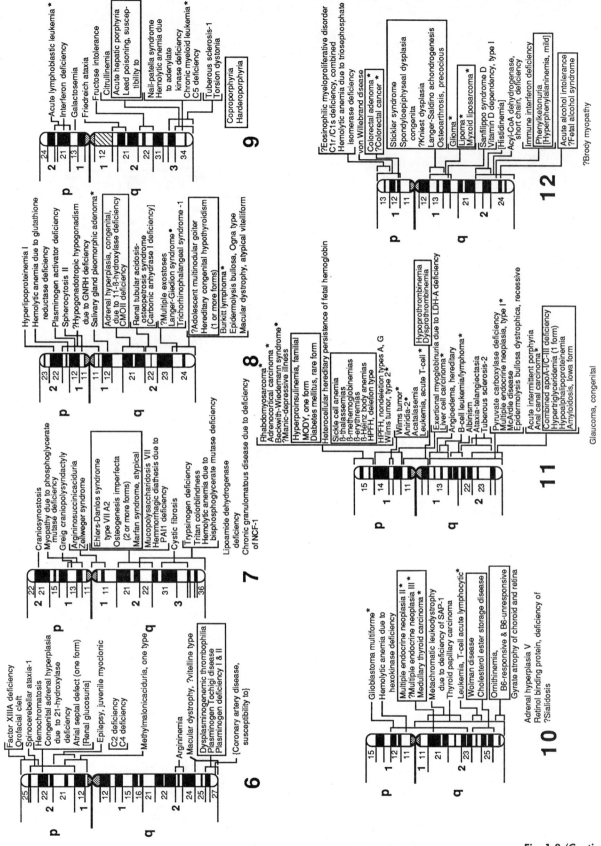

Fig. 1-9 *(Continued)*

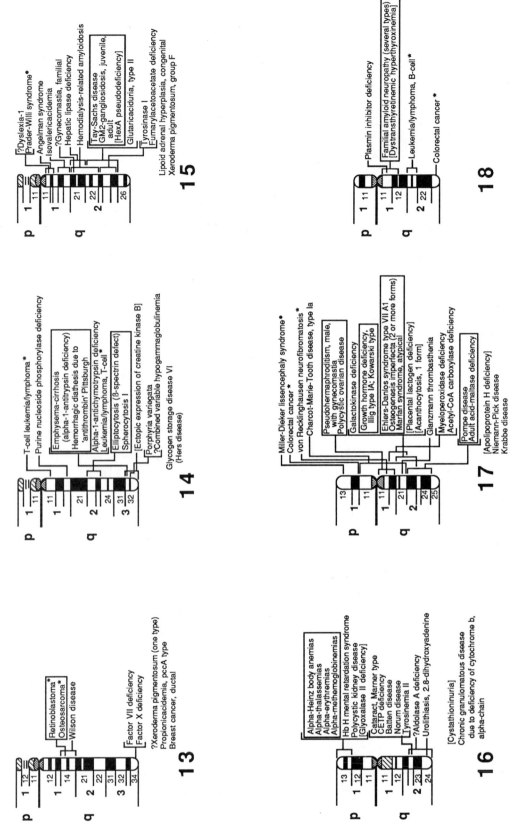

Fig. 1-9 *(Continued)*

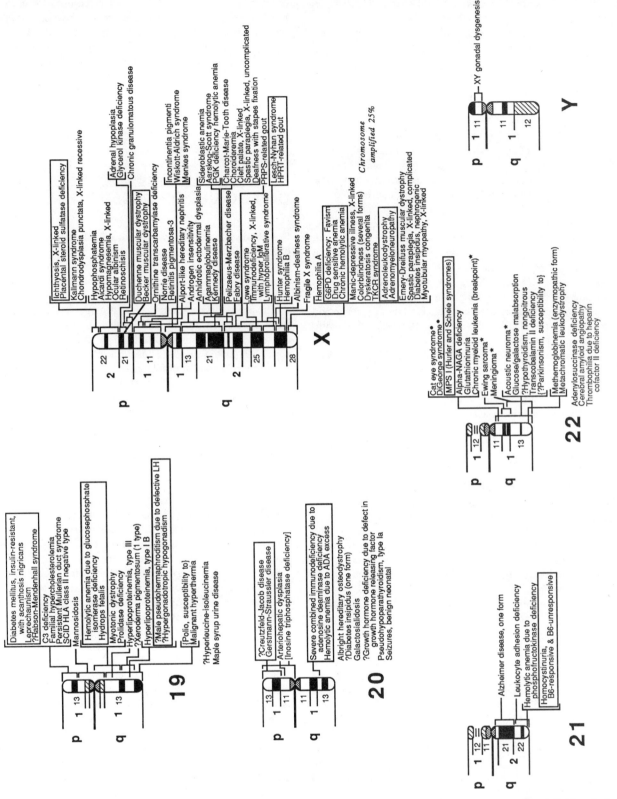

Fig. 1-9 *(Concluded)*

that if two genes are close together on the same chromosome, they do not assort independently at meiosis but are transmitted to the same gamete more than 50 percent of the time. Such genes are said to be *linked*. When two genes on a single chromosome are far apart, they are not genetically linked, even though they are physically linked by being on the same continuous chromosome. This lack of linkage is due to the phenomenon of *crossing-over*.

During the process of meiosis when homologous chromosomes are paired, bridges frequently form between corresponding regions of the chromosome pair. These bridges, or *chiasmas*, are regions in which the two chromosomes break at identical points along their length and subsequently rejoin, the distal segments having been switched from one homologous chromosome to the other. During this process of crossing-over, no net change in the amount of genetic material occurs. However, a *recombination* of genes does occur. For example, consider a chromosome with two loci, A and B, located at opposite ends of the same chromosome. On this particular chromosome, the A locus has a rare *x* allele and the B locus has a rare *y* allele. Without the phenomenon of recombination, every offspring that inherited the *x* allele at the A locus would also inherit the *y* allele at the B locus. However, if recombination occurs, the A locus with the *x* allele would then be on the opposite chromosome from the B locus with the *y* allele. In this case, any offspring that inherited the *x* allele at the A locus could not inherit the *y* allele at the B locus.

Crossing-over in humans occurs with great frequency in every meiosis, and the resultant recombination of genes may occur at any point on a chromosome. The farther apart two genes are on the same chromosome, the greater is the likelihood that a crossing-over will occur in the space between them. When two genes are on the opposite ends of a long chromosome, the probability of recombination is so great that their respective alleles are transmitted to offspring almost independently of one another, just as if the two gene loci were on different chromosomes. On the other hand, gene loci that are close together on the same chromosome are said to be *linked*, so that there is a great likelihood that offspring will inherit the same combination of alleles that is present on the parental chromosome.

Figure 1-9 and its accompanying key give the chromosomal assignments of hundreds of autosomal loci, with indications of the confidence of the assignment. In addition, some 120 loci are known from pedigree studies to be located on the X chromosome. As illustrated in Fig. 1-9, the mapping of genes on virtually all the chromosomes is now quite extensive, and an entire introductory chapter is devoted to how the human gene map can be used in medicine (Chap. 6).

Assignment of a locus to a specific chromosome is based on a variety of methods that have been reviewed in detail by McKusick and Ruddle.[92–94] Many genes have been mapped by linkage of traits in large families with multiple alleles at two loci (e.g., linkage of the nail-patella syndrome and the ABO blood group). Somatic cell hybrids have been used extensively to assign genes to particular chromosomes based on the concordance of the presence of the human gene product with the presence of the human chromosome (e.g., thymidine kinase segregates with chromosome 17). More recently many genes are mapped following the isolation of cDNA or genomic DNA clones. The cloned DNA can be used with a hybrid cell panel to assess the concordance of the DNA hybridizing sequence with a particular chromosome. Alternatively, the cloned DNA

can be used for synthesis of probes to be used for *in situ* hybridization with human chromosomes. The opportunity for linkage studies has been greatly enhanced by the availability of numerous polymorphic DNA probes, and the genes for many common human diseases have been mapped to specific chromosomes using this strategy (e.g., assignment of Huntington disease to chromosome 4 using an anonymous probe to detect an RFLP.[47]) A very large number of the disorders discussed in this text have been mapped to specific human chromosomes. Examples can be found in the summary table at the end of this chapter.

CATEGORIES OF GENETIC DISORDERS

Genetic diseases generally fall into one of three categories. (1) *Chromosomal disorders* involve the lack, excess, or abnormal arrangement of one or more chromosomes, producing large amounts of excessive or deficient genetic material and affecting many genes. (2) *Mendelian or monogenic disorders* are determined primarily by a single mutant gene. Accordingly, these disorders display simple (Mendelian) inheritance patterns that can be classified into autosomal dominant, autosomal recessive, or X-linked types. (3) *Multifactorial disorders* are caused by an interaction of multiple genes and multiple exogenous or environmental factors. Although many of these multifactorial disorders, such as diabetes mellitus, gout, and cleft lip and palate, are said to run in families, the inheritance pattern is complex and the risk to relatives is much less than that seen in the single gene (Mendelian) disorders. Each of the above three categories of genetic disease presents different problems with respect to causation, prevention, diagnosis, genetic counseling, and treatment.[95]

Although it is useful to consider these categories of genetic disorders, this classification necessarily represents an oversimplification. For example, small chromosomal deletions may cause the simultaneous presence of multiple Mendelian or monogenic disorders (contiguous gene syndromes). This is exemplified by the occurrence of patients with visible deletions in the short arm of the X chromosome in association with Duchenne muscular dystrophy, chronic granulomatous disease, retinitis pigmentosa, and the McLeod phenotype.[96] These deletions may be submicroscopic and yet be large enough to cause the simultaneous presence of phenotypes such as Duchenne muscular dystrophy, ornithine transcarbamylase deficiency, and glycerol kinase deficiency (Chaps. 9 and 36). Deletions of the retinoblastoma locus on chromosome 13 may be visible or submicroscopic and may extend to nearby loci such as esterase D (Chap. 9). Thus, these defects bridge the gap between chromosomal and monogenic disorders. The phenotype caused by chromosomal disorders obviously is due to the altered expression of single genes within the abnormal region. Chromosomal translocations may interrupt single genes as exemplified by some females with X autosomal translocations causing Duchenne muscular dystrophy (see Chaps. 9 and 118).

The phenotypes of many of the monogenic disorders discussed in this text are modified by the genes at other loci and by environmental factors. Figure 1-10 emphasizes the effect of nongenetic factors and modifying genes on monogenic phenotypes. There are relatively few monogenic disorders where the single locus *entirely* determines the disease phenotype. Simi-

0

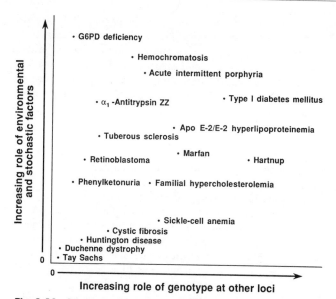

- G6PD deficiency
- Hemochromatosis
- Acute intermittent porphyria
- α₁-Antitrypsin ZZ
- Type I diabetes mellitus
- Apo E-2/E-2 hyperlipoproteinemia
- Tuberous sclerosis
- Marfan
- Retinoblastoma
- Hartnup
- Phenylketonuria
- Familial hypercholesterolemia
- Sickle-cell anemia
- Cystic fibrosis
- Huntington disease
- Duchenne dystrophy
- Tay Sachs

Increasing role of environmental and stochastic factors (vertical axis)

Increasing role of genotype at other loci (horizontal axis)

Fig. 1-10 Depiction of estimated roles of modifier genes and nongenetic factors in influencing the phenotypes for "monogenic" disorders. These are crude estimates meant to depict the range of contributions which might occur.

larly, there are relatively few environmental insults where the genotype does not in some way modify the risk. For example, the genotype undoubtedly influences which infants will survive in a famine. In theory, some disorders might be polygenic, which would imply an effect of multiple genes without a major contribution by exogenous or environmental factors. In practice, the majority of polygenic disorders are very likely to be subject to exogenous factors and are therefore multifactorial. The monogenic disorders have provided an excellent starting point for attempts to understand human genetic disease. The future will increasingly involve the greater challenge of understanding the much more common multifactorial disorders.

Frequency of Genetic Disease

Genetic disease accounts for a significant proportion of hospitalized children in referral centers. In studies in Montreal, Baltimore, and Newcastle, from 6 to 8 percent of diseases among hospitalized children were attributable to single gene defects and from 0.4 to 2.5 percent to chromosomal abnormalities; another 22 to 31 percent were considered gene influenced.[97,98] The overall frequency of monogenic disorders is about 1 percent.[97] About 5.3 percent of live-born individuals below age 25 can be expected to have disease with an important genetic component (single gene, chromosomal, and multifactorial).[99] If multifactorial disorders of late onset are included, about 60 percent of individuals have genetically influenced diseases.[99,100] One recent study[101] evaluated survival of adoptees relative to the survival of their biologic and adoptive parents. The results indicated that premature death in adults has a strong genetic component for death from all causes, for natural causes, for infections, and for cardiovascular causes. Premature death of a biologic parent (less than age 50) resulted in a relative risk of death in the adoptees of 1.71 (95 percent confidence interval, 1.14 to 2.57). More detailed information on the frequency of diseases within categories is provided below.

Chromosomal Disorders

The *karyotype* of an individual (i.e., the number and structure of the chromosomes) can be ascertained from readily accessible body cells, such as peripheral blood lymphocytes or skin fibroblasts, by growing them in tissue culture until active proliferation occurs and then preparing single metaphase cells for examination of chromosomes by microscopy. By the 1970s it became possible to identify each individual chromosome by special staining of DNA sequences, by the affinity of fluorescent dyes (such as quinacrine hydrochloride) for certain chromosomal segments that can be visualized by fluorescence microscopy, and by treatment of the chromosomes with dyes (Giemsa) after treatment with proteolytic enzymes (trypsin). These techniques produce characteristic *banding patterns* for each chromosome (Fig. 1-11). The number of chromosomes in normal individuals is 46, of which 44 are the 22 pairs of *autosomes* and the other 2 are the *sex chromosomes*. Females have two X chromosomes (XX), and males have one X chromosome and one Y chromosome (XY). Each of the 22 pairs of autosomes and the 2 sex chromosomes can be distinguished on the basis of size, location of the centromere (which divides the chromosome into arms of equal or unequal length), and the unique banding pattern (Fig. 1-11). More details regarding cytogenetic methodology are available elsewhere.[95]

Most chromosomal disorders found in humans can be classified into one of four groups: (1) excess or loss of one or more chromosomes (*aneuploidy*); (2) breakage and loss of a piece of a chromosome (*deletion*); (3) breakage of two chromosomes, with transfer and fusion of parts of the broken fragments onto each other (*translocation*); and (4) abnormal splitting of the centromere during mitosis so that one arm is lost and the other is duplicated to form one symmetric chromosome with two genetically identical arms (*isochromosome formation*). In addition, chromosomal *mosaicism* may occur such that a single individual may possess two cell lines, or *clones*, each differing in its chromosomal constitution. For example, many patients with the Turner syndrome have been shown to possess some

Fig. 1-11 A trypsin G-banded normal human female karyotype. (Courtesy of David H. Ledbetter.)

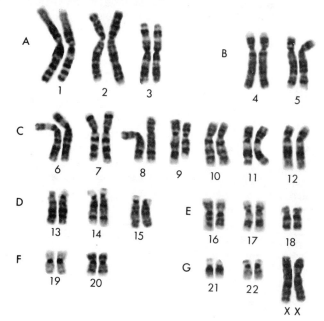

cells with a 45,X constitution and other cells with a normal 46,XX. Their karotype is symbolized 45,X/46,XX

The *autosomal* trisomies responsible for specific clinical syndromes include: (1) trisomy 21 (Down syndrome or mongolism, Chap. 7), characterized by mental retardation, a characteristic facies, marked hypotonia, and many other abnormalities; (2) trisomy 13, characterized by ocular defects, cleft lip and palate, polydactyly, and an average life span of less than 1 year; and (3) trisomy 18, characterized by micrognathia, severe failure to thrive, multiple malformations, and a life span of less than 3 months.

The numeric aberrations of the sex chromosomes include three disorders with 47 chromosomes (47,XXY; 47,XYY; and 47,XXX) and one disorder with 45 chromosomes (45,X). The XXY karyotype is found in patients with the Klinefelter syndrome, who are phenotypic males with testicular dysgenesis, infertility, gynecomastia, tall stature, and behavioral changes. Most individuals with a 47,XYY karyotype are normal fertile males; however, some may be unusually tall and show tendencies to criminality or other behavior abnormalities. Most individuals with the 47,XXX karyotype are clinically normal females, but some may be mentally retarded and deficient in secondary sexual development. The 45,X karyotype is found in about one-half of patients with the Turner syndrome, who are phenotypic females with ovarian dysgenesis, failure of secondary sexual development, short stature, renal anomalies, and pterygium colli. Patients with the Turner syndrome who do not have a 45,X karyotype may have either mosaicism (45,X/46,XX or 45,X/46,XY) or a structural abnormality of the X chromosome, such as an isochromosome X.

Little is known about the factors that cause chromosomal disorders in humans. The most important finding is the association between increasing maternal age and nondisjunction syndromes such as Down syndrome (trisomy 21) and the other autosomal trisomies. A possible etiologic role for other factors, such as genetic predisposition, autoimmune disorders (involving the thyroid gland, in particular), viruses, chemical mutagens, and radiation, has also been suggested.[95]

Chromosomal aberrations are common. The detected frequency of chromosomal aberrations in karyotypes of unselected newborn infants is 1 in 200 (0.5 percent), while among recognized first-trimester spontaneous abortions the frequency of chromosomal defects is as high as 50 percent. Given a 20 percent rate of spontaneous abortion in recognized conceptions, at least 10 percent of all conceptions result in chromosomal aberrations. The vast majority of affected fetuses do not survive the apparently intense in utero selection and are lost early in gestation. Despite this, a high frequency of chromosomal aberrations has been observed in patients with several clinical abnormalities, including (1) multiple congenital malformations (2 to 20 percent); (2) infertility and sterility (1 to 10 percent); (3) mental retardation (1 to 3 percent); and (4) certain forms of malignancy, such as chronic myelogenous leukemia, in which the long arm of chromosome 22 is translocated to one of the larger chromosomes, most often to the long arm of chromosome 9, producing the so-called *Philadelphia* chromosome (a shortened chromosome 22).

Chromosomal aberrations occur with extremely high frequency in various malignancies. In these instances, the constitutional karyotype is usually normal, but the tumor cells show abnormal findings as mentioned above for the Philadelphia chromosome. Numerous chromosomal translocations are now known to be found with some specificity for a variety of tumors.[102–104] In some instances, a constitutional genetic abnormality may represent a first step in a two-step process leading to malignancy. The second step in this process occurs in a single somatic cell and may often be a gross chromosomal aberration which contributes to the development of a tumor. This is best documented for retinoblastoma (Chap. 9), but also occurs in Wilms tumor (Chap. 9), polyposis of the colon,[105] Von Hippel-Lindau disease,[50] and other disorders. The locus involved in hereditary tumors is often also involved in sporadic tumors, as documented for colon tumors, retinoblastoma, renal cell carcinoma, and other tumors (Chap. 9).[106–107]

Chromosomal disorders often occur as new mutations. Both parents are usually normal, and the risk of recurrence in sibs is low. However, when the aberration involves an unbalanced translocation, one parent is a balanced translocation carrier in about a third of the cases. In this instance the recurrence risk for subsequent children may be as high as 20 percent, and additional members of the extended family may also be carriers at high risk for having an offspring with an unbalanced chromosomal complement. Table 1-3 lists the most frequently encountered chromosomal abnormalities occurring among live-born infants.

One important disorder involving a fragile site on the X chromosome is often considered with chromosomal abnormalities, although it may represent a monogenic disorder. Fragile sites are regions of chromosomes which are subject to narrowing or breakage when cells are cultured under conditions which slow or inhibit DNA replication. The fragile X mental retardation syndrome is a common important form of mental retardation associated with the occurrence of a fragile site at Xq28. The disorder has come to attention relatively recently, but enough has been learned to justify a chapter on the subject in this edition (Chap. 8). The disorder shows unusual features of inheritance (see Chap. 8 for details) with a high frequency of clinical expression in hemizygous males and a lower frequency of clinical expression in heterozygous females.

The indications for complete chromosomal analysis have expanded with the growth of information and with the improved resolution of the analysis. Chromosome analysis is clinically indicated in the following situations: (1) in children with two or more major malformations including prenatal or postnatal growth failure as a major malformation; (2) in children with

Table 1-3 Frequency of Chromosomal Disorders among Live-born Infants

Disorders	Frequency
Autosomal abnormalities	
Trisomy 21 (Down syndrome)	1 in 600
Trisomy 18	1 in 5000
Trisomy 13	1 in 15,000
Sex chromosome abnormalities	
Klinefelter syndrome (47,XXY)	1 in 700 males
XYY syndrome (47,XYY)	1 in 800 males
Triple-X syndrome (47,XXX)	1 in 1000 females
Turner syndrome (45,X or 45X/46XX or 45X/46,XY or isochromosome Xq)	1 in 1500 females
Fragile X mental retardation	1 in 2000 males
	1 in 3000 females

SOURCE: Data modified from Vogel and Motulsky,[95] Galjaard,[97] and Chap. 8.

mental retardation of unknown cause with or without malformations; (3) in all children with features of recognized chromosomal syndromes including trisomies, fragile X, and deletions; (4) in couples with a poor reproductive history (infertility, increased numbers of spontaneous abortions, or stillbirths); (5) in antecendents and offspring of individuals with chromosomal translocations; (6) in individuals with sexual malformations or abnormalities of sexual development; and (7) in patients with various malignancies (analysis of tumor cells). The quality of chromosome analysis is important, and attention must be given to special conditions required for detection of the fragile X abnormality. Subtle deletions occur in conditions such as hereditary retinoblastoma, Prader-Willi syndrome, Miller-Dieker syndrome, and other conditions, such that high resolution analysis for a specific region can be requested if particular diagnoses are suspected (see Chap. 9). Analysis of malignancies also requires the use of special techniques. The role of chromosomal analysis in malignancy is growing rapidly.[102-104] Cytogenetic changes in tumors may assist in establishing diagnostic categories, in devising treatment protocols, and in long term follow-up. The role of chromosome analysis in prenatal diagnosis has grown such that the number of analyses performed on prenatal samples now exceeds the number of analyses performed on postnatal samples in most western countries. While prenatal cytogenetic analysis may be performed because of the previous occurrence of cytogenetic abnormalities or because of known familial translocations, the majority of studies are performed for advanced maternal age. There is a progressive trend toward increased utilization of cytogenetic analysis for prenatal diagnosis which can now be carried out using amniocentesis or chorionic villus sampling as discussed below.

For a more complete discussion of the etiology and clinical features of chromosome abnormalities affecting humans, refer to the *Clinical Atlas of Human Chromosomes*[108] and the *Catalogue of Unbalanced Chromosome Aberrations in Man.*[109]

Monogenic Disorders

Having already acknowledged that very few phenotypes are entirely determined by a single locus, it is still very useful to discuss so-called monogenic disorders. Disorders caused by single mutant genes show one of three simple (or Mendelian) patterns of inheritance: (1) autosomal dominant, (2) autosomal recessive, or (3) X-linked. With few exceptions, each of the approximately 3000 Mendelian diseases is rare. As a group, these disorders constitute an important cause of morbidity and death, accounting directly for more than 5 percent of all pediatric hospital admissions.[97] The overall population frequency of monogenic disorders is about 10 per 1000 livebirths, with about 7 in 1000 dominants, about 2.5 in 1000 recessives, and about 0.4 in 1000 X-linked conditions.[97] Table 1-4 lists some of the most common Mendelian disorders.

If a particular disease shows one of the three Mendelian patterns of inheritance, its pathogenesis, no matter how complex, must be due to an abnormality in a single protein molecule. For example, in sickle-cell anemia, the entire clinical syndrome, including such seemingly unrelated disturbances as anemia, pain crises, nephropathy, and predisposition to pneumococcal infections, is the physiological consequence of having a single base change at a specific site in the gene that codes

Table 1-4 Frequency of Some Common Monogenic Disorders among Live-born Infants

Disorder	Estimated frequency*
Autosomal dominant	
Familial hypercholesterolemia	1 in 500
Adult polycystic kidney disease	1 in 1250
Huntington chorea	1 in 2500
Hereditary spherocytosis	1 in 5000
von Willebrand disease	1 in 8000
Marfan syndrome	1 in 20,000
Achondroplasia	1 in 50,000
Autosomal recessive	
Sickle-cell anemia	1 in 655 (U.S. blacks)
Cystic fibrosis	1 in 2500 (Caucasians)
Tay-Sachs disease	1 in 3000 (Ashkenazi Jews)
α_1-Antitrypsin ZZ genotype	1 in 3500
Phenylketonuria	1 in 12,000 (average)
Mucopolysaccharidoses (all types together)	1 in 25,000
Glycogen storage diseases (all types together)	1 in 50,000
X-linked	
Duchenne muscular dystrophy	1 in 7000 males
Hemophilia A	1 in 10,000 males
Fragile X mental retardation	See Table 1-3

*The frequency of some disorders varies widely between ethnic groups (e.g., sickle-cell anemia, cystic fibrosis, Tay-Sachs, α_1-antitrypsin, and phenylketonuria) but is less variant for others, perhaps particularly when new mutations are frequent (e.g., achondroplasia, Duchenne dystrophy, and hemophilia A).
SOURCE: Data modified from Galjaard,[97] Carter,[110] Motulsky,[111] and various chapters in this book.

for the β chain of hemoglobin, producing a substitution of a valine for a glutamic acid in the sixth amino acid position in the protein sequence.

In many Mendelian disorders, it is not yet possible to demonstrate directly the protein that is altered by the mutation. In such cases only the distal physiological effects of the mutation are recognizable. Nevertheless, it is safe to assume that a single primary defect exists whenever a disease is transmitted by a single gene mechanism, and the various manifestations of the disease can all be related to the mutational event by a more or less complicated "pedigree of causes." In recent years, reverse genetic techniques and other molecular methods have led to the cloning of many disease genes, in all cases confirming the monogenic interpretation.

The basic biochemical lesions in monogenic disorders involve defects in a wide variety of proteins, including enzymes, receptors, transport proteins, peptide hormones, immunoglobulins, collagens, and coagulation factors. There are now over 300 human diseases whose biochemical defects have been defined. The majority involve abnormalities in enzymes, but the ability to identify defects in other types of proteins is improving. Most of these disorders are discussed in detail in this book and are tabulated at the end of this chapter. Although genetic defects could involve genes which do not encode a protein (e.g., defects in genes for transfer RNA), none has been identified in humans to date.

The impact of Mendelian disease on human health has been reviewed in detail.[90] It was found that 25 percent of disadaptive Mendelian phenotypes were apparent at birth and over 90 percent by the end of puberty. Slightly more than half of phenotypes involved more than one anatomic or functional sys-

Phenotypic Expression by Systems
(Percent of Phenotypes with System Affected)

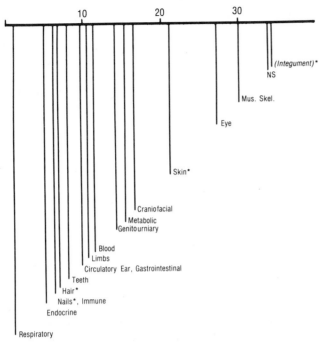

Fig. 1-12 Rank order (abscissa is percentage of phenotypes involving system) for the involvement of a particular anatomic/functional system by Mendelian disease in humans (see Ref. 90 for likelihood that more than one system is involved). Skin, hair, and nails are shown both individually and as a group designated *integument*. Mus Skel = musculo-skeletal; NS = nervous system. *(From T. Costa et al.[90] Used by permission.)*

tem. Life span was reduced in 57 percent of disorders, more often in autosomal recessive and X-linked diseases. Reproductive capacity was reduced in 69 percent of phenotypes. Most phenotypes compatible with prolonged survival were associated with handicaps which limited access to schooling and work. The distribution of phenotypes by systems affected is presented in Fig. 1-12, which indicates, in particular, a high frequency of central nervous system involvement.

Significance of Dominant or Recessive. The distinction between *dominant* and *recessive* is very useful for pedigree analysis but does not imply a fundamental difference in genetic mechanism. The terms are used slightly differently in descriptions of medical disorders than in classical genetics. In classical genetics, alleles are dominant or recessive only if the heterozygote is phenotypically indistinguishable from one or the other homozygote. The dominant allele is the one whose phenotype prevails in the heterozygote. Alleles are codominant if the heterozygote shows an intermediate phenotype. In medicine, the term *dominant* implies that a clinical phenotype will be manifest when an individual has a single copy of the mutant allele (i.e., is *heterozygous* for it), while *recessive* implies that a clinical phenotype occurs only when both alleles are defective (i.e., *homozygosity* or *compound heterozygosity*). These distinctions are extremely useful for clinical diagnosis, for genetic linkage analysis, and for genetic counseling. However, a number of subtleties about the use of the terms dominant and recessive to describe human disorders must be recognized. There is usually no requirement that the phenotype of the het-

erozygote resemble that of either homozygote particularly in the case of dominant disorders. Homozygotes for dominant disorders are identified relatively rarely, but when recognized, their disease is often much more severe than for heterozygotes (e.g., familial hypercholesterolemia, achondroplasia, and some forms of porphyria). When homozygotes are clinically indistinguishable from heterozygotes for dominant disorders, the condition may be described as a *true dominant*. Huntington disease has been suggested as such an example.[112] The terms *homozygous* or *homozygote* are widely used in reference to the phenotype and in a loose sense to imply an individual with two mutant alleles at a locus without knowledge of whether the two mutations are identical. In a strict sense the term implies that an individual has two identical alleles at a particular locus and should be distinguished from a compound heterozygote who is an individual with two different mutant alleles at the locus.

While the distinction of dominant disorders and recessive disorders is useful for classifying clinical phenotypes, there are additional subtleties and complexities to consider. The implication that heterozygotes for a recessive disorder are asymptomatic is an oversimplification. Heterozygotes for at least some recessive disorders may have subtle differences in phenotype which may be accentuated by environmental factors. These subtle phenotypic consequences may be advantageous or disadvantageous. Despite their overall clinical "normality," individuals who are heterozygous for recessive genes often have demonstrable biochemical differences. Many of these complexities are exemplified by sickle-cell anemia, which is best considered to be a recessive disorder for clinical purposes in that the heterozygotes are essentially normal healthy individuals. At a molecular level, the genes are not dominant or recessive, but both genes express their product in what might be described as a *codominant* manner. Both gene products can be demonstrated by hemoglobin electrophoresis in heterozygotes. Despite the general lack of phenotypic effect in heterozygotes, a selective advantage for resistance to malaria is well documented in heterozygotes (Chap. 93). Heterozygotes are also known to have subtle physiological abnormalities affecting renal concentrating ability and cardiopulmonary physiology at high altitudes (Chap. 93). These phenotypic effects in heterozygotes for recessive disorders may be more common than is generally recognized and may contribute to phenotypes more often considered to be of multifactorial etiology. It has been suggested that heterozygotes for ataxia telangectasia are at increased risk of malignancy.[113] Heterozygosity for known recessive disorders contributes to the biochemical and medical individuality of humans.

In other instances, the phenotypic consequences of being heterozygous may be inconsistent, resulting in uncertainty as to whether a disorder is better considered as dominant or recessive. If occasional heterozygotes show clear disease manifestations, a disorder is generally considered dominant. There are dominant disorders where a substantial proportion of heterozygous individuals are asymptomatic as exemplified by some forms of von Willebrand disease (Chap. 87) and some forms of porphyria (Chap. 52). In these instances, homozygous individuals may have heterozygous asymptomatic parents giving rise to an apparent recessive disorder, but these are probably best classified as examples of homozygous dominant disorders. *This exemplifies that the distinction between dominant and recessive disorders is an arbitrary division of a continuum rather than a sharp demarcation.* Clinicians tend to classify a disorder as dominant if most of the symptomatic individuals coming to attention are heterozygotes and as recessive if most of the symptomatic individuals are homozygotes. The distinction of dominant and recessive disorders is additionally complicated for X-linked loci by the mechanism of random X inactivation as discussed under X-linked disorders below.

Whether a mutation generates a dominant or recessive disorder is determined by two factors: (1) the effect of the mutation on the function of the gene product, and (2) the tolerance of the biologic system to a functional perturbation of that particular gene product. In this reductionist time, it is important to realize that gene products work in systems and that the phenotype—be it normal development and physiological homeostasis or maldevelopment and dyshomeostasis—is, at first approximation, the result of the normal or abnormal function of the systems (e.g., the blood glucose homeostatic system or the connective tissue extracellular matrix system). Tolerant systems tend to result in recessive phenotypes; less tolerant systems tend to result in dominant phenotypes. Loci which encode enzymes usually result in recessive phenotypes because of the catalytic nature of enzymes and because enzymes are usually present in amounts considerably in excess of that required to maintain a relatively normal phenotype. Kacser and Burns[114] described the sensitivity coefficient as the fractional change in flux in a pathway over the fractional change in enzyme activity. This quantitative approach demonstrates that a large change in enzyme activity results in a negligible change in flux for most pathways, explaining why most enzyme mutants are recessive. Some mutations at loci encoding enzymes generate dominant phenotypes (many porphyrias, see Chap. 52). Dominant negative mutations can result when a mutant gene product interferes with function of normal molecules produced by the normal allele in a heterozygote.[115] In this way, a product deficiency which might usually be associated with a recessive disorder might occur as a dominant disorder. Different mutations at the same locus may give rise to dominant or recessive disorders depending on the exact nature of the mutation as exemplified by the osteogenesis imperfecta phenotypes resulting from mutations at the loci for the chains of type I collagen (Chap. 115). Although we refer to dominant or recessive "disorders," in reality it is the mutation or allele which is dominant or recessive. Thus, it is possible to have different mutations at a single locus causing a phenotype which is dominant in some families and recessive in others. Some additional aspects of the mechanisms underlying dominant and recessive phenotypes are discussed under the specific categories below. All these complexities notwithstanding, it remains extremely useful to discuss monogenic disorders under separate patterns of inheritance.

Autosomal Dominant Disorders. Dominant diseases are manifest in the heterozygous state, i.e., when only one abnormal gene (*mutant allele*) is present and the corresponding partner allele on the homologous chromosome is normal. By definition, the gene responsible for an autosomal dominant disorder must be located on one of the 22 autosomes; hence, both males and females can be affected. Since alleles segregate independently at meiosis, there is a 1 in 2 chance that the offspring of an affected heterozygote will inherit the mutant allele.

Figure 1-13 shows typical pedigrees involving an autosomal dominant trait. The following features are characteristic: (1) each affected individual has an affected parent (unless the con-

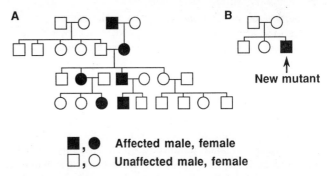

■,● Affected male, female
□,○ Unaffected male, female

Fig. 1-13 Pedigree pattern for an autosomal dominant trait. Note the *vertical* pattern of inheritance; compare new mutation and inherited pedigrees.

dition arose by a new mutation in the sperm or ovum that formed the individual or unless the mutant allele is present but without phenotypic effect in the affected parent as discussed under penetrance, below); (2) an affected individual will bear, on the average, both normal and affected offspring in equal proportions; (3) normal children of an affected individual will have only normal offspring; (4) males and females are affected in equal proportions; (5) each sex is equally likely to transmit the condition to male and female offspring, with male-to-male transmission occurring; and (6) vertical transmission of the condition through successive generations occurs, especially when the trait does not impair the reproductive capacity.

NEW MUTATIONS. While there is a 50 percent risk that the offspring of an individual with an autosomal dominant condition will inherit the disease, it is not necessarily true that each affected person must have an affected parent. In every autosomal dominant disease, a certain proportion of affected persons owe their disorder to a new mutation rather than to an inherited one. Since a rough estimate of the frequency of mutation is 5×10^{-6} mutations per gene per generation and since a dominant trait, by definition, requires a mutation in only one of a pair of alleles, one would expect that about 1 in 100,000 newborn persons would possess a new mutation at any given genetic locus. Many of these mutations either will not impair the function of the gene product or will involve a recessive function, so that the mutation will be clinically silent. Others, however, will cause a defective gene product that gives rise to a dominant trait. The parent in whose germ cells the mutation arose will be clinically normal. The sibs of the affected individual usually will be normal since the mutation will affect one or only a few of the germ cells. Given the nature of germ cell proliferation, it is most probable that a mutation will occur at one of the later cell divisions since they are more numerous, but there may be variable numbers of gametes descended from a single mutational event. Since these mutant gametes still are likely to represent a small minority, and since humans have few offspring, the probability of a recurrence of the disorder among the siblings of a new mutation individual is quite low. Sibs with new mutations can occur, and it is now feasible to document these at a molecular level. The presence of the identical mutation in sibs when neither parent has the mutation in somatic cells can occur (see discussions of osteogenesis imperfecta and Duchenne muscular dystrophy in Chaps. 115 and 118). It will be possible to assess the proportion of gonadal mosaicism by molecular analysis of sperm in some cases. Individuals affected with new mutations are able to transmit the disease, and their offspring are at 50 percent risk for the condition.

The proportion of patients with dominant disorders that represent new mutations is inversely proportional to the effect of the disease on biologic fitness. The term *biologic fitness* refers to the ability of an affected individual to produce children who survive to adult life and reproduce. In the extreme case, if a dominant mutation produced absolute infertility, then all observed cases would, of necessity, represent new mutations, and it would be impossible to prove the genetic transmission of the trait. Molecular analysis could document such mutations. In less severe disorders, as in tuberous sclerosis, the severe mental retardation reduces biologic fitness to about 20 percent of normal, and the proportion of cases due to new mutations is about 80 percent.[116] In dominant disorders such as familial hypercholesterolemia, in which there is negligible if any reduction in biologic fitness, virtually all affected persons have a family pedigree showing classic vertical transmission (Chap. 48). The incidence of a dominant disorder is dependent on the biologic fitness and on the mutation frequency for the locus, which is widely variable. Although the proportion of cases due to new mutation is directly related to biologic fitness, genetic counseling and reproductive planning now can alter this proportion.

Many new mutations appear to occur in the germ cells of fathers who are of relatively advanced age.[95,117] Such a "paternal age effect" is seen, for example, in Marfan syndrome, in which the average age of fathers of sporadic or "new mutation" cases (37 years) is in excess of the mean age of fathers generally (30 years) and also in excess of the age of fathers who transmit Marfan disease due to an inherited mutation (30 years).[118] The increased mutation rate associated with advanced paternal age may be due to the large number of gene replications required for sperm production over many years. Differences in mutation rates for male and female gametes are discussed further below under X-linked disorders.

Before one concludes that a dominant disorder in a given patient with unaffected parents is the result of a new mutation, it is important to consider two other possibilities: (1) the gene may be carried by one parent, in whom the mutant allele is not penetrant (discussed below), and (2) nonpaternity may have occurred (i.e., the father is someone other than the putative father), since this is found in about 3 to 5 percent of randomly studied children in many cultures.

PENETRANCE AND EXPRESSIVITY. These terms are frequently the subject of confusion and slight variations in usage. In the autosomal dominant medical context, penetrance is the proportion of heterozygotes for a given mutation that present with *any* of the phenotypic features of the disorder induced by the mutation. In the medical context, the concept of penetrance can be usefully distinguished in both a clinical and a molecular way. Penetrance is the question at issue when the apparently unaffected offsprings of an affected individual wish to know the probability that they might still carry the mutant gene and bear an affected offspring. The mutant gene is not penetrant if an individual carrying the mutant gene shows absolutely no phenotypic effects. In molecular terms, the presence or absence of the mutant gene can be determined, and a person without the mutant gene can be distinguished from one carrying the mutant gene with lack of penetrance. In this medical and genetic counseling context, the ability to determine penetrance is dependent on diagnostic methods. For example, a new magnetic resonance imaging technique might demonstrate findings not previously recognizable. In the biologic context, the gene can be considered penetrant if it affects the function of the individual.

Expressivity or variability in clinical expression is a concept which describes the range of phenotypic effects in individuals with a mutant genotype. This variability can include the type and severity of symptoms and also can include variation in the age of onset of symptoms. Variability in clinical expression is illustrated dramatically by the multiple endocrine adenoma-peptic ulcer syndrome.[119] Patients in the same family inheriting the same abnormal gene may have hyperplasia or neoplasia of one or all of a wide variety of endocrine tissues, such as the pancreas, parathyroid glands, pituitary gland, or adipose tissue. The resulting clinical manifestations are extremely diverse; different members of the same family may develop peptic ulcers, hypoglycemia, kidney stones, multiple lipomas of the skin, or bitemporal hemianopsia. Because of this variability, the recognition that each family member suffers from the same genetic abnormality can be difficult. There is evidence that some of the variability in this disorder can be explained by chance second somatic mutations at the locus for the disorder on chromosome 11.[120]

Variation in age of onset is seen in disorders such as Huntington chorea and adult polycystic kidney disease. These disorders often do not become manifest clinically until adult life, even though the mutant gene is present from the time of conception. Consideration of variation in age of onset as one form of variation in expression is somewhat arbitrary. In one sense, it cannot be said finally that the mutant gene was never penetrant in an individual until the individual has had a maximal clinical evaluation, completed life, and died from other causes. Lack of penetrance can be considered as the absolute mildest end of the spectrum of expression such that no phenotypic effects whatsoever are observed. In the clinical context, variation in expression can be distinguished from penetrance as the question at issue when an affected individual wishes to know whether his or her offspring will have mild or severe symptoms if born affected. In molecular terms, analysis of the single gene locus will not answer this (i.e., predict variation in expression within a family) but can determine whether the mutant gene is present and not penetrant. Thus, molecular and biochemical analysis of the monogenic locus can uncover lack of penetrance but cannot predict variability in expression within a family with a dominant disorder. Variability in clinical expression between families may be due to allelic heterogeneity which can be defined by molecular methods.

The factors underlying lack of penetrance and variability in expression are similar and fall into three main categories: (1) the genotype at other loci, (2) exogenous or environmental factors, and (3) stochastic factors. The relevant genes at other loci are sometimes called *modifier genes* and probably play a large role in determining phenotypic expression. Despite their presumed importance, good examples are difficult to cite among dominant disorders, although the genotype at the α-globin locus affecting the sickle cell anemia phenotype[88,89] and the genotype at various loci affecting the monogenic hyperlipidemias (see Chap. 47) are examples of effects by modifier genes. The phenotypes in monogenic hyperlipidemias, the porphyrias, and hemochromatosis are affected by diet, alcohol use, smoking, and exercise; these are examples of the impact of environmental and exogenous factors. Stochastic factors are important in at least some instances as exemplified by the severity and distribution of lesions among identical twins with disorders such as retinoblastoma, neurofibromatosis, or tuberous sclerosis. Differences in phenotypic expression due to variable X inactivation among identical twin females heterozygous for an X-linked disorder represent another example of a stochastic effect. Although the issues of penetrance and expressivity are most easily discussed in the context of autosomal dominant disorders, these principles are relevant to chromosomal disorders, autosomal recessive disorders, X-linked disorders, and multifactorial disorders as well.

BIOCHEMICAL BASIS OF DOMINANT TRAITS. Historically, the biochemical bases for recessive disorders were frequently identified as enzyme deficiencies, while the biochemical defects for dominant disorders remained enigmatic. Subsequently, this has changed as the biochemical defects for disorders such as familial hypercholesterolemia, amyloidosis, hereditary spherocytosis, osteogenesis imperfecta, and hereditary retinoblastoma are being determined. A number of mechanisms can account for an abnormal phenotype in the presence of one normal gene and one mutant gene. One mechanism is simply that a half-normal level of gene product is insufficient to maintain a normal phenotype. This is likely to be true when the gene product is a major determinant of the metabolic phenotype in a complex network,[114] such as membrane receptors and rate limiting enzymes in biosynthetic pathways under feedback control (e.g., familial hypercholesterolemia and dominant porphyrias, Chaps. 48 and 52). Another mechanism involves abnormalities of structural proteins where a complex network of direct protein interactions is involved (e.g., collagens in osteogenesis imperfecta and erythrocyte cytoskeleton proteins in spherocytosis and elliptocytosis, Chaps. 95 and 115). Dominant negative mutations are instances where the molecules of mutant gene product interfere with the function of the molecules of normal gene product.[115] Although specific human examples are not well identified, this mechanism may occur for some collagen abnormalities (Chap. 115). In transgenic mice, as little as 10 percent gene expression of a mutant collagen gene can disrupt normal collagen function.[121] Another mechanism for dominant phenotypic effects results when heterozygous defects become homozygous at a single cell level owing to second somatic mutations (e.g., hereditary retinoblastoma, Chap. 9). These defects may be considered dominant at pedigree level and recessive at the single cell level. Conceptually, it is useful to distinguish dominant mutations which generate a product with a new biologic property creating a harmful effect (e.g., amyloidosis, Chap. 97) from those which merely represent a deficiency of normal gene product (e.g., familial hypercholesterolemia and porphyrias, Chaps. 48 and 52). In the former group, restoration of a normal level of gene product would not negate the effect of the mutant gene.

Autosomal Recessive Disorders. Autosomal recessive conditions are those that are clinically apparent only in the homozygous or compound heterozygous state, i.e., when both alleles at a particular genetic locus are mutant alleles. By definition, the gene responsible for an autosomal recessive disorder must be located on one of the 22 autosomes; thus, both males and females can be affected.

Figure 1-14 shows two pedigrees for families with an autosomal recessive trait. Monoplex families (pedigree A) are the most common, but families with multiple affected individuals occur, and the following features are characteristic: (1) the parents are clinically normal; (2) only sibs are affected, and

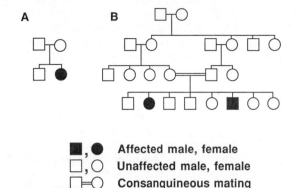

	Affected male, female
	Unaffected male, female
	Consanguineous mating

Fig. 1-14 Pedigree pattern for an autosomal recessive trait. Note the *horizontal* pattern of inheritance and consanguinity in the multiplex pedigree *(B)* in comparison to the more common monoplex pedigree *(A)*.

vertical transmission does not occur; and (3) males and females are affected in equal proportions.

CHARACTERISTICS OF AUTOSOMAL RECESSIVE TRAITS. The relative infrequency of recessive genes in the population and the requirement for two abnormal genes for clinical expression combine to create special conditions for autosomal recessive inheritance: (1) the less frequent the mutant gene in the population, the stronger the likelihood that affected individuals are the product of consanguineous matings (see "Consanguinity," below); (2) if both parents are carriers for the same autosomal recessive gene, the probability for disease is 0.25, for a heterozygote (carrier) is 0.50, and for a noncarrier normal is 0.25; (3) if an affected individual mates with a heterozygote (as may occur with a common mutant gene or a consanguineous marriage), there is a 50 percent probability of disease for each child, and a pedigree simulating dominant inheritance will result; and (4) if two individuals with the same recessive disease mate, all their children will be affected.

The clinical picture in autosomal recessive disorders tends to be more uniform than that of dominant diseases, and onset often occurs early in life. As a general rule, recessive disorders are more commonly diagnosed in children, while dominant diseases have a trimodal age of symptomatology and are more frequently encountered in adults.[90]

In recessive inheritance the probability is that only one in four children in a sibship will be affected; hence, multiple cases in a family may not occur. This is especially true in a society in which small families are common. Consider, for example, 16 families in which both parents are heterozygous for the same recessive disorder, such as cystic fibrosis. If each family has 2 children, the probability is that 9 of the 16 families will have no affected children, 6 will have 1 affected and 1 normal child, and only 1 of the 16 families will have 2 affected children. Because of the tendency toward small families in many contemporary societies, physicians usually see sporadic or isolated cases of a recessive disease without an affected sib to alert them to the possibility of a genetic disorder. Fortunately, because of the relatively uniform clinical picture of recessive disorders and because many can be diagnosed directly by biochemical tests, the diagnosis of a genetic disease can usually be made even when no other members of a family are clinically affected.

BIOCHEMICAL DEFECTS. Basic biochemical lesions underlying many autosomal recessive disorders have been identified. Mutations that give rise to recessive diseases often involve enzymatic proteins, as opposed to nonenzymatic proteins. In these conditions, recessive inheritance occurs because a mutation that destroys the catalytic activity of an enzyme generally does not impair the health of a heterozygote (i.e., an individual who has one mutant allele specifying a functionless enzyme and one normal allele on the partner chromosome specifying a normal enzyme). In this situation, each cell in the body usually produces about 50 percent of the normal number of active enzyme molecules. However, normal regulatory mechanisms function to avert any clinical consequences of this 50 percent deficiency, and so heterozygotes for enzyme defects usually are clinically normal.[122] Frequently such compensation involves nothing more complicated than a simple two- to threefold increase in the substrate concentration for the enzyme. The concentration of a substrate is usually maintained at a point below saturation for the enzyme that metabolizes it. When the enzyme level is reduced 50 percent, as in a heterozygote for a functionless gene at that locus, the residual 50 percent of enzyme molecules can be made to function twice as fast as normal, simply by allowing the substrate concentration to increase twofold. If the twofold increase in substrate does not otherwise affect metabolism adversely, the heterozygote is clinically normal. On the other hand, when an individual inherits functionless alleles at both loci specifying an enzyme, the reduction in enzyme activity is too great for a compensatory mechanism to overcome the deficiency, and a disease results.

The genetic enzyme deficiencies that produce recessive diseases tend to involve enzymes that participate in catabolic pathways. Frequently these enzymes degrade organic molecules that are ingested in the diet, such as galactose (galactosemia), phenylalanine (PKU), and phytanic acid (Refsum syndrome). A special class of such catabolic diseases is one in which the deficiency affects an acid hydrolase that occurs within lysosomes. In these *lysosomal storage disorders*,[123–125] the substrate, usually a complex lipid or polysaccharide, accumulates within swollen lysosomes in specific organs, giving the cells a foamy appearance. Examples of such lysosomal diseases include the mucopolysaccharidoses such as Hurler syndrome (α-iduronidase deficiency) and the sphingolipidoses such as Gaucher disease (glucocerebrosidase deficiency).

POPULATION GENETICS. In general, recessive diseases are rare because the reduced biologic fitness of homozygotes acts to remove the mutant gene from the population. A few lethal recessive disorders, such as cystic fibrosis and sickle-cell anemia, are common. To explain this paradox, it has been postulated that the biologic fitness of heterozygotes is greater than that of noncarriers for these genes. In such a case, the frequency of the gene in the population depends on the balance between the increased fitness of the relatively numerous heterozygotes and the reduced fitness of the less common homozygotes. A small selective advantage of the heterozygote over the normal person results in a high gene frequency and hence a high birth frequency of homozygotes even when the disease is lethal.[126] Thus, about 1 in 20 to 25 Caucasians is heterozygous (a carrier) for the genetically lethal disease cystic fibrosis, and the disease occurs in about 1 in 2500 Caucasian births. In order to maintain such a high gene frequency, heterozygotes for cystic fibrosis may have a selective advantage over noncarriers, but the nature of such a potential advantage is unknown. A selective advantage for the mutant gene might involve the viability of heterozygotes for a reproductive advantage. There

could be a slight meiotic drive, i.e., gametes carrying the mutant gene could have a slightly greater probability of achieving fertilization compared to gametes with the normal gene.[127] It has been argued that disorders might achieve a frequency as high as that seen with cystic fibrosis occasionally without a selective advantage, i.e., by chance. There is evidence from linkage disequilibrium that most or all cystic fibrosis genes are descended from a single mutational event,[128] but this does not resolve why the mutant gene is so frequent. In sickle-cell anemia, another recessive disorder with high frequency among certain populations, heterozygotes are known to have increased resistance to malaria (Chap. 93).

CONSANGUINITY. By definition, a recessive disease requires the inheritance of a mutant allele at the same genetic locus from each parent. When the genes are rare, the likelihood of any two parents being carriers for the same defect is small. If the parents have a common ancestor who carried a recessive gene, then the likelihood that two of the descendants would each have inherited the gene becomes relatively great. The less frequent the recessive gene, the stronger becomes the likelihood that an affected individual may have resulted from such a consanguineous mating. On the other hand, certain recessive genes are so common in the population that the likelihood of two random parents being carriers is great enough to minimize the role of consanguinity. For common traits such as sickle-cell anemia, PKU, cystic fibrosis, and Tay-Sachs disease, all of which have a high carrier frequency in certain populations, consanguinity is usually not present in the parents.

NEW MUTATION. Although new mutations for recessive disorders occur, they rarely can be identified in a clinical setting. This is because a new mutation usually will generate only an asymptomatic heterozygote. Only generations later will the descendants of that mutation be involved in a mating where both parents are heterozygotes. In addition, the selective pressure to eliminate deleterious recessive traits from the population is less because these traits are easily passed on in heterozygous form. A large portion of recessive disease is due to mutations that occurred many, many generations ago; this is becoming clear from studies of phenylketonuria, β thalassemia, and cystic fibrosis (see Chaps. 15, 93, and 108).

X-Linked Disorders. The genes responsible for X-linked disorders are located on the X chromosome; therefore, the clinical risk and severity of the disease are different for the two sexes. Since a female has two X chromosomes, she may be either heterozygous or homozygous for a mutant gene, and the trait may therefore demonstrate either recessive or dominant expression. Expression in females is often variable and heavily influenced by random X inactivation. Males, on the other hand, have only one X chromosome, so they can be expected to display the full syndrome whenever they inherit the gene regardless of whether the gene produces a recessive or dominant trait in the female. Thus, the terms *X-linked dominant* and *X-linked recessive* refer only to the expression of the gene in women.

The distinction of dominant and recessive X-linked disorders is complicated by the effect of X inactivation. This has led to some arbitrary and inconsistent assignments. Ornithine transcarbamylase deficiency (Chap. 20) has often been described as an X-linked dominant, while Fabry disease (Chap. 70) has often been described as an X-linked recessive. Phenotypic abnormalities occur relatively frequently in heterozygotes for either disorder, particularly if the heterozygotes are examined in an informed manner. Since there is no clear convention, it may be best to consider such disorders as simply X-linked without a dominant or recessive designation. The recessive or dominant descriptors are more useful for X-linked disorders where, respectively, heterozygotes are quite consistently asymptomatic (e.g., X-linked recessive Hunter disease, Chap. 61) or are quite consistently symptomatic in a manner similar to hemizygous males (e.g., X-linked dominant hypophosphatemic rickets, Chap. 105).

An important feature of all X-linked inheritance is the absence of male-to-male (i.e., father-to-son) transmission of the trait. This follows because a male must always contribute his Y chromosome to his sons; hence, he can never contribute his X chromosome. On the other hand, a male contributes his sole X chromosome to all his daughters, and so all daughters of a male with an X-linked trait must inherit the mutant gene.

X-LINKED PEDIGREES. The pedigrees in Fig. 1-15 illustrate some of the characteristic features of X-linked inheritance. (1) In contrast to the vertical distribution in dominant traits (parents and children affected) and the horizontal distribution in autosomal recessive traits (sibs affected), the pedigree pattern in X-linked recessive traits tends to be oblique; that is, the trait occurs in the maternal uncles of affected males and in male cousins who are descended from the mother's sisters who are carriers (Fig. 1-15A). (2) Male offspring of carrier females have a 50 percent chance of being affected. (3) All female offspring of affected males are carriers, and affected males do not transmit the disease to their sons. (4) Unaffected males do not transmit the trait to any offspring. (5) Affected homozygous females occur only when an affected male fathers the child of a carrier female.

Examples of X-linked recessive disorders in humans include the Lesch-Nyhan syndrome, glucose-6-phosphate dehydrogenase deficiency, testicular feminization, and Hunter mucopolysaccharidosis. Color blindness is also inherited as an X-linked recessive trait, but it is sufficiently frequent (occurring in about 8 percent of Caucasian males) that the occurrence of homozygous color-blind females is no rarity.

A pedigree for an X-linked disorder with variable symptomatology in females is depicted in Fig. 1-15B. Heterozygous females with and without symptoms occur in the same family. X-linked diseases may occur on the basis of new mutation as

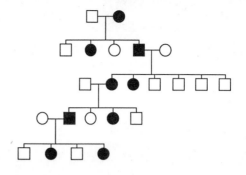

■ Affected hemizygous male
● Affected heterozygous female
□,○ Unaffected male, female

Fig. 1-16 Pedigree pattern of an X-linked dominant trait.

shown by the pedigree in Fig. 1-15C (see "New Mutation and Heterozygote Detection," below).

X-linked dominant inheritance is illustrated by the pedigree in Fig. 1-16. Its characteristic features are as follows: (1) females are affected about twice as often as males; (2) an affected female has a 50 percent probability of transmitting the disorder to her sons or daughters; (3) an affected male transmits the disorder to all his daughters and to none of his sons; and (4) the syndrome may be more variable and less severe in heterozygous affected females than in hemizygous affected males. One common trait, the Xg(a+) blood group, is inherited as an X-linked dominant trait, as are a few diseases, such as hypophosphatemic rickets.

Some rare conditions may be inherited as X-linked dominant traits in which there is lethality in the hemizygous male. The characteristics of this form of inheritance are illustrated by the pedigree in Fig. 1-17. (1) The disorder occurs only in females who are heterozygous for the mutant gene; (2) an affected mother has a 50 percent probability of transmitting the trait to her daughters; (3) an increased frequency of abortions occurs in affected women, the abortions representing affected male fetuses. An example of a condition that is transmitted by this mode of inheritance is incontinentia pigmenti.

X-LINKED DISORDERS AND X INACTIVATION. Understanding of the mechanisms of expression of X-linked traits in females has been greatly advanced by knowledge of the phenomenon of random X inactivation, or the so-called Lyon effect.[129] Early in embryonic development, one of the two X chromosomes in each somatic cell of a female is irreversibly inactivated. The inactivation process is random, so that for each cell there is an equal probability that the paternally or maternally derived X chromosome will be inactivated. The inactivated X chromosome is rendered permanently nonfunctional, so that all progeny of the initial cell inherit the same active and inactive X chromosomes. Thus, each female is a mosaic; on the average, half of her cells express the X chromosome of the father, and half express the X chromosome of the mother. If a mutation in a gene is carried on one of her X chromosomes, about one-half of the cells in each tissue will be normal and the other half will manifest the mutant phenotype. Chance or preferential survival of one clone of cells may disturb these proportions in any given individual. Depending on the proportions of mutant and normal X chromosomes that are active in each tissue, a genetically heterozygous female may be clinically normal or she may have mild or severe manifestations of the disease.

Fig. 1-15 Pedigree pattern for an X-linked trait. A. Note the oblique pattern of inheritance. B. Note the occurrence of symptomatic and asymptomatic heterozygous females in the same pedigree. Heterozygotes are consistently asymptomatic in some disorders (recessive) and are variably symptomatic in other disorders (see text). C. New mutations can give rise to affected males and can give rise to heterozygous females.

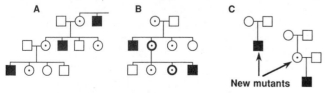

New mutants

■ Affected hemizygous male
⊙ Asymptomatic heterozygous female
◉ Symptomatic heterozygous female
□ Unaffected male
○ Noncarrier female

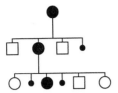

●,○ **Affected and unaffected female**
□ **Unaffected male**
♦ **Spontaneous abortion**

Fig. 1-17 Pedigree pattern of an X-linked dominant trait lethal in the hemizygous male.

In each female cell the nonfunctional X chromosome can be identified as a condensed clump of chromatin—the Barr body. The inactive X chromosome is late replicating, and its DNA is more highly methylated. Methylation of DNA is thought to play a role in maintenance of X inactivation.[130]

Random X inactivation appears to be the single most important determinant of expression in females for many X-linked disorders. There can be a wide range of expression in females with many individuals being asymptomatic, while other individuals have only mild symptoms, and other individuals have very severe symptoms. The recognized frequency of detectable phenotypic alterations in the heterozygote depends on how carefully the women are examined and in some instances on the age at examination. Ornithine transcarbamylase deficiency represents an excellent example of a highly variable phenotype in heterozygotes. Many heterozygous females are asymptomatic, some have minimal protein intolerance, and others experience intermittent episodes of hyperammonemic coma with numerous examples of fatal outcome. For many of these disorders, the hemizygous males are more consistently and more seriously symptomatic than are heterozygous females. Other examples where clinical expression occurs only occasionally in females include Duchenne muscular dystrophy and hemophilia A, while symptoms occur with higher frequency in Fabry disease. As discussed above, it may be easier to describe these as X-linked disorders without applying the dominant or recessive descriptor since the literature has been inconsistent.

NEW MUTATION AND HETEROZYGOTE DETECTION. New mutation in X-linked genes is a particularly important problem in families ascertained because of an isolated affected male (monoplex families). In these families, the mother may be a noncarrier and may have contributed an egg with a new mutation. The father cannot contribute the new mutation, since he contributes a Y chromosome. Alternatively, the mother may be a carrier and may have herself been conceived from a gamete with a new mutation from either her father or her mother. If the new mutation rate for male gametes is greater than for female gametes, as seems likely in some instances, then a larger fraction of mothers of isolated male patients will be carriers. This is because male gametes carrying a new mutation can only give rise to carriers and cannot be contributed to a male offspring. If the mutation rates for male and female gametes are identical, approximately two-thirds of mothers of isolated male patients are expected to be carriers. This proportion increases, if the mutation rate for male gametes exceeds that for female gametes. There is evidence of advanced paternal age in the maternal grandfathers of isolated male patients of some X-linked disorders such as hemophilia A.[131]

Detection of heterozygous females can sometimes be achieved using biochemical methods. These methods have varying degrees of accuracy and are useful in Lesch-Nyhan syndrome, Fabry disease, Hunter syndrome, hemophilia A, hemophilia B, ornithine transcarbamylase deficiency, and Duchenne muscular dystrophy. These biochemical methods are seldom completely accurate because random X inactivation may lead to a relatively normal biochemical result. Accuracy can be increased to some extent by sampling relatively clonal cell sources such as hair roots or cloned skin fibroblasts. Molecular methods can circumvent some of the problems of biochemical analysis of the gene product, particularly when the mutation can be detected directly. Detection of gene deletions or of mutations which alter restriction enzyme sites is very powerful in this regard. RFLP analysis without direct detection of the mutation generally will indicate whether descendants of carriers are themselves carriers or not but generally will not determine whether antecedent individuals in the pedigree are carriers or not (see "Molecular Techniques for Clinical Diagnosis," below). For Duchenne muscular dystrophy, molecular techniques currently allow for detection of gene deletions in the majority of families, making this the preferred method for prenatal diagnosis and carrier detection when informative.[45]

GENETIC HETEROGENEITY

Genetic heterogeneity may result from the existence of a series of different mutations at a single locus (*allelic heterogeneity*) or from mutations at different genetic loci (*nonallelic heterogeneity*). For example, phenotypes such as Charcot-Marie-Tooth neurogenic atrophy, congenital sensorineural deafness, and retinitis pigmentosa all have autosomal dominant, autosomal recessive, and X-linked forms (nonallelic heterogeneity). A clinically similar bleeding disorder can be caused by mutations at either of two loci on the X chromosome, one leading to a deficiency of factor VIII (classic hemophilia, hemophilia A) and the other causing a deficiency of factor IX (Christmas disease, hemophilia B). That both allelic and nonallelic heterogeneity may underlie a clinical phenotype is exemplified by the syndrome of hereditary methemoglobinemia, which was once regarded as a homogeneous clinical entity. The disorder is the result of at least 10 different mutations occurring at three distinct gene loci: two at the locus coding for the α chain of hemoglobin, three at the locus coding for the β chain of hemoglobin, and at least five at the NADH dehydrogenase locus (Chaps. 92 and 93). It is likely that most, if not all, hereditary diseases, when carefully analyzed, will be shown to be genetically heterogeneous.[132,133]

The extent of allelic heterogeneity is particularly impressive and is being rapidly defined at a molecular level. As discussed in the section on mutations above, hundreds of different mutations (hemoglobinopathy and thalassemia) have been described at the β-globin locus, and similar molecular heterogeneity may exist at many if not most loci. Numerous different mutations have been delineated for the low density lipoprotein receptor (Chap. 48) and for phenylalanine hydroxylase (Chap. 15). Considerable clinical heterogeneity can be explained by the occurrence of different mutations at a single locus. With detailed molecular information, it becomes clear that many, if not most, patients with autosomal recessive disorders are in fact compound heterozygotes rather than true homozygotes in the strict sense. Compound heterozygotes have different mutations in the two abnormal genes as exemplified by an individual with SC hemoglobinopathy. Exceptions to this generalization would be when a patient is the product of a consanguineous mating or when a particular mutant allele achieves a high frequency in the population, e.g., sickle-cell anemia.

The extent of clinical heterogeneity that can occur secondary to allelic heterogeneity is particularly impressive for autosomal recessive disorders. For example, Hurler mucopolysaccharidosis and Scheie mucopolysaccharidosis were judged to be different genetic conditions based on the severe, lethal phenotype in Hurler disease compared with the much milder phenotype of bone and joint disease in Scheie disease (Chap. 61). These conditions were ultimately found both to be due to deficiency of L-iduronidase. Description of presumed Hurler-Scheie compound heterozygotes based on the existence of intermediate phenotypes served to emphasize the phenomenon of compound heterozygotes in the 1970s. Similarly the severe Duchenne muscular dystrophy and milder Becker muscular dystrophy are now known to be allelic disorders, both of which, surprisingly, can be caused by sizable gene deletions. Numerous other examples of widely different clinical phenotypes due to allelic heterogeneity are found throughout this text. In many instances there is a classic phenotype in which no functional gene product is produced. Many different alleles (presumably all those which encode no functional gene product) may cause this most severe phenotype. There is frequently a continuum of milder expression arising from mutations which do not totally eliminate the functional gene product. The complexity of the clinical continuum is contributed to by the occurrence of compound heterozygotes. At the mild end of the continuum are those mutant alleles which encode a product which leads to a nearly normal clinical phenotype or to one which is normal under most environmental circumstances. This continuum then extends into detectable biochemical variation which is ordinarily not associated with clinical effect. Hyperphenylalaninemia of mild degree (Chap. 15), mild ("benign") methylmalonic acidemia,[134] and Hartnup disorder (Chap. 101) are examples of this mild biochemical phenotype. Obviously the amount of functional gene product required to prevent clinical symptoms is dependent on other genetic factors and on exogenous factors such as diet and catabolic events. An individual with benign methylmalonic acidemia must be considered to be at greater risk than other individuals in the face of major catabolic episodes so that the benign designation is merely conditional. The individual with Hartnup disorder is at some risk for a "pellagra" complication, and even that risk can be anticipated (Chap. 101). This type of genetic heterogeneity forms one part of the border between monogenic disorders and multifactorial diseases.

MULTIFACTORIAL GENETIC DISEASES

The common chronic diseases of adults (such as essential hypertension, gout, coronary heart disease, diabetes mellitus, peptic ulcer disease, and schizophrenia), as well as the common birth defects (such as cleft lip and palate, spina bifida, and congenital heart disease), have long been known to "run in families." These disorders are described as *multifactorial genetic diseases*. It is useful to distinguish first, however, the ex-

istence of heterogeneity within the etiology for these disorders. For cleft lip and palate, some cases are due to single gene defects, some cases are due to chromosome abnormalities, and the majority of cases appear to be due to multiple genetic and environmental factors. The implication is that multiple factors enter into the etiology of a *single case* in the majority of circumstances. Similarly the etiology of coronary artery disease can be considered to be heterogeneous with a small proportion due primarily to single gene defects (e.g., familial hypercholesterolemia) while the majority of cases are multifactorial (i.e., multiple factors contribute to the etiology of individual cases). Multifactorial etiology implies the interaction of multiple genes with multiple environmental factors in the etiology of individual cases to produce familial aggregation without a simple Mendelian pattern.[135,136]

In the multifactorial genetic diseases, there are *constitutional (polygenic) components* consisting of multiple genes at independent loci whose effects interact in a cumulative fashion. An individual who inherits a particular combination of these genes has a relative risk which may combine with an *environmental component* to cross a "threshold" of biologic significance such that an individual is affected with a multifactorial disease.[135,136] In order for another individual in the same family to express the same syndrome, a similar combination of genes must be inherited. Since sibs share half of their genes, the probability of a sib inheriting the same combination of genes is $(\frac{1}{2})^n$, where n is the number of genes required to express the trait (assuming that none of the genes is linked).

Inasmuch as the precise number of genes responsible for polygenic traits is unknown, the risk of inheritance for a relative of an affected individual is difficult to calculate, and the standard is based on empiric risk figures (i.e., a direct tally of the proportion of affected relatives in previously reported families). In contrast to the monogenic disorders, in which 25 or 50 percent of the first-degree relatives of an affected proband are at genetic risk, multifactorial genetic disorders are generally observed empirically to affect no more than 5 to 10 percent of first-degree relatives. Moreover, in contrast to Mendelian traits, the recurrence risk of multifactorial conditions varies from family to family, and its estimation is significantly influenced by two factors: (1) the number of affected persons already present in the family, and (2) the severity of the disorder in the index case. The greater number of affected relatives and the more severe their disease, the higher the risk to other relatives. For example, the risk of cleft lip in the sibs of a child with unilateral cleft lip is about 2.5 percent, but if the lesion in the index case is bilateral, the risk in the sibs rises to 6 percent.[135,136]

Multifactorial etiology is thought to be important for many diseases which occur beyond adolescence, and diseases with later age of onset may have decreased heritability on average.[137] Review of nine multifactorial diseases provided evidence compatible with a decline in the impact of the genes on disease with increasing age.

The hypothesis of a polygenic component in the inheritance of multifactorial diseases has been given a sound basis in recent years by the demonstration that at least 28 percent of all gene loci harbor polymorphic alleles that vary among individuals (discussed above). Such a large degree of variation in normal genes undoubtedly provides the substrate for variations in genetic predisposition with which environmental factors can interact. So far, the genetic loci most strikingly associated with predisposition to specific diseases are those that constitute the major histocompatibility locus or HLA (human leukocyte antigens) system (Chap. 4). The HLA gene complex is located on the short arm of chromosome 6. It consists of multiple closely linked but distinct loci (A, B, DR, DQ, and DP). The products of these genes are proteins that are found on the surface of body cells and that enable an individual's immune system to distinguish its own cells from those of someone else. Each HLA locus in the population consists of multiple alleles, each of which produces an immunologically distinct protein. For example, an individual may inherit any 2 of 36 alleles at the HLA-B locus. The inheritance of certain alleles predisposes to the development of certain diseases when the individual is exposed to an environmental challenge. For a more detailed discussion of the HLA locus and its role in disease suceptibility, the reader is referred to Chap. 4.

Multifactorial disorders are heterogeneous in etiology in the sense that the relative contribution of the polygenic factors ("risk genes") and environmental factors will vary greatly from patient to patient. As discussed above, among common phenotypes which are largely multifactorial, a small proportion of cases may be due to monogenic or chromosomal abnormalities. For example, although coronary heart disease is usually of multifactorial etiology, about 5 percent of subjects with premature myocardial infarctions are heterozygotes for familial hypercholesterolemia, a single-gene disorder that produces atherosclerosis in the absence of an extraordinary environmental factor (Chap. 48). However, even in a single gene disorder such as familial hypercholesterolemia, other loci (e.g., the genes for apolipoprotein B and apolipoprotein E) could easily influence the phenotype, and nongenetic factors (diet and smoking) certainly modify the risk. The complexity of the etiology for coronary artery disease is detailed in part in Table 1-5. Numerous interrelated biochemical and genetic factors, as well as numerous nongenetic factors, affect the risk. An appreciation of this etiologic heterogeneity and careful investigation of each patient are necessary prerequisites for counseling families at risk for these disorders.

INTERACTION BETWEEN SINGLE GENETIC AND ENVIRONMENTAL FACTORS

In addition to polygenic states, many single-gene mutations are known to create abnormal responses to environmental factors. Some of the best examples of this interaction between genes and environmental factors are those monogenic disorders which produce clinically significant and often life-threatening idiosyncratic responses to drugs.

Table 1-6 lists the most important of these *pharmacogenetic* disorders, which encompass all three of the Mendelian modes of inheritance.[95,138] Perhaps the most common is glucose-6-phosphate dehydrogenase deficiency, an X-linked trait in which a variety of drugs may precipitate a hemolytic anemia (Chap. 91). Plasma pseudocholinesterase deficiency and hepatic transacetylase deficiency are examples of autosomal recessive traits that alter drug catabolism so that when the muscle relaxant suxamethonium or the antituberculous drug isoniazid is administered, apnea or peripheral neuropathy, respectively, may ensue. Malignant hyperthermia is an autosomal dominant trait in which acute hyperpyrexia, muscle rigidity, and hyperkalemic cardiac arrest may be induced by administration of any one of several anesthetic agents. Acute intermittent porphyria is another example of a single-gene disorder that is exacerbated by drugs such as barbiturates (Chap. 52).

Misinterpretation of adverse drug reactions may result in serious harm to patients. In general, all unusual idiosyncratic reactions should be considered to be genetically determined until proven otherwise. Fortunately, the pharmacogenetic disorders are a group of diseases for which therapy is straightforward: avoidance of the noxious drug by the patient and relatives.

In addition to drugs, other factors in the environment may aggravate specific genetic traits. Cigarette smoke may have deleterious effects on persons homozygous (and possibly heterozygous) for α_1-antitrypsin deficiency, who are predisposed to the development of emphysema (Chap. 96). Patients with xeroderma pigmentosum are unusually sensitive to sunlight and high temperatures (Chap. 120). Avoidance of milk at an early age prevents many of the complications ordinarily seen in persons with galactosemia (Chap. 13). Unfortunately a modern society is also subjected to an endless array of novel environmental exposures. The recent widespread utilization of aspartame is an example of a special risk for PKU patients (Chap. 15).

Genetic-environmental interactions are particularly important in pregnancy. Women who are affected with PKU may develop high plasma phenylalanine levels during pregnancy, and thus their offspring may suffer from phenylalanine-induced birth defects even though the offspring may not themselves have PKU (Chap. 15). Other examples of diseases resulting from an adverse genetic relation between the mother and fetus include erythroblastosis caused by Rh incompatibility and diabetic embryopathy, a series of major birth defects occurring in about 5 percent of the offspring of women who are clinially diabetic during pregnancy.

PATHOGENESIS OF GENETIC DISEASES

Every genetic disease results from a primary alteration in DNA structure. This DNA change leads to the production of an abnormal mRNA or to a change in the amount of normal mRNA. The alteration in mRNA produces a disturbance in the amount of protein or in protein structure and function. This disturbance in turn leads to a disruption of cell and organ function. Three general mechanisms of pathogenesis can be distinguished: (1) Proteins may have a relatively direct effect on a biologic system, often by affecting functionally related proteins. (2) Proteins may affect the metabolism of other molecules (often small metabolites) which are intermediates in the

Table 1-5 Risk Factors for Atherosclerosis and Coronary Artery Disease

LDL receptor genotype	Aging
Apolipoprotein E genotype	Male sex
Familial hypertriglyceridemia	Smoking
Familial combined hyperlipidemia	Hypertension
Lipoprotein Lp(a)	Obesity
Apolipoprotein RFLP associations?	Diet
Rarer gene disorders	Diabetes mellitus
Increased LDL	Inactivity?
Decreased HDL	Stress?

NOTE: See Chapters 10, 44 to 51, 64, and 70 for discussion of various genetic risk factors.

Table 1-6 Examples of Pharmacogenetic Disorders

Disorder	Abnormal protein	Mode of inheritance	Frequency	Drugs producing the abnormal response	Clinical effect
Slow inactivation of isoniazid	Isoniazid acetylase in liver	Autosomal recessive	Approximately 50% of U.S. population	Isoniazid, sulfamethazine, sulfamaprine, phenelzine, dapsone, hydralazine, procainamide	Polyneuritis (isoniazid); lupuslike reaction (hydralazine)
Suxamethonium sensitivity or atypical pseudocholinesterase	Pseudocholinesterase in plasma	Autosomal recessive	Several mutant alleles; most common allele occurs 1 in 2500	Suxamethonium or succinylcholine	Apnea
Warfarin resistance	? Altered receptor or enzyme in liver with increased affinity for vitamin K	Autosomal dominant	Rare	Warfarin (coumadin)	Inability to achieve anticoagulation with usual doses of drug
Glucose-6-phosphate dehydrogenase deficiency	Glucose-6-phosphate dehydrogenase in erythrocytes	X-linked recessive	Approximately 100 million affected in world; occurs in high frequency where malaria is endemic; multiple alleles	Analgesics, sulfonamides, antimalarials, nitrofurantoin, other drugs	Hemolysis
Malignant hyperthermia	Unknown	Autosomal dominant	Approximately 1 in 20,000	Various anesthetics, especially halothane	Severe hyperpyrexia, muscle rigidity, death
Drug-sensitive hemoglobins					
Hemoglobin Zurich	Arginine substitution chain histidine at the 63d position of the β of hemoglobin	Autosomal dominant	Rare	Sulfonamides	Hemolysis
Hemoglobin H	Hemoglobin composed of four β chains; α chains missing	Autosomal dominant	Rare	Many different drugs	Hemolysis

SOURCE: Data modified from Vesell.[138]

pathogenesis. (3) Proteins may regulate the expression of other genes. These conceptual separations may not always be complete. In addition there is great heterogeneity in the exact nature of the structural and functional abnormalities of individual proteins. Some examples of mechanisms of pathogenesis are listed in Table 1-7.

Proteins with Direct Actions

Even in instances where the pathogenesis involves a direct action of the protein, proteins are interacting in complex systems, and there will be secondary effects on other molecules. Disorders of globin chains may lead to direct effects on the ability to transport oxygen, as in the case of certain hemoglobinopathies, or may lead to abnormalities of red cell maturation or stability, as occurs in the thalassemias and in sickle-cell anemia (Chap. 93). Disorders of the plasma proteins involved in the coagulation system also lead to relatively direct biologic effects, but these proteins do act in a cascade which leads ultimately to a carefully regulated coagulation process (Chaps. 84 to 90). Inherited abnormalities of α_1-antitrypsin cause a series of relatively direct defects which are due in part to hepatic injury secondary to accumulation of abnormal protein in hepatocytes and in part to the lack of action of the protein at peripheral sites such as the lung, but this is an example where understanding of pathogenesis is incomplete (Chap. 96). Abnormalities of the red cell cytoskeleton are thought to have a direct effect on red cell shape and function

(Chap. 95). For amyloidosis, the presence of an altered peptide chain leads to extracellular deposition with distortion of architecture within various organs (Chap. 97). Abnormalities of surface proteins are thought to lead directly to the cellular dysfunction in leukocyte adhesion deficiency (Chap. 114). Abnormalities of collagen chains lead to relatively direct effects on extracellular matrix, but clearly there are associated secondary effects involving calcium and bone density in osteogenesis imperfecta (Chap. 115).

Proteins Affecting the Metabolism of Small Molecules

The pathogenesis of the majority of disorders discussed in this book involves secondary effects on metabolism of small molecules. In some instances, the pathogenesis involves *deficiency of products* whose synthesis or transport is impaired. In other instances the pathogenesis involves the harmful *accumulation of metabolites* due to impaired metabolism or transport. The details of pathogenesis are often poorly understood as in phenylketonuria, where it is clear that lowering phenylalanine intake is an effective form of treatment, but the biochemical mechanisms by which phenylalanine accumulation causes mental retardation are incompletely understood (Chap. 15). In the glycogen storage diseases, the phenotypes represent mixed effects of accumulation of excessive and/or abnormal glycogen in the tissues and deficiency of glucose to be derived from glycogen (Chap. 12). For many of the amino acid and organic

Table 1-7 Examples of Pathogenesis of Genetic Disease

Disorder	Mechanism	Chapter
A. Proteins with relatively direct biologic effects		
1. Globin abnormalities	Altered oxygen transport	
	Alteration of cell shape or viability	93
2. Coagulation factor abnormalities	Increased or decreased coagulation cascade	84–90
3. Spherocytosis	Altered cell shape and membrane stability	95
4. Amyloidosis	Deposition of abnormal peptide in extracellular spaces	97
5. Leukocyte adhesion deficiency	Absence of cell adhesion protein impairs leukocyte motility and attachment	114
6. Osteogenesis imperfecta	Abnormal collagen chains impair extracellular matrix function	115
7. Kartagener syndrome	Alteration of organelle structure	112
B. Proteins affecting the metabolism of other (often small) molecules		
1. Altered flux through metabolic pathways		
a. Phenylketonuria	⎰ Accumulation of toxic precursor ⎱	15
b. Lysosomal storage diseases	⎱ (catabolic pathway) ⎰	61–72
c. Thyroxine synthetic defects	Deficiency of product (anabolic pathway)	73
d. Gout with altered PP-ribose-P synthetase	Overproduction of product (anabolic pathway)	37
2. Disordered feedback regulation of synthetic pathways		
a. Acute intermittent porphyria	⎧ Overproduction of	52
b. Lesch-Nyhan	products owing to decreased	38
c. Familial hypercholesterolemia	synthesis or availability of feedback regulator	48
3. Disordered transport		
a. Cystinuria	Impaired renal reabsorption	99
b. Glucose-galactose malabsorption	Impaired gastrointestinal absorption	98
c. Cystinosis	Impaired lysosomal transport	107
4. Effects on other proteins		
a. Mucolipidosis II	Abnormal processing of lysosomal enzymes	62
b. Biotinidase deficiency	Deficiency of cofactor for various enzymes	83
C. Proteins regulating the expression of other genes (possible)		
1. XY females	Deficiency of sex-determining factor, ? failure of product to regulate other genes	(Ref. 8)
2. Testicular feminization	? Failure of testosterone receptor to regulate other genes	75

acid disorders, the pathogenesis appears to involve accumulation of substrates and their metabolites secondary to an enzyme deficiency rather than to lack of products of the reactions. This is reflected by the fact that many of these disorders can be treated by restriction of dietary products which feed into the pathway which is blocked. Disorders of vitamin metabolism often have secondary effects on multiple enzymes which function in the amino acid and organic acid pathways.

Other examples of secondary involvement of small molecules include the porphyrias and disorders of bilirubin metabolism, where the toxic effects of accumulated substrates and related metabolites appear to represent a major pathogenic mechanism, although product deficiency may also be important in some porphyrias. Disorders of copper and iron metabolism also appear to involve toxic effects of accumulated metals in some instances, but the details of pathogenesis are often poorly delineated. The lysosomal storage diseases represent a group of disorders where accumulation of various macromolecules is thought to have a detrimental effect on cell and organ function (Chaps. 61 to 72). Again the details of the biochemical mechanisms underlying these cellular disturbances are incompletely understood.

The disorders of hormone synthesis provide a contrast in that these usually involve deficiencies of the products of reactions rather than harmful effects of accumulated substrates (Chaps. 73 to 80). The details of pathogenesis in these instances are largely related to the understanding of the action of the various hormones. This mechanism of pathogenesis

lends itself to treatment by replacement of the deficient hormone.

Disorders of membrane transport affect the compartmentation of small molecules (Chaps. 98 to 108). This can lead to gastrointestinal malabsorption, excessive urinary losses, or abnormalities of transport within cells as in the case of cystinosis. The pathogenesis of lipoprotein disorders is complex and variable. Even in instances such as LDL receptor deficiency where considerable information is available, the details of how excessive LDL accumulation leads to increased atherosclerosis are not entirely clear. These mechanisms certainly involve secondary effects on lipoproteins and lipid metabolism.

Regulatory Proteins

Although human mutations have yet to be definitively identified in proteins which regulate other genes, it seems likely that they exist. DNA is the "substrate" for these variant proteins. There are extensive data indicating that trans-acting proteins bind to DNA sequences which are cis to the structural genes, as discussed under "Control of Gene Expression," above. There is ample evidence that many hormone and ligand binding proteins represent regulatory gene products including the glucocorticoid receptor, the estrogen receptor, the progesterone receptor, the thyroid hormone receptor (c-*erb*-A), the vitamin D receptor, and the mineralocorticoid receptor.[74,75] Human defects in some of these genes may ultimately prove to represent control gene mutations. In fact, deletion of the sex-determining region of the Y chromosome in XY females may prove to be a good example.[8] There is evidence that the sex-determining region encodes a protein which binds to DNA in a sequence specific manner, and may regulate transcription. Disorders of the androgen receptor (Chap. 75) may prove to represent defects in a protein which regulates transcription.

The Nature of Protein Abnormalities

The pathogenesis of a disease may be influenced by the exact nature of the mutation. A protein may be totally absent, may be produced but have no functional activity, or may be produced and have altered functional properties. In the case of enzymes, residual activity may be associated with decreased affinity for substrates or cofactors. Reduced activity may also result from instability of the protein. In other instances, a reduced amount of normal protein may be synthesized, as in the case of a splicing mutation where a small proportion of mRNA molecules is spliced normally. Often, residual levels of protein function or enzyme activity can be correlated with milder phenotypes, but lack of correlation between in vitro and in vivo activity frequently prevents reliable prognostication based on in vitro results. Proteins may be defective in posttranslational modification as in the case of the Z allele for α_1-antitrypsin deficiency. Many proteins are targeted to mitochondria, lysosomes, other compartments, or the extracellular space, and they may be mutated in ways that affect the targeting mechanisms (Chap. 3). Thus a mutation in the locus for a lysosomal enzyme may lead to no protein production, to production of a protein which never reaches the lysosome, or to production of a protein which reaches the lysosome but is unstable or catalytically impaired. Nonenzymatic proteins may show a variety of defects including an enhanced tendency to aggregation (sickle-cell disease) or defective ligand binding (familial hypercholesterolemia and testicular feminization).

TECHNIQUES FOR STUDYING METABOLIC DISEASES

Originally, inborn errors of metabolism attracted Garrod's attention because of the deficiency of a product (melanin in albinism) or the urinary excretion of an excess amount of a precursor (pentosuria, cystinuria, and alkaptonuria). Identification of the specific metabolite depended on the existence of qualitative chemical tests. This approach is still the basis for the detection of most biochemical genetic defects, although more complex analytic methods have been introduced. The reverse genetics approach is an entirely different strategy which is assuming a prominent role.

Initial Biochemical Clues: Accumulated or Missing Metabolites, Histochemistry, and Clinical Features

The majority of biochemical genetic defects are known today because of initial observations made with simple chemical tests or because a biochemical or medical test which was in widespread use detected unusual results in some individuals. Typical examples would include the detection of abnormal phe-

nylalanine metabolites in PKU, elevated uric acid in Lesch-Nyhan syndrome, and elevated cholesterol in familial hypercholesterolemia. Simple screening procedures such as the ferric chloride test for detection of phenylalanine metabolites, the use of nitrosonaphthol for detection of tryosyl compounds, tests for reducing agents, and the dinitrophenylhydrazine reaction for detection of keto acids were very useful in the past. Screening tests for detection of mucopolysaccharides and the use of nitroprusside for detection of disulfides such as cystine or homocystine remain valuable. Paper chromatography and subsequently thin layer chromatography were used to identify the majority of amino acid disorders known presently. Currently, quantitative analysis of amino acids using ion-exchange chromatography, high performance liquid chromatography (HPLC), or gas chromatography has replaced the semiquantitative methods for analysis of plasma, serum, urine, or cerebrospinal fluid in most metabolic centers. The use of gas chromatography and mass spectroscopy (GC/MS) for detection of organic acids has been applied primarily to the urine for detection of numerous new biochemical genetic disorders (see organic acidemias, Chaps. 27 to 36). Fast atom bombardment has proven particularly useful for analysis of acyl carnitines in the urine (Chap. 33). Analysis of very long chain fatty acids in the plasma has contributed to the recognition of a number of peroxisomal disorders (Chaps. 57 to 60). With the application of each new technology, new classes of disorders are detected. Hence there are separate sections in this text for organic acidemias and for peroxisomal disorders.

Other conditions have been recognized as part of routine medical procedures. The presence of jaundice, excessive bleeding, recurrent infections, muscle weakness, fragile connective tissues, or evidence of hormonal insufficiency may offer broad clues to the underlying biochemical genetic defect. When electrophoretic procedures were adopted, direct detection of protein abnormalities occurred relatively incidentally, as in the case of many hemoglobinopathies, α_1-antitrypsin deficiency, analbuminemia, and adenosine deaminase deficiency. Accumulated metabolites were discovered for many disorders using pathologic and histochemical analyses as exemplified by the detection of glycogen in the glycogen storage diseases, the recognition of various lipids and glycoproteins in many lysosomal storage diseases, the presence of excess iron in hemochromatosis, and the unusual staining properties of tissues in amyloidosis.

In contrast to the examples where phenotypic features may suggest a particular biochemical area, the current level of knowledge frequently does not allow for any anticipation of the biochemical defect which might underlie a phenotype as exemplified by the Lesch-Nyhan syndrome, galactosemia, gyrate atrophy of the retina, and many other disorders. This inability to suspect the biochemical defect in the majority of monogenic disorders presumably will be increasingly circumvented by the reverse genetic approach. Despite the many mechanisms for identifying biochemical defects, the underlying abnormality in the majority of disorders listed in McKusick's *Mendelian Inheritance in Man*[4] remains unknown.

The clinical approach to diagnosis of inborn errors of metabolism relies heavily on a large fund of knowledge on the part of the diagnostician because of the large number of disorders. Some phenotypes are very distinctive (e.g., self-mutilation in Lesch-Nyhan syndrome), and some are very nonspecific (e.g., developmental delay in PKU). Good detection of inborn errors of metabolism relies in part on screening programs but depends primarily on a high index of suspicion and access to expert laboratory services. Detailed strategies for diagnosis and selection of laboratory tests are available.[139]

Direct Analysis of Enzymes and Proteins

When a biochemical pathway is known, chemical identification of an accumulated metabolite frequently leads directly to recognition of the site of the metabolic derangement and to confirmation by direct assay for activity of the suspect enzyme. When the steps in a metabolic pathway are not well understood, full disclosure of the biochemical abnormality frequently has to await the elucidation of the normal pathways of synthesis and degradation of the compound. Indeed, metabolic errors have served as a stimulus and a source of insight for biochemists in defining pathways of normal metabolism, as in the case of the gangliosidoses. In many cases, the accumulation of a metabolite in a patient with an enzyme deficiency provides the first clue to the existence or importance of a pathway.

Diagnosis of an enzymatic defect may be made by direct assay of blood or tissue obtained by biopsy. Direct demonstration of abnormality or deficiency of the gene or gene product is the preferred diagnostic approach. This can frequently be accomplished using blood samples. A particularly useful technique is enzyme assay using white blood cells which are easily isolated from normal and affected individuals. Leukocytes can be used to demonstrate the defect in a variety of disorders, such as maple syrup urine disease, methylmalonic acidemia, some forms of glycogen storage disease, and almost all lysosomal storage diseases. Plasma or serum may be used for many enzyme diagnoses as exemplified by Tay-Sachs disease and biotinidase deficiency. Erythrocytes provide a convenient source of enzyme for analysis as in Lesch-Nyhan syndrome, galactosemia, and deficiencies in many of the enzymes involving glycolytic and oxidative pathways of glucose metabolism. In some instances, cultured skin fibroblasts or cultured lymphoblasts may be the preferred tissue for enzymatic diagnosis or may represent a convenient source of viable cells which can be sent to consultant laboratories. Of course, abnormalities of coagulation and of hemoglobin can be studied using blood samples. In some instances, electrophoretic abnormalities of proteins rather than measurement of enzyme activity provide the diagnosis, as in the case of α_1-antitrypsin deficiency.

Samples from blood and cultured skin fibroblasts are preferred for diagnosis because of the less invasive nature of the sampling process, although tissue biopsy is necessary in some circumstances. Biopsies of liver, intestinal mucosa, muscle, and thyroid may usually be obtained at low risk and can provide critical information in some instances in which such information would have been unobtainable in any other way. In many instances, it is possible to use blood samples for enzymatic assay even though the major pathology involves specialized tissues as in Tay-Sachs disease. An important aspect of the clinical practice of metabolic disease involves the proper selection of diagnostic samples. If diagnosis can be accomplished by DNA analysis as discussed below, any source of DNA such as that from leukocytes can avoid the need for more invasive procedures. This is true for Duchenne muscular dystrophy where gross deletions can be demonstrated by DNA analysis in the majority of patients,[45] thus circumventing any need for muscle biopsy in the diagnosis of many patients.

Cell Culture Studies

The technology of cell culture has been standardized so that it is routine to grow somatic cells in vitro. The most readily cultured cells, skin fibroblasts and Epstein-Barr (EB) virus transformed lymphoblasts, have been exploited widely in the study of human genetic disorders. Single cells can be isolated and cloned. Biochemical studies of varying levels of complexity can be performed on the cells. Important advantages of cultured cells include: (1) the ability to incorporate radioactive precursors, (2) the ability to perform repeated studies without recourse to the patient, and (3) relative ease with which comparative studies can be done on different patients. Radioisotopic precursors can be used to follow the fate of metabolites in pathways. Studies of biosynthesis and posttranslational processing can be accomplished by incorporation of radioactive amino acids into newly synthesized proteins followed by immunoprecipitation and polyacrylamide gel electrophoresis. Such studies have been very valuable for analysis of lysosomal storage diseases (e.g., Tay-Sachs), mitochondrial protein disorders (e.g., ornithine transcarbamylase deficiency), and disorders of cell surface proteins (e.g., familial hypercholesterolemia and leukocyte adhesion deficiency). Hundreds of strains of mutant human fibroblasts and lymphoblasts are available on request from repositories around the world. A very large proportion of all biochemical genetic research conducted during the 1970s and 1980s has used cultured fibroblasts or lymphoblasts as a primary methodology.

The use of cell culture proved essential in the elucidation of the biochemical defects for several metabolic disorders. The underlying defects in the mucopolysaccharidoses were first revealed in the now classic "cross-correction" studies of Neufeld and Fratantoni.[140] These workers found that the medium in which fibroblasts from a patient with the Hurler syndrome had grown was able to correct the defect in the cells from a patient with the Hunter syndrome. This was because the Hurler cells excreted induronate sulfatase, the lysosomal enzyme that was deficient in the Hunter cells. Conversely, the medium from the Hunter cells contained α-iduronidase, which corrected the defect of the Hurler cells. These observations were the first to indicate the nature of the biochemical defects in these two syndromes, viz., in each case a deficiency of a different enzyme involved in mucopolysaccharide catabolism (Chap. 61). Moreover, these experiments provided the first indication that lysosomal enzymes could exchange between cells, a finding that later led to the elucidation of the pathway for receptor-mediated endocytosis of lysosomal enzymes (Chap. 62).

In addition to the mucopolysaccharidoses, the use of cultured cells provided the first clue to the elucidation of the biochemical defects in several other genetic disorders, including familial hypercholesterolemia (Chap. 48), I-cell disease (Chap. 62), and xeroderma pigmentosum (Chap. 120).

The fibroblast culture technique, unfortunately, is not applicable to the study of all inborn errors, since the metabolic activity at fault may not be expressed in the fibroblast. For example, phenylalanine hydroxylase activity is confined to the hepatic parenchymal cell. However, many specialized cell culture systems have proven useful for study of genetic disorders. The gene for chronic granulomatous disease was cloned using a myeloid leukemia cell line (HL-60 cells).[44] The Duchenne muscular dystrophy gene product is expressed in cultured myoblasts.[141] T-cell receptors were cloned using established T-cell lines. The ion channel abnormalities in cystic fibrosis are being studied using primary tracheal epithelial cultures and primary sweat gland cultures (Chap. 108). Many other specialized cell cultures are of use including erythroleukemia cells and hepatoma cell lines. Cultured embryonic stem cells from mice have been used to select mutations in vitro and then generate a mouse from these mutant cells.[142,143] Hypoxanthine-guanine phosphoribosyltransferase (HPRT)-deficient mice have been obtained in this manner.

With the techniques of molecular biology, it is possible to analyze genomic DNA in cultured cells, even when the gene product is not synthesized in the cells (see below and Chap. 2). Although cultured fibroblasts are adequate for isolation of DNA, cultured lymphoblasts are even more attractive because the cell lines are immortal, large numbers of cells are easily grown, and only a blood sample rather than a tissue biopsy is required to initiate the culture.

Cells in culture offer unique opportunities for testing genetic mechanisms. X-linked mutations have been used in cell cultures to text the X-inactivation hypothesis of Lyon. Studies of at least five X-linked loci, including the loci for glucose-6-phosphate dehydrogenase, hypoxanthine-guanine phosphoribosyltransferase (Lesch-Nyhan syndrome), phosphoglycerate kinase, ceramide trihexose α-galactosidase (Fabry disease), and phosphorylase-b-kinase (glycogen storage disease, type VIII), have shown random X inactivation of the paternal or maternal X chromosome in each cell of heterozygous females.[144] Similar inactivation does not occur in autosomal loci. Nor does it appear that inactivation of one X is necessarily complete at all loci. Present evidence suggests that in the case of at least three X-linked loci—the Xg(a) locus,[145] the steroid sulfatase locus,[146] and the MIC2X locus[147]—both alleles are expressed in cells of heterozygous females.

Somatic cell hybrids whose nuclei contain genomes from different species, including serially propagated hybrids of mouse and human fibroblast cells, have been prepared in a number of laboratories.[148–150] Following hybridization, there is a gradual reduction in chromosome number in which human chromosomes are preferentially eliminated. As mentioned earlier, this technology has been responsible for much of the genetic mapping of the human autosomes.

The cell hybridization technique has also been useful in defining heterogeneity of a number of inborn errors by complementation analysis.[149,150] Cultured fibroblasts from two affected individuals with a similar phenotype are fused to form heterokaryons with the use of either Sendai virus or polyethylene glycol. Generally, if the abnormal phenotype of the two parental strains is corrected in the heterokaryon, the defects must involve different genes, although intraallelic complementation also can occur. On the other hand, a negative complementation test suggests that the defects in the two parental strains involve allelic mutations that are not mutually corrective. This approach has been skillfully used in the analysis of heterogeneity in several inborn errors, including xeroderma pigmentosum (Chap. 120), the methylmalonic acidemias (Chap. 29), the propionic acidemias (Chap. 29), the G_{M2} gangliosidoses (Chap. 72), and galactosialidosis (Chap. 71).

Recombinant DNA Techniques

The most powerful new techniques for studying human biochemical genetics are those of recombinant DNA technology.

They are described in broad terms in Chap. 2 and in specific detail in relevant chapters. These techniques include restriction enzyme digestion, cDNA cloning, genomic DNA cloning, DNA sequencing, Southern blotting for analysis of DNA, Northern blotting for analysis of RNA, and the polymerase chain reaction for amplification of DNA and RNA sequences. Molecular techniques allowed initially for the cloning of cDNAs and genomic DNAs for numerous well characterized gene products such as globin chains, phenylalanine hydroxylase, and HPRT (Chaps. 93, 15, and 38 respectively). Innumerable mutations were characterized at a nucleic acid level, and RNA splicing mutations were identified. The ability to associate unique mutations with haplotypes of RFLPs has provided insight into the history of the mutations currently contributing to allelic heterogeneity (e.g., thalassemia, PKU, and cystic fibrosis). This analysis of the gene and of mutations has been extended to most of the clotting factors (Chaps. 84 to 90), to the collagen genes (Chap. 115), and to most of the lipoprotein disorders (Chaps. 44 to 49). Study of mutations often contributes to the understanding of functional aspects of the corresponding gene product, as exemplified by the LDL receptor where mutations in various domains affect processes such as LDL binding or receptor internalization (Chap. 48). Molecular studies of apolipoprotein B allowed for determination of the structure of this gene product which was extremely difficult to analyze at a protein level. In addition, a remarkable new mechanism probably involving a single base alteration in mature mRNA to produce two mRNAs and two polypeptide products (apo B-48 and apo B-100) from a single gene was identified (Chap. 44B). Classic mutations in disorders such as Gaucher disease and Tay-Sachs disease are being delineated at the molecular level (Chaps. 67 and 72). In some cases, the molecular definition and biologic definition of conditions are approximately concurrent, as in the case of deficiency of a leukocyte adhesion subunit in leukocyte adhesion deficiency (Chap. 113).

Recombinant DNA techniques have opened the possibility for major new adventures such as reverse genetics as described in Chap. 2. The genes for retinoblastoma, chronic granulomatous disease, and Duchenne muscular dystrophy[44–46] (Chaps. 9, 114, and 118, respectively) have been cloned without prior knowledge of the gene product. Recombinant DNA techniques allowed the unraveling of the complex processes of genomic DNA recombination for production of immunoglobulins and T-cell receptors. The feasibility of a detailed human gene map based on RFLPs (Chap. 6) was a direct outgrowth of recombinant DNA techniques.

The use of a polymerase chain reaction technique (PCR) for amplification of DNA or RNA has become a powerful new tool. Using this technique, a small amount of genomic DNA, mRNA, or other nucleic acid can be amplified thousands or even millions of times to yield an abundant product for easy analysis.[151–153] The procedure can be automated using a heat stable *Taq* (from *Thermus aquaticus*) polymerase which survives the series of temperature changes necessary for the cycles of polymerization, denaturation, and oligonucleotide hybridization. The advantage of this procedure is the ability to prepare DNA within a single day from tiny amounts of whole blood or even dried blood.[153,154] The amplified product can be analyzed rapidly using restriction enzymes, hybridization with oligonucleotides, or direct DNA sequencing. This method has been used for rapid prenatal diagnosis of sickle-cell anemia[153] and hemophilia A.[155] The method has also been used for direct sequencing of mutations in genomic DNA.[156–158] It is now practical to use this method to sequence directly amplified cDNA, as has been demonstrated for HLA gene products beginning with RNA from peripheral leukocytes. This has been done for a number of individuals with insulin dependent diabetes and for controls.[159] The ability to automate the PCR method may allow for major new applications for population screening for human genetic variation.

Molecular Techniques for Clinical Diagnosis

Biochemical analysis in the form of enzyme assay and protein electrophoresis is a long-standing method for clinical diagnosis and heterozygote detection. Molecular diagnostic techniques gather small bits of genotypic information, and the interpretation of results is usually quite straightforward. The strategies for family analysis and interpretation are sometimes more complex. Multiple approaches for clinical application of molecular techniques should be clearly distinguished: (1) Molecular methods can be used to achieve *direct detection of the mutation*. (2) Diagnosis can be established using *linkage with negligible recombination*, usually using the cloned gene as the probe. (3) Diagnosis can also be achieved using *linkage with detectable recombination*, usually using linked RFLPs. (4) Although less common, diagnostic information can be based on *linkage disequilibrium* between genetic markers and a disease mutation.

Direct Detection of Mutations. Direct detection of mutations can be carried out if a restriction enzyme detects the gain or loss of a cutting site due to the mutation. Direct detection of a mutation can also be accomplished using standard Southern blotting analysis in combination with oligonucleotide probes which specifically hybridize with the normal or mutant sequence (allele specific oligonucleotides or ASOs).[160] The restriction enzyme method and the oligonucleotide method can be combined with the polymerase chain reaction to shorten the time required and increase the sensitivity of these methods. All these methods have been applied for detection of the sickle-cell mutation.[153,160,161] Direct detection of mutations is also possible in the instance of deletions or major gene rearrangements. This is particularly simple in instances where a probe is available which detects an abnormal junction fragment at the site of the rearrangement. In the instance where an entire gene is deleted and no junctional probe is available, dosage analysis may be required to identify heterozygotes for the deletion.[162] Dosage analysis requires great caution and appropriate use of control probes, and should be supplemented by use of RFLPs and junctional probes where possible. In general, direct detection of mutations is amenable to simple interpretation because the genotype of each individual is determined in regard to the mutation in the family. The only disadvantage of direct detection of mutations is the specificity of the process which means that slightly different tests must be used to detect alleleic heterogeneity from family to family or even from chromosome to chromosome in a compound heterozygote. Direct detection of a mutation is particularly powerful when the same mutation affects very large numbers of individuals in the population, as in the case of the sickle-cell mutation and as may prove to be the case for disorders such as cystic fibrosis and Huntington disease.

Linkage with Negligible Recombination. The general concepts for genetic recombination and linkage are discussed earlier in this chapter and in Chap. 6. Genetic diagnosis by linkage is utilized when it is not possible to demonstrate by direct analysis the mutation or the mutant gene product. For clinical linkage analysis, it is essential that some genetic marker near the disease locus (or near the mutation if the locus is very large) be *informative*. The genetic marker is informative if an individual who is heterozygous for the disease locus is also heterozygous for the marker. Linkage analysis is appropriate when an individual carries one mutant gene and one normal gene, and the goal is to determine which has been transmitted to the next generation. Most analyses can be made informative since RFLPs are frequent, and since it is usually possible to identify useful polymorphisms near genes causing diseases. A second requirement for linkage analysis is that of *phase* information between the two loci for genetic analysis. If an individual is heterozygous for an RFLP (genotype 1/2) which is tightly linked to a mutation, it must be determined whether allele 1 for the RFLP is on the chromosome with the disease gene or on the chromosome with the normal gene, assuming that allele 2 for the RFLP would be on the chromosome with the alternate gene. When the genetic marker is informative and the phase is known, genetic diagnosis can be carried out in the form of heterozygote detection, presymptomatic diagnosis, detection of lack of penetrance, and prenatal diagnosis. When the DNA probe is a portion of the gene which is mutated, crossing-over between the genetic marker (often an RFLP) and a mutation is usually negligible. Duchenne muscular dystrophy is an exception with an extremely large gene where crossing-over within the gene does occur at a detectable frequency.

A hypothetical series of families with a recessive disorder is illustrated in Fig. 1-18 demonstrating some questions of informativeness and phase. For these examples, it is assumed that the cloned gene is available as a probe. For family 1 the analysis is informative, and the phase can be deduced; both parents are heterozygous for an RFLP, and the first affected child indicates that the 5-kb fragment is on the same chromosome as the disease gene in both parents. For family 2, the analysis is informative only for the father. For family 3, both parents are heterozygous for the RFLP, but the phase cannot be determined adequately, and the analysis is only partially informative. Family 3 is described as having an intercross result. For families 2 and 3, prenatal diagnosis can still be of some value since there is a 50 percent probability that a fetus will be predicted to be unaffected and a 50 percent probability that a fetus will be predicted to be at 50 percent risk. For family 4, the analysis is entirely uninformative, since both parents are homozygous for the RFLP. For family 5, complete information can be obtained using two RFLPs, since the father is informative for one analysis and the mother is informative for the other analysis. Because more than one RFLP is potentially informative, most families are fully informative, and prenatal diagnosis can be provided to the majority of families with a previously affected child.

Numerous examples of molecular diagnosis by linkage, where there is negligible recombination between the loci, are presented in Fig. 1-19. Genetic marker data are presented as letters which might represent simple RFLP alleles or haplotypes of RFLPs. Phase can usually be determined from a single index case for autosomal recessive disorders (Fig. 1-19A).

TECHNIQUES FOR STUDYING METABOLIC DISEASES **37**

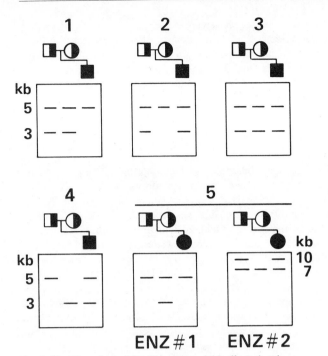

Fig. 1-18 Hypothetical families with a child affected with an autosomal recessive disorder. Simplified but realistic examples of Southern blot analysis using the cloned cDNA for the mutant gene are depicted. Families are numbered above, and restriction fragment sizes are indicated in kilobases; see text. *(From A. Beaudet.[217] Used by permission.)*

Phase can also be determined for recessive disorders in the absence of an index case if a reliable biologic or biochemical heterozygote test is available as might occur for β thalassemia (Fig. 1-19B). Fetuses of AA genotype are predicted to be affected for panels A and B. For autosomal dominant disorders, linkage phase usually cannot be determined from a single affected individual (Fig. 1-19C). Exceptions would occur in retinoblastoma or polyposis of the colon, when analysis of tumor DNA may distinguish the allele on the abnormal chromosome (often retained in the tumor) from the allele on the normal chromosome (often lost in the tumor). Linkage phase for autosomal dominant disorders can be determined from two appropriate individuals; it is not essential that both be affected (Fig. 1-19D and E). Fetuses of AB genotype are predicted to be affected for panels D and E. For X-linked disorders, phase information is most readily obtained from a single affected male individual (Fig. 1-19F). In general, linkage information can be used to determine the genotype of offspring of individuals of known genotype. Linkage information generally cannot be used consistently to determine the genotype of antecedents of individuals of known genotypes because of the possibility of new mutation from one generation to the next. This is exemplified for an X-linked disorder where linkage information will not clarify if the mother of an isolated affected male is a heterozygote or not (Fig. 1-19G). This represents an important difference between direct detection of a mutation and linkage analysis. Occasionally, linkage analysis can suggest the genotype of an antecedent. Note for panel G that the mutation arose on the chromosome from the unaffected maternal grandfather, and it can be stated that the maternal grandmother and the maternal aunt of the index case do not carry the mutation and that either the mother or the index case is the recipient of

the new mutation. The situation is similar in panel H, except that the mutation is on the chromosome from the maternal grandmother, and the site of the new mutation is unknown and could go back further in the family. Still by linkage analysis, the maternal aunt is not a carrier of the mutation. The genotype of an antecedent also can be inferred when a woman has two sons with the same DNA marker, one son being affected and one son being unaffected with the X-linked disorder (Fig. 1-19I). In this instance, the data indicate that the mother is not a heterozygote for the X-linked disorder, although the possibility of gonadal mosaicism is not eliminated.

Linkage with Detectable Recombination. Linkage analysis using a genetic marker which shows detectable recombination with a disease mutation has the same requirements for informativeness and phase as discussed above. However, the analysis is further complicated by the possibility of recombination at each meiosis in the family. For purposes of discussion, it is convenient to consider a genetic marker which has a recombination fraction of 0.1 with a disease mutation (Fig. 1-20). The immediate implication is that genetic diagnosis will be only 90 percent accurate using this single marker, even if complete informativeness and phase are available. If a second genetic marker is available at a similar distance on the *opposite* side of the disease mutation (flanking markers), the two can be used to increase greatly the accuracy of diagnosis, if no crossover occurs between the two markers. However, the information would be almost useless in about 20 percent of fam-

Fig. 1-19 Examples of molecular diagnosis by genetic linkage with negligible recombination between the DNA probe and the disease locus. Letters indicate haplotypes for RFLPs. Panels A and B depict autosomal recessive disorders; C through E depict autosomal dominant disorders; and F through I depict X-linked disorders. The phase is presented with the A haplotype on the same chromosome as the mutant allele in all cases where it can be determined; see text for discussion.

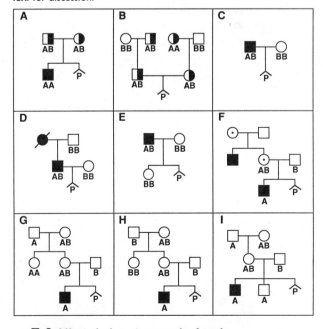

■,● Affected phenotype; male, female
◨,◖ Heterozygote for autosomal recessive disorder
⊙ Obligate heterozygote for X-linked disorder
□,○ Normal phenotype

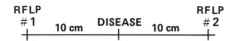

ONE MARKER INFORMATIVE

- 100% OF FAMILIES, 90% ACCURATE

TWO MARKERS INFORMATIVE

- 81% OF FAMILIES, 99% ACCURATE
- 19% OF FAMILIES, NO DIAGNOSIS

Fig. 1-20 Demonstration of the effect of flanking linked genetic markers; see text for discussion. (From A. Beaudet.[217] Used by permission.)

ilies who would have at least one crossover between the flanking markers. The determination of phase is also complicated by the possibility of recombination. If phase is deduced from the offspring of an affected individual, a larger number of offspring increases the certainty of the phase information. Continuing to assume a recombination fraction of 0.1 between a genetic marker and a disease mutation, the phase in an individual with a dominant disorder can be deduced with a probability of 0.90 from a single offspring but with a probability of 0.99 from two offspring of affected or unaffected status (Fig. 1-21, compare panels A and B). In some families with a dominant disorder, the phase can be deduced with complete certainty from antecedent data such as when an affected individual must have inherited the disease gene and a particular genetic marker from an affected parent (Fig. 1-21C). Fetuses of the AB genotype have probabilities of being affected of approximately 0.81, 0.89, and 0.90 for panels A, B, and C,

respectively, since crossovers may occur in the meioses leading to conception of the fetus. For autosomal recessive disorders, the considerations are analogous. If prenatal diagnosis is based on phase data from a single previous affected offspring, there are four meioses which would affect the prediction (Fig. 1-21D). For example, using a single genetic marker at a recombination fraction of 0.02, there would be approximately an 8 percent chance that a prediction of an affected fetus would be erroneous, since a single crossover at any of the four meioses would cause a diagnostic error. For X-linked disorders phase can be deduced from offspring of heterozygous females, but more definitive phase information can often be obtained by analysis of the fathers of heterozygous females. In Fig. 1-21E and F, the same family is depicted with and without data from the maternal grandfather. If an unwise counselor (panel E) fails to obtain a sample from the maternal grandfather, the data suggest that the A marker is on the chromosome with the disease gene in the pregnant woman. The phase is known with only 90 percent certainty, and prenatal diagnosis would provide accuracy of approximately 81 percent because of the possibility of crossing-over in either of the meioses leading to the offspring of the heterozygous mother. If a wiser counselor (panel F) recognizes the absolute necessity of a sample from the maternal grandfather, the phase in the heterozygous mother becomes known with certainty, and it becomes obvious that the affected son represents a crossover between the genetic marker and the disease mutation. Prenatal diagnosis now becomes 90 percent accurate, but, more important, the prediction of disease or non-disease has been reversed for the presence of a given marker in a male fetus. If phase is to be determined for heterozygous females based on their offspring, the accuracy of phase information increases with increasing numbers of offspring as for the autosomal disorders.

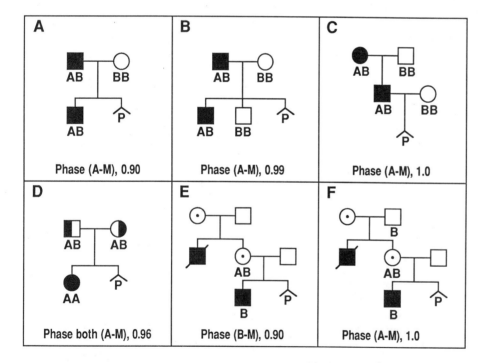

Fig. 1-21 Examples of molecular diagnosis using genetic linkage with detectable recombination between the DNA probe and the disease locus. Letters indicate haplotypes detected with RFLPs. Panels A through C depict autosomal dominant disorders; panel D depicts an autosomal recessive disorder; and panels E and F depict X-linked disorders. The probability of phase at the bottom of each panel indicates the probability that a given haplotype is on the chromosome with the mutant allele (M) in the parent(s) of the pregnancy (P). For example, phase (A-M), 0.90, in panel A indicates that the probability is 0.90 that the A haplotype is on the chromosome with the mutant allele and the B haplotype is on the chromosome with the normal allele in the father of the pregnancy. The recombination fraction is presented as 0.1 for all cases except in panel D where a recombination fraction of 0.02 is assumed; see text for discussion.

■,● Affected phenotype; male, female
◧,◑ Heterozygote for autosomal recessive disorder
⊙ Obligate heterozygote for X-linked disorder
□,○ Normal phenotype

Linkage Disequilibrium. Linkage disequilibrium refers to the fact that certain alleles at two nearby loci may be found together more often than would be predicted from their frequency in the general population. For purposes of genetic diagnosis, this is most readily discussed in terms of a genetic marker and a disease mutation. Linkage disequilibrium reflects the rarity of crossing-over in the historical meioses between the present and the origin of the more recent of the two genetic variations under study. For linkage disequilibrium to be present, the two genetic markers must be quite tightly linked. In addition, there must be one or only a few origins for the disease mutations, or the mutations will be found relatively randomly with various alleles for the marker gene. Either extensive crossing-over or frequent occurrence of new mutations would lead to relatively random occurrence of the mutation with marker genotypes.

Linkage disequilibrium is extensive within the HLA complex, and numerous diseases are found in association with various HLA haplotypes (see Chap. 4). Although it is unclear whether some associations such as that with ankylosing spondylitis represent causation by genetic variation in the HLA loci themselves or represent linkage disequilibrium, it is more definite that the finding of certain HLA haplotypes with mutant genes for 21 hydroxylase deficiency represents linkage disequilibrium (Chap. 74). It is also likely that the association of particular HLA haplotypes with hemochromatosis also represents linkage disequilibrium (Chap. 55). For offspring of individuals with hemochromatosis, one mutant gene is inherited from the affected parent, since this is a recessive disorder. The possibility that the unaffected parent has contributed the hemochromatosis gene can be calculated taking into account the HLA haplotypes inherited from the unaffected parent and the appropriate data on linkage disequilibrium. A striking example of linkage disequilibrium is found for the Z allele at the α_1-antitrypsin locus where a particular allele for an RFLP is found almost uniquely with the Z allele (Chap. 96). This instance is unusual, since the presence of the allele at the RFLP and the presence of the Z allele correlate almost completely. This is different from the usual circumstance where a particular mutation is often found with a unique haplotype of RFLPs, but the RFLP haplotype associated with the mutation may also be found with normal copies of the gene (PKU and β thalassemia).

Recently, RFLPs showing strong linkage disequilibrium with cystic fibrosis were identified. This result indicates that the DNA markers are extremely close to the cystic fibrosis (CF) locus and that a single mutation accounts for most or all of the mutant CF genes in the population. The linkage disequilibrium information can be used in a variety of ways for genetic counseling in cystic fibrosis. Linkage disequilibrium can be used to estimate phase in parents who have an affected but deceased offspring. Linkage disequilibrium can be used to adjust the probability of a cystic fibrosis mutation on a chromosome contributed by an individual with no prior family history of CF. This can be used to modify risk calculations for pregnancies of aunts, uncles, and sibs of CF patients in defined populations. Linkage disequilibrium has played a limited role in genetic diagnosis in the past, and its role is likely to remain limited, since it is found with unique mutations which could be directly detected once they are characterized.

Molecular diagnosis is assuming an increasingly important role in medical genetics. Selected examples of current applications are listed in Table 1-8. The cystic fibrosis gene was cloned and the common mutation identified in late 1989.[218–221]

DIAGNOSIS AND PREVENTION OF GENETIC METABOLIC DISEASES

The present trend for couples to have smaller families has heightened the concern that children should be healthy and free of genetic diseases. Primary-care physicians are called upon to play a more active role in the prevention and treatment of hereditary diseases. In many clinical situations, genetic advice can be given by the primary physician once the relatively simple principles of medical genetics and genetic

Table 1-8 Examples of Role of Molecular Analysis for Diagnosis of Genetic Disease

Disease	Detection of mutation*	RFLPs with gene probe	RFLPs with linked marker	Comments
Sickle-cell anemia	+ + + +			*Mst* II analysis
β Thalassemia	+ +	+ +		Very heterogeneous
α Thalassemia	+ + +	+		Many deletions
Hemophilia A	+	+ +	+	
Hemophilia B	+	+ +	+	
Phenylketonuria	+	+ + +		
α₁-Antitrypsin ZZ	+ + +	+		
Antithrombin III deficiency	+	+ +		Biologic tests valuable
Familial hypercholesterolemia	+ +	+ +		Biologic tests valuable
Growth hormone deficiency	+			Rare form
Lesch-Nyhan syndrome	+ +	+ +		Heterozyote detection
Retinoblastoma	+ + +	+		Inherited form
Huntington disease			+ + +	Delay over ethical concerns
Myotonic dystrophy			+ +	
Adult polycystic kidney disease			+ + +	
Ornithine transcarbamylase deficiency	+	+ + +		Prenatal and heterozygote
Tay-Sachs disease	+ + +	+		Enzyme diagnosis
X-linked retinitis pigmentosa			+ + +	
Fragile X syndrome			+ + +	
Cystic fibrosis	+ + +	+	+	See ref. 218–221

* + = relative importance of an approach as of early 1990, and the status for disorders could change rapidly.
NOTE: See Appendix 1-1 for greater detail.

counseling have been mastered. In other situations, the complexities may make referral to a genetic specialist a necessity, but a good genetic history is essential even for identification of families for appropriate referral. For a more in-depth discussion of these principles, the reader is referred to Vogel and Motulsky's textbook *Human Genetics: Problems and Approaches.*[95] Genetic counseling may be provided because of the occurrence of an affected individual (index case) in a family. Other types of programs are population based and may include newborn screening, heterozygote screening, prenatal screening, and screening for disease in later life.

Genetic Counseling with an Index Case

The prevention of genetic diseases requires the advance identification of matings that are capable of producing genotypes associated with medical disorders. These may involve matings in which one of the two individuals is carrying a dominant or X-linked gene mutation or a balanced translocation, or matings in which both individuals carry a deleterious recessive gene at the same locus. Such individuals are usually identified through the birth of an affected child or near relative, in which case retrospective genetic counseling can be provided.

When advising family members about the risk of transmitting a disorder that has already affected someone in the family, the counselor's first step is to be certain of the *correct diagnosis*—in particular, to make certain that the problem in question is really of genetic origin. This is especially important in disorders that may have either a genetic or a nongenetic etiology, such as deafness or mental retardation. Second, if the disease has a hereditary element, the possibility of genetic heterogeneity must be considered.

Estimation of the *recurrence risk* of a disease requires knowledge of the genetic mechanisms controlling the relevant disorder. When more than one genetic mechanism exists, or when environmental factors can cause clinically indistinguishable traits, the *relative probabilities* of the different mechanisms operating in the particular family are computed. For conditions determined by simple Mendelian inheritance, there is no difficulty in predicting the probability of an offspring's being affected, provided the genotypes of the parents can be recognized. Identification of the parental genotype is easiest if a biochemical or molecular test is available to detect the mutant gene.

For autosomal dominant disorders, identification of the parental genotype is often more difficult because of the occurrence of *lack of penetrance* and *variation in expression*. In counseling a family in which one relative is affected with a dominant disorder, it is important that appropriate clinical examination of all first-degree relatives and appropriately selected distant relatives be carried out. If relatives appear unaffected, there is the possibility that the gene is present but not penetrant or the possibility of delayed age of onset or mild expression. When no relatives are affected, the possibility of a new dominant mutation must be entertained. Presumably it will become increasingly feasible to determine genotypes using biochemical and molecular methods in such circumstances.

When advising families about multifactorial genetic diseases, such as diabetes mellitus, in which the inheritance pattern is not clear-cut, the physician must resort to empiric risk estimates that have been derived from retrospectively assembled data.[95]

Once the parental genotypes are determined, the genetic prognosis is usually presented in terms of probability that a given couple will produce an affected offspring. The physician providing genetic counseling must make certain that the couple understands not only the meaning of such absolute risk figures but also the severity of the disease and the variability in clinical expression. In other words, in dealing with a disorder such as α_1-antitrypsin deficiency, it is important for the parents to realize not only that they have a 25 percent risk of producing a child with this disorder but also that a certain proportion of children with the disorder have severe disease with both liver and pulmonary manifestations, a certain portion have mild disease with only pulmonary manifestations, etc. They should also have an understanding of the potential impact of the disease on their family. A disease that is lethal at birth might be classified by some as more "severe" than one that is lethal at age 16, but the latter is likely to have a much more profound impact on the family. There is evidence that the relative burden of a disorder is an important factor in the decision-making process for couples with increased genetic risks.[163]

Heterozygote Detection

Heterozygote testing is one form of genetic screening. The efficiency of a genetic screening test is related to its sensitivity (detection rate) and its false positive rate (equivalent to 1 minus specificity).[164] *Sensitivity* is defined as the ability of the test to identify those with the mutant phenotype. Such persons yield either a positive test (with frequency a) or a normal (false negative) test (with frequency b). Sensitivity (detection rate) is thus $a/(a + b)$. *Specificity* is defined as the ability to exclude those with the normal genotype (with frequency d) from a false positive classification (with frequency c); specificity of the screening test is thus $d/(c + d)$ [the false-positive rate is 1 minus specificity or $c/(c + d)$]. Binary discrimination yields perfect specificity and sensitivity (value = 1 for each). In practice, discrimination of most tests is statistical (i.e., dependent on the distribution of metric parameters); hence specificity and sensitivity are less than perfect. There is thus no overlap of values between classes (e.g., heterozygotes and normals) for a binary test, but there are overlapping values for a statistical test.

Detection of heterozygotes is an important part of counseling families where a known genetic disorder has occurred. This arises most frequently in the case of X-linked disorders or autosomal recessive traits, but analogous questions arise in the case of autosomal dominant disorders where an enzyme assay is available, and the phenotype is not always obvious clinically (e.g., acute intermittent porphyria). The ideal method for heterozygote detection is the direct demonstration of the mutant gene or gene product (i.e., binary discrimination with a specificity and sensitivity both with a value of 1). This is possible for some disorders using protein electrophoresis as for hemoglobin or α_1-antitrypsin. This is also possible when the disease mutation can be directly detected by molecular techniques. As discussed above, heterozygote detection is also possible using linkage analysis, in which case the accuracy will depend on the possibility of recombination between the linked marker and the disease mutation.

Another method for heterozygote detection involves the detection of half-normal levels of the mutant gene product. In such a statistical discrimination, the values for specificity and sensitivity are both less than 1. This approach usually involves enzyme assay on blood or tissue samples. The ability to separate heterozygotes from normal individuals is extremely dependent on the coefficient of variation for the determination in question, as demonstrated in Fig. 1-22. A high degree of variation may be due to unavoidable biologic variation in the human population. In many instances the variation can be reduced by appropriate strategies. For example analysis of mixed leukocytes may give a wide variation because of heterogeneity in differential white blood cell count, while analysis of a specific leukocyte population such as granulocytes or lymphocytes may reduce the variation. For many enzyme assays causing inborn errors of metabolism, the data sets for determining the normal and heterozygote ranges are suboptimal, in part due to lack of adequate numbers of obligate heterozygote samples and in part due to infrequent demand for the procedures. In the case of Tay-Sachs disease, the ability to distinguish heterozygotes by enzyme assay is unusually good. This is due in part to the excellent data sets available, but perhaps also in part to the intrinsic circumstances where the deficiency of α subunits both reduces hexosaminidase A activity and increases hexosaminidase B activity through the formation of β_2 dimers. Heterozygote detection tests are frequently interpreted as positive or negative, and this is appropriate for a relatively absolute or binary test such as hemoglobin electrophoresis. When significant doubt is present, it would be preferable to use the results to modify the probability that an individual is a carrier based on the range of values observed in heterozygotes and normal individuals.[165] Again, the data are frequently inadequate to pursue this optimal approach, but it should be recognized that many enzyme determinations for heterozygote detection do not provide absolute diagnoses. These same issues apply when diagnosing affected individuals with autosomal dominant enzyme disorders such as acute intermittent porphyria. As more molecular tests become available, heterozygote detection may move increasingly from a statistical to a binary discrimination.

In the case of X-linked disorders, heterozygote detection is complicated by the Lyon mechanism for random X inactivation as discussed above. Strategies for circumventing the problems of X inactivation include analysis of clonal cell populations which can include individual hair roots, randomly isolated cultured cell clones, and cell clones isolated by selection methods. In the case of the Lesch-Nyhan syndrome, toxic purine antimetabolites such as thioguanine or azaguanine can be used to select for, and thereby demonstrate the presence of, deficient cells in a mixed population from a heterozygote female.

Heterozygote detection can also be based on various metabolic studies. In general, these tests (again statistical discriminations) which are more removed from the defective gene are less reliable. For example, in heterozygotes for cystinuria, the excretion of dibasic amino acids in the urine is elevated, but not as much as in the patient with the homozygous disease (Chap. 99). Appropriate measurements of the ratio of blood phenylalanine to tyrosine provide a useful heterozygote test for phenylketonuria (Chap. 15). In the case of ornithine transcarbamylase deficiency, urinary excretion of orotic acid and orotidine is significantly increased in heterozygotes after a protein loading test or after administration of allopurinol (Chap. 20). These metabolic heterozygote tests for ornithine transcarbamylase deficiency are quite accurate, although molecular data offer a binary discrimination when informative.

Antenatal Diagnosis of Genetic Disease

During the 1960s, transabdominal amniocentesis came into widespread use for the purpose of diagnosis of certain genetic diseases at a stage early enough to permit parents the option of terminating the pregnancy and preventing the birth of a defective child. This procedure gives high-risk couples the opportunity to have unaffected children provided they are willing for the pregnancy to be terminated in the event that an abnormal fetus is detected. Since the 1960s, there has been a progressive expansion of prenatal diagnostic techniques with improved resolution by prenatal ultrasound, measurement of amniotic fluid α-fetoprotein, fetal blood sampling, and the development of transcervical and transabdominal chorionic villus sampling.

Amniocentesis consists of the transabdominal aspiration of amniotic fluid from the uterus. The procedure involves minimal risk. Maternal mortality has not been observed, and morbidity has been minor. Fetal loss (due to death or spontaneous abortion) is minimally different from that in controls matched for maternal age, gravidity, parity, race, religion, socioeconomic group, gestational age, and other features.[95,166–169] If a diagnostic amniocentesis is performed at the fifteenth week of gestation, the 4-week delay required for culture of an adequate number of cells for biochemical or cytogenetic study brings one only to the twentieth week, when pregnancy may still be terminated safely.

Direct examination of the amniotic fluid itself may be diagnostic. For example, an elevated level of α-fetoprotein is a relatively good indicator of the presence of spina bifida or some other related neural tube abnormality.[170] More frequently, prenatal diagnosis requires culture of the fetal cells in vitro, as mentioned above. By this means, the karyotype of the fetus can be determined to ascertain fetal sex and to detect various chromosomal aberrations such as Down syndrome.

Transcervical or transabdominal chorionic villus sampling (CVS) can be used to obtain tissue of fetal origin.[171–174] Transcervical CVS can be performed at 9 to 12 weeks gestation (only 5 to 8 weeks after the first missed menstrual period), and transabdominal CVS can be performed similarly early in gestation. Chorionic villi can be analyzed directly using cytogenetic, biochemical, or molecular techniques. In addition, cells can be cultured from chorionic villi and again subjected

Fig. 1-22 The relevance of the coefficient of variation using a quantitative trait such as enzyme activity for diagnosis of heterozygotes and homozygotes.

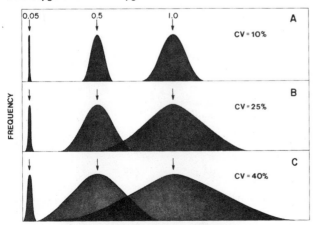

RELATIVE ENZYME ACTIVITY

to any of these forms of analysis. The major advantage of CVS is the earlier sampling time and the availability of larger amounts of tissue which allow for direct analysis, so that a woman undergoing CVS at 9 weeks gestation might have final diagnostic information at 10 weeks gestation in comparison to approximately 20 weeks gestation for amniocentesis. The earlier results are substantially more attractive to many high-risk families. The safety of CVS is still under evaluation through collaborative studies in various countries, but the risk of fetal loss above the background risk appears to be between 1 and 3 percent, which may be acceptable to families facing a high genetic risk.

Virtually all cytogenetic disorders can be detected using either amniocentesis or CVS. Many biochemical genetic disorders can be detected by suitable assays of specific enzyme activities in cultured fetal cells or in chorionic villi. In general, most of the disorders which can be detected by enzyme assay in cultured amniotic fluid cells can also be detected using CVS, but the relative expression of genes in these tissues differs slightly, and the reliability of each cell type for each enzymatic assay must be documented carefully.[175] DNA can be obtained from any of the cell sources, and molecular diagnosis is assuming an expanding role using direct detection of the mutation, linkage where recombination is negligible, and linkage where recombination is measurable. Increasingly, the cloned gene itself is used as the diagnostic molecular probe. Molecular diagnosis does not require that the gene product be expressed in the fetal cells. Table 1-9 lists numerous biochemical genetic disorders for which prenatal diagnosis is currently feasible. Many different circumstances are included in Table 1-9. For some disorders, such as Tay-Sachs disease, Lesch-Nyhan syndrome and sickle cell anemia, prenatal diagnosis is extremely reliable. In some instances, diagnosis has traditionally been accomplished by enzyme assay, and molecular diagnosis is becoming a useful alternative. In some instances, molecular diagnosis may be available only for a proportion of families, because of incomplete informativeness and inability to detect all possible mutations directly (currently exemplified by hemophilia A). Fetal blood sampling is useful for prenatal diagnosis of hemophilia if molecular analysis is not informative (Chap. 86). In other instances, prenatal diagnosis is complex, as in the case of fragile X syndrome where cytogenetic diagnosis is of partial value, and linkage analysis is complicated by incomplete information and crossing-over in some cases. It is virtually certain that the range of disorders which can be diagnosed will continue to expand rapidly and that the accuracy of diagnosis will improve in instances where it is still troublesome. Specific details for prenatal diagnosis can be found in chapters throughout this book.

Population Based Genetic Screening

Genetic screening represents the search in a population for persons possessing certain genotypes that are known to be associated with or to predispose to disease in the individuals or their descendants.[164,176] Screening is also employed for research purposes in order to ascertain distributions of traits, e.g., polymorphisms, not known to be associated with disease. In this section, we are concerned only with the identification of deleterious genes in individual members of populations.

Population based genetic screening will be considered under the headings of newborn screening (usually for disease), heterozygote screening, prenatal screening, and screening for disease later in life. Newborn screening involves the identification of genetic disease in an infant to allow the institution of a

Table 1-9 Overview of Prenatal Diagnosis of Genetic Disorders

Chromosomal
  Most routine cytogenetic analysis
  Fragile X, possible but complex, cytogenetic and
    linkage
Carbohydrate disorders
  Glycogen storage II, III, and IV by enzyme
  Galactosemia by enzyme
Amino acid disorders
  Majority possible by enzyme, e.g., maple syrup
    urine disease, citrullinemia, ornithinemia
  Some by DNA, e.g., PKU, ornithine
    transcarbamylase
Organic acidemia
  Most possible by enzyme, e.g., methylmalonic
    acidemia, isovaleric acidemia
Purine and pyrimidine disorders
  Most possible by enzyme with DNA possible also,
    e.g., HPRT, adenosine deaminase
Lipoprotein disorders
  Familial hypercholesterolemia by receptor assay or
    DNA
  DNA increasingly feasible for apolipoproteins
Porphyrias and heme disorders
  Many porphyrias by enzyme, DNA feasible
Disorders of metal metabolism
  Menkes by copper in cells
Peroxisomal disorders
  Most possible by lipid and enzyme analysis
Lysosomal disorders
  Virtually all possible by enzyme assay, DNA
    increasingly feasible, e.g., Tay-Sachs deletions
    and mutations

Disorders of hormone synthesis
  21-Hydroxylase deficiency by metabolites, HLA
    linkage, and DNA
  Steroid sulfatase by enzyme and DNA
  Testicular feminization by receptor assay
Vitamin disorders
  Biotinidase by enzyme
  Cobalamins by bioassays
Blood disorders
  Most proteins by DNA, e.g., hemophilias,
    α_1-antitrypsin, amyloidosis
  Most hemoglobins by DNA
Disorders of membrane transport
  Cystinosis by cystine content
  Cystic fibrosis by DNA
Disorders of immune defense
  Many feasible by fetal blood analysis
  Chronic granulomatous disease and leukocyte
    adhesion deficiency by DNA
Disorders of connective tissue
  Hypophosphatasia and carbonic anhydrase II
    deficiency by enzyme, DNA feasible for latter
  Collagen disorders by protein analysis and DNA
Muscle disorders
  Duchenne dystrophy by DNA
  Myotonic dystrophy by linkage
Skin disorders
  Xeroderma pigmentosa by bioassay
Intestinal disorders
  Analysis of enzymes in amniotic fluid feasible

prophylactic or therapeutic program to prevent injury to the child. Heterozygote screening and prenatal screening are designed to identify couples at high risk of transmitting a serious genetic disease in order to provide the couple with the option to forestall the birth of affected children. Reproductive options for carrier couples detected by heterozygote screening are numerous and include avoidance of pregnancy, adoption, artificial insemination by noncarrier donor, selective abortion after prenatal diagnosis, and acceptance of the birth of affected infants. Screening for disease is designed to detect individuals in the population under circumstances where some prophylactic or therapeutic program may avert or reduce the burden of the disease. This strategy is similar to newborn screening but is applied later in life.

Detailed discussions of genetic screening are available in a report published by the United States National Academy of Sciences in 1975[176] and in the report of an international workshop held in 1982.[164] Recommendations from the workshop are:[164]

1. The specific rationale for genetic screening should be defined, namely, whether the goal is medical intervention, family planning, or research.

2. Population screening for medical intervention should not be performed outside an integrated program capable of information dispersal, screening, retrieval of persons with positive tests, diagnosis, counseling, medical management, and outcome evaluation.

3. The screening procedure should maximize specificity (by counting false positive tests), sensitivity (by counting false negative tests), and predictive efficiency (ratio of true positive to false positive tests) of the test. Proficiency testing should be implemented to monitor performance. (See explanation of specificity and sensitivity, above, under "Heterozygote Detection.")

4. The contribution of ethnic and geographic factors to variation of phenotype should be considered when designing and implementing programs.

5. Participation should be informed and in keeping with the relevant mores of the society; participants should acquire accurate information relevant to their needs.

6. Information about the rationale and goal of the program and the meaning of test results should be available to participants, physicians, and all other personnel affected by the program.

7. Outcome and impact of the program, whether for service or research in medical, economic, social, and legal contexts, should be evaluated. Policy should be sufficiently flexible so that practice can be modified in keeping with developments and findings.

Newborn Screening. The goal of newborn screening is almost always to make a specific diagnosis for the purpose of providing medical intervention to avoid or ameliorate symptoms. Newborn screening first evolved to identify PKU in infants in time to institute a low phenylalanine diet and thus prevent the devastating effects of the untreated disease.[177] Newborn screening for PKU is discussed in detail in Chap. 15. Subsequently newborn screening has been implemented for many other disorders including aminoacidopathies, galactosemia, congenital hypothyroidism, sickle-cell anemia, cystic fibrosis, α_1-antitrypsin deficiency, and Duchenne muscular dystrophy. Almost all disorders detected by newborn screening represent Mendelian conditions, except congenital hypothyroidism,

which has a heterogeneous etiology. For some disorders, the evidence for efficacy of medical intervention is overwhelming as in the cases of PKU, galactosemia, and congenital hypothyroidism. In other instances, the benefits of medical intervention are less dramatic but probably significant. Examples include sickle-cell anemia, cystic fibrosis, and α_1-antitrypsin deficiency. In the case of Duchenne muscular dystrophy, no significant medical intervention is available. Prenatal diagnosis is more widely accepted and practiced for the disorders where intervention is most beneficial (Table 1-10). There are some genetic counseling benefits for early detection of disorders such as Duchenne muscular dystrophy.

Heterozygote Screening. The general recommendations for genetic screening in populations cited above apply to heterozygote screening as well. The usual goal for heterozygote screening in this context is to provide options for family planning. The specificity and sensitivity of the heterozygote test are important variables. Qualitative or binary tests such as hemoglobin electrophoresis for sickle-cell anemia provide relatively absolute diagnosis, while quantitative or statistical tests may provide lower specificity and sensitivity as discussed under "Heterozygote Detection," above.

TAY-SACHS DISEASE. The carrier frequency of this lethal disorder is 1 in 30 to 1 in 60 in the Jewish population of northeastern European ancestry, approximately tenfold higher than in the population at large. Detection of Tay-Sachs heterozygotes is accomplished by quantitative analysis of hexosaminidase A in serum, plasma, or leukocytes using a ratio to hexosaminidase B (Chap. 72). Tay-Sachs disease is an ideal disorder for screening for reproductive counseling for the following reasons: (1) it is limited mainly to a defined population; (2) there is a simple, reliable, automated, and relatively inexpensive test for identifying the carrier state; (3) there are positive reproductive alternatives for couples, both of whom are carriers, because the disorder can be diagnosed antenatally at a time when induced abortion can be safely performed. Thus, such couples can plan to have unaffected children while avoiding having children with the disease. Heterozygote screening has led to a marked reduction of the frequency of Tay-Sachs

Table 1-10 Frequency of Some Inborn Errors of Metabolism for Which Newborn Screening Tests Are Available

Disorder	Average frequency in liveborn infants*
Cystic fibrosis	1 in 2500
Congenital hypothyroidism	1 in 6000
Cystinuria	1 in 7000
α_1-Antitrypsin deficiency	1 in 8000
Phenylketonuria	1 in 12,000
Histidinemia	1 in 17,000
Iminoglycinuria	1 in 20,000
Hartnup disorder	1 in 26,000
Hyperprolinemia	1 in 40,000
Galactosemia	1 in 57,000
Biotinidase deficiency	1 in 60,000
Adenosine deaminase deficiency	<1 in 100,000
Maple syrup urine disease	1 in 200,000
Homocystinuria	1 in 200,000

*These frequencies often vary widely among ethnic groups, e.g., about 1 in 5000 in Dublin compared with 1 in 200,000 in Japan for phenylketonuria (see Ref. 164 for details).
SOURCE: Data from Galjaard[97] and various chapters in this text.

disease in the Jewish and French Canadian populations as detailed in Chap. 72.

The advent of reliable screening procedures for heterozygote detection and antenatal diagnosis is particularly valuable in Tay-Sachs disease, in which 80 percent of cases are first cases. But amniocentesis also enables the prevention of the birth of a second affected child in a family in which one Tay-Sachs case has appeared and in which both parents are therefore known heterozygotes.

SICKLE-CELL DISEASE. Many heterozygotes for sickle-cell anemia are being diagnosed as a relatively incidental component of newborn screening programs designed to detect homozygotes. In addition, heterozygote screening programs are being offered in many cities in the United States and elsewhere.[178] The most reliable procedure for heterozygote detection is hemoglobin electrophoresis, which will also screen for other hemoglobinopathies. Molecular techniques have made prenatal diagnosis for sickle-cell anemia completely reliable. The three favorable features of screening for Tay-Sachs disease listed above apply here also. There is a major difference however in regard to the severity and burden of sickle-cell anemia in comparison to Tay-Sachs disease. There is considerable variation in expression for sickle-cell disease, and some individuals experience mild disease which is compatible with a long and productive life. In addition, there are major cultural, educational, and socioeconomic differences between the Jewish population and the black population in the United States and elsewhere. Because of some combination of these reasons, perhaps primarily due to the milder expression, heterozygote screening and prenatal diagnosis have not been used in combination to reduce the frequency of sickle-cell anemia to anywhere near the extent that this approach has been applied for Tay-Sachs disease. While heterozygote screening for sickle-cell anemia may be successful at an educational level or for individual couples, it has not reduced substantially the burden of disease in the population up to the present time. This may provide important lessons for milder disorders such as α_1-antitrypsin deficiency and familial hypercholesterolemia where individuals in the population may be more attracted to therapeutic strategies and may show little interest in preventive approaches which make extensive use of selective abortion.

OTHER DISEASES. Heterozygote screening programs for β thalassemia have been extremely successful in various parts of the Mediterranean and North America. Major reductions in the frequency of β thalassemia have been achieved.[179,180] Heterozygote screening programs for β thalassemia and α thalassemia may be appropriate in various parts of Asia as other health care needs are met with further economic development. The prospects for population based heterozygote screening for cystic fibrosis appear excellent, since there is now evidence from linkage disequilibrium that the majority of heterozygotes carry the same mutation. Reproductive decisions regarding risks for cystic fibrosis will be complex, since the disorder has a wide range of expression, intelligence is normal, and supportive treatment continues to improve. It is possible that further developments involving the automation of molecular diagnosis, particularly using the polymerase chain reaction, could increase the technical feasibility for heterozygote detection for disorders such as PKU, cystic fibrosis, α_1-antitrypsin deficiency, and other conditions. Population based carrier testing for cystic fibrosis is now possible using mutation analysis, and its utilization is being debated.[221]

Prenatal Screening. Major forms of population based prenatal screening in use today include cytogenetic prenatal diagnosis for advanced maternal age, maternal serum α-fetoprotein analysis, and routine prenatal ultrasound. These methods represent a growing approach to monitor the health of the fetus prior to delivery, usually in conjunction with the option of elective abortion of abnormal fetuses. Utilization of cytogenetic prenatal diagnosis for women of advanced maternal age has grown steadily since it became generally available in the 1960s. The procedure is widely used, but utilization is quite variable depending on urban compared to rural location, educational level, and religious preference.[181] Maternal serum α-fetoprotein screening was instituted with the goal of prenatal detection of anencephaly and meningomyelocele.[170,182] Subsequently it was recognized that low levels of maternal serum α-fetoprotein may be associated with increased risk of Down syndrome. This has led to strategies which calculate the risk of Down syndrome based on maternal age in combination with the maternal serum α-fetoprotein level to determine who should be offered cytogenetic prenatal diagnosis.[183] Fetal ultrasound studies during the second trimester have become widespread and are routine in some settings. Careful ultrasound evaluation can detect a very broad range of fetal anatomic abnormalities.[184] Although heterozygote screening would optimally be implemented prior to conception, such testing is frequently delayed until the time of pregnancy. Strategies for prenatal screening are likely to continue to expand.

Screening for Disease in Later Life. Screening for genotypes that are associated with increased risk of disease in the individual or in their offspring or relatives is assuming many different forms. Newborn screening programs are detecting individuals who will have major disease risks later in life (e.g., sickle-cell anemia and cystic fibrosis). Screening institutionalized populations for genetic disorders can lead to genetic counseling for relatives. For example, detection of fragile X syndrome, chromosomal translocations, or Lesch-Nyhan syndrome can lead to anticipatory genetic counseling for numerous relatives.

However, the primary focus of screening for disease later in life would be to detect adults or children for whom medical intervention would be beneficial. Widespread use of laboratory screening in adult populations is leading to the identification of numerous individuals with disorders such as hyperlipidemia. Identification of disorders such as heterozygous familial hypercholesterolemia has both major therapeutic implications for the individual detected and implications for disease risk in offspring. The impetus to screen for diseases increases as therapeutic options improve. Genetic screening of individuals in the workplace is beginning to occur and may become more frequent. It is appropriate to consider whether individuals with heterozygous or homozygous α_1-antitrypsin deficiency should work in environments with pulmonary risks (e.g., coal mines). Genetic screening of populations carries many potential risks and benefits for the future.

TREATMENT OF GENETIC DISEASE

Genetic disease is the result of inherited abnormalities in the complex systems which program normal development and physiological homeostasis. Environmental factors contribute variably to the disease phenotype by stressing these defective systems. Treatment of genetic disorders requires accurate diagnosis, early intervention, and knowledge of the biochemical basis of the disorder, i.e., the pathophysiology. The current explosion of information concerning the molecular basis of genetic diseases plus continued technological advances in the analysis of biological samples (e.g., gas chromatography/mass spectrometry and fast-atom bombardment mass spectrometry) have greatly enhanced the capabilities for rapid and specific diagnosis.

While our understanding of the corresponding pathophysiology is increasing more slowly, the development of noninvasive metabolic monitoring techniques, such as positron emission tomography[185] and topical nuclear magnetic resonance spectrometry,[186] offer promising new approaches to this problem. Meanwhile, incomplete knowledge of pathophysiology hampers our attempts at therapeutics. For example, we still lack a clear understanding of the mechanism(s) and developmental timetable of the neural damage in phenylketonuria, and we are unsure if toxic precursors and/or deficiencies of downstream metabolites are the major pathologic factor(s) in the defects of fatty acid oxidation.

Evaluation of therapy of genetic disease is another difficult problem. Two general questions must be asked: (1) does the treatment improve the patients' condition and (2) does the treatment restore the patients to full physiological normality—as if they did not have the disease. These questions are relevant to the treatment of any medical disorder, but they have special significance for genetic diseases which often are predictable and preventable.

A recent study systematically evaluated the impact of therapy of 351 representative monogenic disorders on three basic variables: life span, reproductive capability, and social adaptation.[1,90] The results showed that available therapy normalized life span in 15 percent of the patients, reproductive capability in 11 percent, and social adaptation in only 6 percent. Only slightly better outcomes were found with a subset of 65 diseases in which the basic defect was known.[1] Because more severe diseases are more quickly recognized, this sample of currently known diseases may be skewed toward the worst. Nevertheless, the results are disappointing, and they highlight both the difficulty in developing effective therapies for genetic diseases and the need for continued work in this area. The results also underscore the value of preventive measures (genetic screening, genetic counseling, and prenatal diagnosis) in the management of genetic disease.

Conventional approaches to therapy of genetic disease can be viewed as a biologic model starting from the clinical phenotype and working back to the level of the defective gene.[187,187a] Table 1-11 lists some therapies currently used.

Treatment at the Clinical Phenotype Level

Therapy at this level covers a variety of conventional medical practices and depends on a thorough understanding of the natural history of the particular disorder. The basic genetic defect is not corrected, but the patients' problems often are ameliorated. Examples include education of patients with pharmacogenetic susceptibilities, instruction to limit sun exposure for patients with the various forms of albinism and xeroderma pigmentosa, administration of β-adrenergic blocking agents to patients with Marfan syndrome to prevent or slow dilatation of the aortic root, and use of anticonvulsants for a variety of

Table 1-11 Some Examples of Proven and Experimental Treatments for Inborn Errors of Metabolism

Level of treatment and method	Disorder
Clinical phenotype	
Patient education	
Avoidance of certain drugs	Pharmacogenetic disorders
Avoidance of sun exposure	Albinism
	Xeroderma pigmentosa
Pharmacologic	
β-Blockers	Marfan syndrome
Anticonvulsants	Neurodegenerative disorders
Surgical	
Orthopedic reconstruction	Chondrodystrophies
Colectomy	Familial polyposis coli
Metabolite	
Substrate restriction	
Phenylalanine	Phenylketonuria
Branched chain amino acids	Maple syrup urine disease
Galactose	Galactosemia and galactokinase deficiency
Alternative pathway	
Benzoate and phenylacetate	Urea cycle disorders
Glycine	Isovaleric acidemia
Carnitine	Organic acidemias
Cysteamine	Cystinosis
Penicillamine	Wilson disease
Metabolic inhibition	
Allopurinol	Gout
Mevinolin	Familial hypercholesterolemia
Replacement of deficient product	
Glucose polymers (cornstarch)	Glycogen storage disease, types I and III
Uridine	Hereditary orotic aciduria
Corticosteroids	Adrenogenital syndromes
Thyroxine	Familial goiter
Biotin	Biotinidase deficiency
Dysfunctional protein	
Activation	
Pyridoxine (Vitamin B$_6$)	Homocystinuria
Thiamine	Maple syrup urine disease
Protein replacement	
Growth hormone	Growth hormone deficiency
Factor VIII	Classic hemophilia
α$_1$-Antitrypsin	α$_1$-Antitrypsin deficiency
Polyethylene glycol–adenosine deaminase	Adenosine deaminase deficiency
Organ transplantation	
As a source for a specific protein	
Allogenic bone marrow	Lysosomal storage diseases β-Thalassemia
Liver	Glycogen storage disease, type 1
	Familial hypercholesterolemia
	Ornithine transcarbamylase deficiency
As a protein source and replacement of a damaged organ	
Liver	α$_1$-Antitrypsin deficiency
	Hepatorenal tyrosinemia
Kidney	Cystinosis

patients with neurogenetic disorders. In addition, a host of surgical interventions can benefit patients with malformations, chondrodystrophies, and disorders with increased risk of malignancy in a particular organ.

Treatment at the Metabolite Level

Therapy at this level often involves nutritional or pharmacological approaches. It is absolutely dependent on some understanding of pathophysiology (Fig. 1-23). Deficient function of a mutant enzyme may cause a disease phenotype because (1) a substrate accumulates to toxic levels (precursor toxicity), (2) an alternative metabolite is produced in excessive amounts (alternative pathway overflow), (3) there is reduced formation of the reaction product or some downstream metabolite (product deficiency), or (4) some combination of these possibilities coexists. Although this paradigm is most easily visualized for enzymes in a metabolic pathway, it holds for all proteins which participate in biochemical interactions with small molecules.

Substrate Restriction. Dietary alterations designed to restrict intake of a particular substrate may be effective if the pathophysiology involves accumulation of a toxic precursor whose major source is nutritional. Inborn errors of essential amino acids and certain sugars are the best examples of this approach. Diets restricted in phenylalanine or the branched chain amino acids are effective in preventing the mental retardation associated with phenylketonuria and maple syrup urine disease, respectively, if the diets are started soon after birth and monitored in such a way that amounts of these substances just sufficient for normal growth are supplied[188] (see Chaps. 15 and 22). Episodes of net protein catabolism (e.g., associated with intercurrent infections or trauma) complicate this therapy by providing large amounts of the offending amino acids from endogenous sources. In the case of maple syrup urine disease, these episodes may require hospitalization for administration of intravenous fluids and even dialysis. In a similar fashion, lifetime restriction of dietary galactose in patients with galactosemia due to deficiency of galactose 1-phosphate uridyl transferase corrects growth failure, prevents cataracts, and reduces but does not seem to prevent completely the impairment of cognitive development (Chap. 13). Despite this improved outcome, the observation that treated galactosemic females exhibit ovarian failure as a long-term complication of their disease[189] indicates that the efficacy of therapy is only partial.

Utilization of Alternative Pathways to Remove Toxic Metabolites. For disorders in which the pathophysiology involves accumulation of a toxic precursor or alternative pathway overflow, it is sometimes possible to promote conversion of the offending metabolite to a readily eliminated substance.[190] The effectiveness of this approach may be limited by the capacity of the converting system and often it must be combined with some dietary restriction of the offending substrate. Administration of benzoate and phenylacetate to patients with inborn errors of ureagenesis is a good example of this approach[191] (Chap. 20). Benzoate and phenylacetate undergo conjugation reactions with glycine and glutamine, respectively, forming hippurate and phenylacetylglutamine. These conjugates are readily excreted and contain more nitrogen than their precursors, thereby providing a means to eliminate excess nitrogen. When used in conjunction with restrictions of dietary protein, this therapy reduces the accumulation of the toxic precursor (ammonium) characteristic of the urea cycle disorders. Similar approaches include the use of glycine to conjugate with isovaleryl CoA in isovaleric acidemia, carnitine to conjugate with accumulated CoA esters in various defects of fatty acid and organic acid metabolism, cysteamine to help eliminate cystine in cystinosis, penicillamine to remove stored copper in Wilson disease, and phlebotomy to remove iron in hemochromatosis (see Chaps. 28, 33, 107, 54, and 55, respectively).

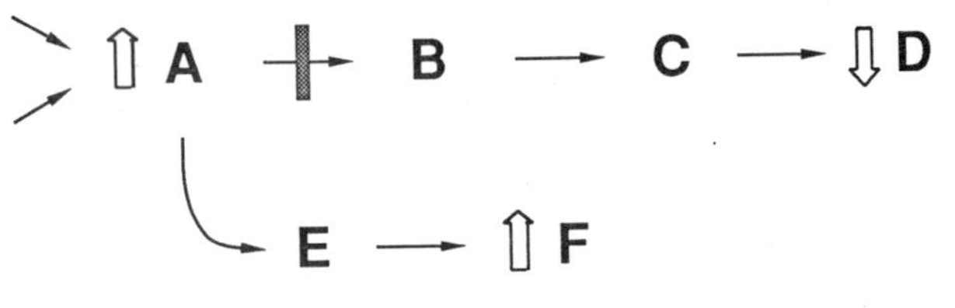

Metabolic Inhibitors. In certain disorders, often those in which the alternative pathway produces a toxic level of a particular metabolite, it is possible to reduce the accumulation by inhibiting a step in the pathway. This may lead to accumulation of upstream substrates which may be better tolerated if this approach is to be successful. Allopurinol, for example, is used to inhibit xanthine oxidase in gout and in a variety of situations characterized by excessive purine degradation and uric acid accumulation (Chaps. 37 and 38). Inhibition of xanthine oxidase lowers the level of uric acid and reduces the risk of uric acid nephropathy and gouty arthritis. Accumulation of xanthine is the biochemical consequence of xanthine oxidase inhibition but, because of its greater aqueous solubility, xanthine accumulation usually is well tolerated. Similarly, heterozygotes for mutations at the LDL receptor locus experience significant reductions in plasma cholesterol when treated with mevinolin, a potent inhibitor of 3-hydroxy-3-methylglutaryl-CoA reductase, which catalyzes an important early and rate limiting step in the synthesis of cholesterol[192] (Chap. 48).

Replacement of Deficient Product. For disorders in which the pathophysiology involves product deficit, nutritional or pharmacological approaches to replenishing this product may be effective. For example, deficient hepatic glucose production in patients with deficiency of glucose 6-phosphatase (glycogen storage disease, type Ia) is treated by frequent feeding with glucose or glucose polymers (Chap. 12). Cornstarch, a slowly digested glucose polymer, acts as a timed-release source of glucose and is helpful to these patients.[193] Similarly, administration of uridine to patients with impaired pyrimidine synthesis due to hereditary orotic aciduria provides a source for the deficient product and corrects the macrocytic anemia caused by pyrimidine deficiency (Chap. 43). Furthermore, the products depress the stimuli for pyrimidine biosynthesis, reducing orotic acid production and decreasing episodes of orotic acid nephrolithiasis.

Many of the inborn errors in hormone biosynthesis respond well to pharmacologic replacement of the deficient hormone. Thyroid hormone replacement for patients with cretinism (Chap. 73), corticosteroid administration to patients with the adrenogenital syndrome (Chap. 74), and biotin treatment of biotinidase deficient patients (Chap. 83) are examples of product replacement therapy. Biotinidase deficiency disrupts recovery of biotin from biotinylated proteins, resulting in in-

Fig. 1-23 Pathophysiological consequences of a genetic defect in a metabolic pathway. Substrate A is converted via a series of intermediates to a final product, D. The enzymes catalyzing these reactions are indicated by the horizontal arrows. A also is converted to F in an alternative pathway. A genetic deficiency in the enzyme converting A to B (indicated by the hatched rectangle) may have pathophysiological consequences related to accumulation of A (precursor toxicity), overflow to F (alternative pathway overflow), reduced formation of D (product deficiency), or some combination of these possibilities.

creased biotin losses and eventually biotin deficiency and impairment of the biotin-dependent carboxylases. The recognition of this cause of mental retardation by Wolf and his colleagues,[194] the development of a presymptomatic screening test,[195] and the ease of replacement therapy with biotin all augur for this being one of the most successfully treated genetic disorders.

Treatment at the Dysfunctional Protein Level

Therapy at this level involves either activation or replenishment of the mutant protein.

Activation with Vitamin Cofactors. Enhancement of the activity of a dysfunctional enzyme may be possible when the protein utilizes a vitamin cofactor which is tolerated by the patient in amounts far exceeding normal. Furthermore, not all mutations of a vitamin-dependent protein will respond. Those that do are likely to be missense mutations which either decrease the affinity of the enzyme for its cofactor or destabilize the protein in a way that can be partially overcome by substantial increments in cofactor concentration in the surrounding milieu. For example, about one-third of the cases of homocystinuria due to deficiency of cystathione β-synthase recover a functionally significant amount of enzyme activity when treated with large doses (50–500 mg/day) of pyridoxine (vitamin B_6) (Chap. 23). The actual increment in enzyme activity is often small but is sufficient to improve or even normalize metabolic flux in the transsulfuration pathway. Since activation of residual activity both reduces precursor accumulation and increases product formation, knowledge of the pathophysiological mechanism is less critical. Other examples of this type of therapy include the use of thiamine in some cases of maple syrup urine disease and thiamine, biotin, or riboflavin for certain forms of lactic acidosis. Thus, vitamin responsive disorders may represent either examples of inborn errors of vitamin metabolism with replacement of deficient product as described for biotinidase deficiency above or examples of enhancement of apoprotein function as described for cystathionine β-synthase deficiency.

Protein Replacement Therapies. Replacement of the mutant protein continues to be an active area of research. To have some hope of succeeding, the protein must be administered directly into or eventually reach its appropriate physiological compartment. Thus, blood proteins or proteins which transverse the vascular compartment (peptide hormones) are good candidates for this approach. Other considerations include the availability, stability, and immunogenicity of the administered protein. In a few instances, recombinant DNA technology is being utilized to supply sufficient amounts of pure protein (e.g., human growth hormone). Other proteins, including factor VIII for the treatment of hemophilia A and α₁-antitrypsin for the treatment of its deficiency,[196] are still being purified from natural sources but may soon be produced by recombinant DNA technology. This advance would ensure adequate supplies and avoid the risk of transmission of contaminating viruses to the recipients.

An innovative approach to the problems of stability and avoidance of immunological recognition has been reported by Hershfield et al.[197] in the treatment of severe combined immunodeficiency caused by adenosine deaminase deficiency

(Chap. 40). These investigators used polyethylene glycol (PEG) cross-linked to bovine adenosine deaminase and administered the product by intramuscular injection to adenosine deaminase deficient patients. The bulky hydrophilic PEG molecules coat the surface of the enzyme and prevent immunologic recognition and rapid clearance of it from the vascular space. Substrates and products diffuse through the PEG layer and reach the active site of the protein. Weekly intramuscular injections are sufficient to maintain high blood adenosine deaminase levels and have resulted in gradual improvement in immunologic function over several months. The long-term consequences of continued exposure to PEG and the feasibility of this sort of approach in patients who are not immunocompromised will require additional study.

Organ Transplantation

Organ transplantation lies on the borderline between therapy at the level of the dysfunctional protein and gene therapy. On the one hand a transplanted organ supplies a deficient protein; on the other, the transplanted tissue also brings new genetic information, although this is not integrated into the recipient's genome. Without resolving the semantic question, transplantation of kidneys, bone marrow, and livers is being applied increasingly to a variety of genetic diseases. The development of more effective and specific immunosuppressants (particularly cyclosporine) and inadequacies of more conventional therapies contribute to the increased interest in this form of treatment. The long-term efficacy and consequences of organ transplantation are unknown.

In some instances, transplantation is done strictly to supply the recipient with a tissue which can provide a missing protein; in others, the transplant also replaces a damaged organ. Examples of the former include bone marrow transplants for lysosomal storage diseases[198] as well as β thalassemia[199] and liver transplantation for type I glycogen storage disease,[200] familial hypercholesterolemia[201] and ornithine transcarbamylase deficiency.[202] Examples of the latter include liver transplants in α₁-antitrypsin deficiency and hepatorenal tyrosinemia[203] as well as kidney transplants in cystinosis. In the future, the distinction may be relevant because, when the intent is simply to provide a source for a deficient protein, it may be possible to perform partial liver transplants or even to infuse hepatocytes into the portal vein or peritoneal cavity. The recipient's liver, which is normal except for the specific deficiency, can then remain in place. Promising results with hepatocytes bound to inert beads injected into the peritoneal cavity of rats with analbuminemia or UDP-glucuronyltransferase deficiency have been reported.[204] Immunosuppression still is required, but the procedure is much less involved than liver transplantation. Perhaps this technique will be improved in the future and combined with a method of storing the donor cells indefinitely (as is done with tissue culture cells) so that frozen normal hepatocytes would be immediately available as a reagent to treat, at least temporarily, a variety of liver specific deficiencies.

A second major consideration when transplantation is performed to provide a tissue source for a deficient protein is whether or not the protein will reach the tissue or organelle of pathophysiological significance. This is of special concern for bone marrow transplantation in the lysosomal storage diseases. The rationale is that the transplanted marrow will provide cells capable of repopulating the recipient's reticuloendothelial system, and the lysosomal enzymes released from the donor cells will enter host cells by systems which deliver the enzyme to the proper subcellular compartments (i.e., lysosomes). Evidence from marrow transplants in patients with mucopolysaccharidosis indicates that both of these desired results occur. It is not clear, however if either transplant derived cells or enzymes can cross the blood-brain barrier. Since central nervous system involvement is a prominent feature of most lysosomal storage diseases, failure to reach this tissue would severely limit the applicability of bone marrow transplantation, particularly in view of the attendant morbidity and mortality. Clinical trials in patients with a variety of lysosomal storage diseases provide no evidence of transfer of donor cells or enzymes across the blood-brain barrier.[198] The one exception is a study done in dogs with α-iduronidase deficiency and a Hurler-Scheie phenotype who had some biochemical and ultrastructural evidence for improvement in the central nervous system 3 to 9 months after transplant.[205] This tantalizing observation requires additional investigation.

Somatic Gene Therapy

While there is great hope that patients with genetic disorders can be treated by somatic gene replacement (Chap. 2), as of early 1988, no patient has benefited from such an approach. Most of the interest has focused on introduction of a competent replacement gene into tissues such as bone marrow stem cells, hepatocytes, or fibroblasts. A number of biologic considerations enter into the feasibility of somatic gene replacement therapy, including the question of whether the addition of normal gene product will be therapeutic. Presumably this would be the case for many or most disorders, but it might not be adequate for a "true dominant" disorder where a mutant gene can negate the presence of normal gene product. The latter instance might require gene specific correction or elimination of the dominant mutation. And how much gene product would indeed be required to ameliorate or totally correct the disease phenotype? In some instances, as little as 1 to 5 percent of normal gene product activity might be virtually curative (e.g., some enzyme activities or clotting factors). The need for tissue specific expression and gene regulation are also important, as are several ethical considerations. Many reviews and commentaries on the potential for somatic gene replacement therapy are available.[206–208] Early efforts at gene therapy have focused attention on tissue which can be removed for purposes of infection and then restored to the patient (Fig. 1-24). This approach is feasible for bone marrow and fibroblasts and perhaps for hepatocytes, epithelial cells, and some other cell types. Disorders which affect bone marrow derived cells merit particular attention, including sickle-cell anemia, thalassemias, adenosine deaminase deficiency, chronic granulomatous disease, and leukocyte adhesion deficiency. It may be possible to use bone marrow–derived cells to achieve expression of gene products which ordinarily would be produced by other tissues. Production of clotting factors, hormones, or enzymes that utilize circulating metabolites might be therapeutic in bone marrow cells even if this were not the natural site for expression. Similar use might be made of cultured fibroblasts or epithelial cells. The feasibility of infecting bone marrow–derived cells, fibroblasts, or hepatocytes in vitro followed by reintroduction of the infected cells into the organism is being explored in various rodents and other animal models.[209–211] Eventually, one goal might be to obtain adequate viral titers

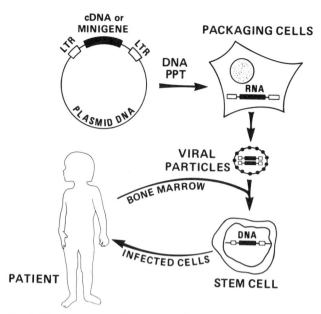

Fig. 1-24 One strategy for attempting gene replacement therapy for bone marrow derived cells. (*From A. Beaudet.[217] Used by permission.*)

and targeting ability to allow direct injection of viral preparations into humans. At the moment, diseases which would require introduction of DNA sequences into the central nervous system would seem to be the most challenging and least feasible.

The need for proper gene regulation is likely to vary considerably from disease to disease. In many instances where there is total absence of gene product, it is probable that any level of expression—from very low to even excessive—would be beneficial. In other instances, relatively precise levels of expression and tissue specificity would be required as in the case of hemoglobin disorders.

Most of the work up to the present has focused on the use of retroviral vectors (derived from components of retroviral genomes). Typically, a cloned cDNA for a human gene product is inserted into a retroviral vector using the long terminal repeat (LTR) of the retrovirus or a regulatory element from another gene as a promoter. Pseudovirus particles are produced by introduction of the vector sequences into packaging cell lines, which are designed to provide the necessary viral gene products in trans without leading to the production of infectious retrovirus particles. Pseudovirus particles encoding the following human gene products have been demonstrated: adenosine deaminase, HPRT, phenylalanine hydroxylase, α_1-antitrypsin, β-glucocerebrosidase, LDL receptor, β globin, and others (see chapters in gene therapy section in Ref. 212). There have been difficulties in obtaining good gene expression after reimplantation of cells into animals, but some limited expression in intact animals is being reported.[209]

Many different diseases have been discussed as candidates for somatic gene therapy. The relative feasibility for disorders being considered takes into account the burden of the disease, the availability of alternative treatment, the disease frequency, the requirement for tissue specificity, the possible need for gene regulation, and the availability of the cloned gene. Some widely discussed examples are listed in Table 1-12, including some examples where feasibility appears quite poor because of the need to reach the central nervous system (e.g., Huntington disease and Tay-Sachs disease).

Table 1-12 Human Diseases as Candidates for Gene Replacement Therapy

Disorders	Burden of disease	Alternative treatment	Disease frequency	Requirement for tissue specificity	Regulation	Relative feasibility*
Hemoglobinopathies	Great	Transfusion, fair to poor	1 in 600 in ethnic groups	Erythroid	Required	+ +
Lesch-Nyhan	Great	Poor	Rare	Brain, ?other	?Not essential	+ +
Adenosine deaminase and nucleoside phosphorylase	Great	Transplant, enzyme replacement, fair to good	Very rare	Bone marrow	?Not essential	+ + +
Leukocyte adhesion deficiency	Great	Transplant, fair to poor	Very rare	Bone marrow	?Not essential	+ + + +
Phenylketonuria	Small to moderate	Diet, good	1 in 11,000	Liver, ?other	?Not essential	+ +
Urea cycle disorders	Moderate to great	Diet, drug, good to poor	1 in 30,000 for all types	Liver, ?other	?Not essential	+ +
α₁-Antitrypsin	Moderate	Poor	1 in 3500	Liver, ?other	?Not essential	+ + +
Hemophilia A & B	Moderate to great	Replacement, fair (AIDS)	1 in 10,000 males	?Any organ, factor VIII	?Not essential	+ + + +
Lysosomal storage diseases	Great	Poor	1 in 1500 for all types	Brain for many	?Not essential	+
Familial hypercholesterolemia	Great	Diet, drug, fair	1 in 500 heterozygotes	Liver, ?other	Some importance	+ +
Cystic fibrosis	Great	Supportive, fair to poor	1 in 2500 whites	?	?	?
Duchenne muscular dystrophy	Great	Poor	1 in 10,000 males	?Muscle	?	?Poor
Tay-Sachs disease	Great	Poor	1 in 3000 Jews	?Brain	?Not essential	?Poor
Huntington disease	Great	Poor	1 in 20,000	?Brain	?	?Poor

*Relative feasibility attempts to take into account requirements for regulation, accessibility of target organ, alternative treatment, and risk-benefit considerations.

ANIMAL MODELS

Numerous examples of genetic diseases in animals are cited throughout this text and elsewhere,[213] including diseases in mice, rats, dogs, cats, sheep, and cattle, among others. Exactly analogous enzyme deficiencies and gene defects are known as well as similar clinical phenotypes such as albinism. Available models include amino acid disorders, urea cycle disorders, numerous lysosomal enzyme deficiencies, receptor deficiencies, bilirubin disorders, and clotting disorders. For example, a mutated canine guanosine triphosphate cyclohydrolase deficiency mimics the human counterpart variant of PKU (Chap. 15). These animal models are likely to become of increasing importance because they facilitate the study of two areas which are particularly poorly developed in biochemical genetics: (1) treatment and (2) understanding of pathogenesis.

Another perspective occurs when diseases are discovered first in animals, and analogous human disorders are then sought. Defects in the gene for myelin basic protein cause the *shiverer* phenotype in mice, and this disorder has been characterized at a nucleic acid and protein level.[214] The discovery of homeotic mutations in *Drosophila* has led to the identification of homologous regions in homeotic genes in mice and humans.[215] Perhaps this will lead to the identification of human genetic disorders involving these homeotic loci.

Animal models are also receiving new impetus from two quarters. First there is the great potential value for trials of somatic gene replacement therapy. Prior to human treatment, there is a need to demonstrate both the safety and efficacy of such procedures. Efficacy can best be judged by correcting an analogous defect in an animal prior to human trials. The second impetus is coming from the potential to generate animal models for human mutations, particularly in mice, rather than simply discovering naturally occurring mutants. This has been achieved in part by intensely mutagenizing mice and screening them for biochemical defects. This has led to the discovery of a series of mutations at the mouse *mdx* locus,[216] which is homologous with the Duchenne muscular dystrophy locus.[9] Another strategy has been to take advantage of the availability of embryonic stem cells which can be cultured and then used to generate chimeric animals and introduce new genotypes into the germ line. This strategy has been used to obtain HPRT deficient mice.[142,143] Many animal models have exactly analogous biochemical defects and phenotypes compared to the human diseases. Interestingly, for the *mdx* mouse and for the HPRT deficient mouse, this is not the case. The *mdx* mouse has no significant muscular disability and the HPRT deficient mouse does not show self-mutilation or obvious neurologic symptoms. While one might be concerned that these then represent poor animal models, they may represent very good models in terms of the potential for understanding pathogenesis and developing therapy, if one can understand the different consequences of the mutations in different species. Attempts to analyze the homeostatic differences between the mouse and human diseases are likely to focus attention on those factors which are instrumental in the primary genetic defect generating the phenotypic abnormalities (i.e., pathophysiology). Understanding the basis of these differences might provide the insights to modify the human circumstance so that it is less symptomatic and more similar to the *mdx* mouse or HPRT deficient mouse.

REFERENCES

1. HAYES A, COSTA, T, SCRIVER CR, CHILDS B: The effect of Mendelian disease on human health. II: Response to treatment. *Am J Med Genet* 21:243, 1985.
2. WILLIAMS RJ: *Biochemical Individuality.* New York, Wiley, 1956.
3. GARROD AE: *Inborn Factors in Disease.* London, Oxford University Press, 1931.

4. MCKUSICK VA: *Mendelian Inheritance in Man*, 8th ed. Baltimore, Johns Hopkins University Press, 1988.

5. FREZAL J: Human gene mapping 9. *Cytogenet Cell Genet* 46:1, 1988.

6. *Mapping and Sequencing the Human Genome*. Washington, DC, National Academy of Sciences, 1988.

7. GARROD A: The lessons of rare maladies. *Lancet* 1:1055, 1928.

8. PAGE DC, MOSHER R, SIMPSON EM, FISHER EM, MARDON G, POLLACK J, MCGILLIVRAY B, de la CHAPPELE A, BROWN LG: The sex-determining region of the human Y chromosome encodes a finger protein. *Cell* 51:1091, 1987.

9. HOFFMAN EP, BROWN RH, KUNKEL LM: Dystrophin: The protein product of the Duchenne muscular dystrophy locus. *Cell* 51:919, 1987.

10. GARROD AE: Inborn errors of metabolism (Croonian Lectures). *Lancet* 2:1, 73, 142, 214, 1908.

11. GARROD AE: *Inborn Errors of Metabolism*, 2d ed. London, Oxford University Press, 1923.

12. GARROD AE: A contribution to the study of alkaptonuria. *Proc R Med Chir Soc* 2:130, 1899.

13. GARROD AE: The incidence of alkaptonuria: A study in chemical individuality. *Lancet* 2:1616, 1902.

14. MENDEL G: *Versuche über Pflanzenhybriden*. Leipzig, Engelmann, 1901.

15. BEARN AG, MILLER ED: Archibald Garrod and the development of the concept of inborn errors of metabolism. *Bull Hist Med* 53:315, 1979.

16. LaDU BN, ZANNONI VA, LASTER L, SEEGMILLER JE: The nature of the defect in tyrosine metabolism in alcaptonuria. *J Biol Chem* 230:251, 1958.

17. JOHANNSEN W: The genotype conception of heredity. *Am Nat* 45:129, 1911.

18. BEADLE GW: Biochemical genetics. *Chem Rev* 37:15, 1945.

19. BEADLE GW, TATUM EL: Experimental control of developmental reactions. *Am Nat* 75:107, 1941.

20. BEADLE GW, TATUM EL: Genetic control of biochemical reactions in *Neurospora*. *Proc Natl Acad Sci USA* 27:499, 1941.

21. EPHRUSSI B: Chemistry of "eye color hormones" of *Drosophila*. *Q Rev Biol* 17:327, 1942.

22. BEADLE GW: Genes and chemical reactions in *Neurospora*. *Science* 129:1715, 1959.

23. TATUM EL: A case history of biological research. *Science* 129:1711, 1959.

24. HOROWITZ NH, LEUPOLD U: Some recent studies bearing on the one gene one enzyme hypothesis. *Cold Spring Harbor Symp Quant Biol* 16:65, 1951.

25. BENZER S: The elementary units of heredity, in McElroy WD, Glass B (eds): *The Chemical Basis of Heredity*. Baltimore, Johns Hopkins University Press, 1957, p 70.

26. JONES ME: Pyrimidine nucleotide biosynthesis in animals: Genes, enzymes, and regulation of UMP biosynthesis. *Annu Rev Biochem* 49:253, 1980.

27. DOUGLASS J, CIVELLI O, HERBERT E: Polyprotein gene expression: Generation of diversity of neuroendocrine peptides. *Annu Rev Biochem* 53:665, 1984.

28. LYNCH DR, SNYDER SH: Neuropeptides: Multiple molecular forms, metabolic pathways, and receptors. *Annu Rev Biochem* 55:773, 1986.

29. SCHIBLER U, SIERRA F: Alternative promoters in developmental gene expression. *Annu Rev Genet* 21:237, 1987.

30. AMARA SG, JONAS V, ROSENFELD MG, ONG ES, EVANS RM: Alternative RNA processing in calcitonin gene expression generates mRNAs encoding different polypeptide products. *Nature* 298:240, 1982.

31. NABESHIMA Y, FUJII-KURIYAMA Y, MURAMATSU M, OGATA K: Alternative transcription and two modes of splicing result in two myosin light chains from one gene. *Nature* 308:333, 1984.

32. BREITBART RE, ANDREADIA A, NADAL-GINARD B: Alternative splicing: A ubiquitous mechanism for the generation of multiple protein isoforms from single genes. *Annu Rev Biochem* 56:467, 1987.

33. CRAIGEN WJ, CASKEY CT: Translational frameshifting: Where will it stop? *Cell* 50:1, 1987.

34. JACKS T, POWER MD, MASIARZ FR, LUCIW PA, BARR PJ, VARMUS HE: Characterization of ribosomal frameshifting in HIV-1 *gag-pol* expression. *Nature* 331:280, 1988.

35. GIBSON QH: The reduction of methaemoglobin in red blood cells and studies on the cause of idiopathic methaemoglobinaemia. *Biochem J* 42:13, 1948.

36. CORI GT, CORI CF: Glucose-6-phosphatase of the liver in glycogen storage disease. *J Biol Chem* 199:661, 1952.

37. JERVIS GA: Phenylpyruvic oligophrenia: Deficiency of phenylalanine oxidizing system. *Proc Soc Exp Biol Med* 82:514, 1953.

38. PAULING L, ITANO HA, SINGER SJ, WELLS IC: Sickle cell anemia: A molecular disease. *Science* 110:543, 1949.

39. INGRAM VM: A specific chemical difference between the globins of normal human and sickle cell anaemia haemoglobin. *Nature* 178:792, 1956.

40. KAN YW, DOZY AM: Polymorphism of DNA sequence adjacent to human β-globin structural gene: Relationship to sickle mutation. *Proc Natl Acad Sci USA* 75:5631, 1978.

41. BOTSTEIN D, WHITE RL, SKOLNICK M, DAVIS RW: Construction of a genetic linkage map in man using restriction fragment length polymorphisms. *Am J Hum Genet* 32:314, 1980.

42. ORKIN SH: Reverse genetics and human disease. *Cell* 47:845, 1986.

43. GEHRING WH, HIROMI Y: Homeotic genes and the homeobox. *Annu Rev Genet* 20:147, 1986.

44. ROYER-POKORA B, KUNKEL LM, MONACO AP, GOFF SC, NEWBURGER PE, BAEHNER RL, COLE FS, CURNUTTE JT, ORKIN SH: Cloning the gene for an inherited human disorder—chronic granulomatous disease—on the basis of its chromosomal location. *Nature* 322:32, 1986.

45. KOENIG M, HOFFMAN EP, BERTELSON CJ, MONACO AP, FEENER C, KUNKEL LM: Complete cloning of the Duchenne muscular dystrophy (DMD) cDNA and preliminary genomic organization of the DMD gene in normal and affected individuals. *Cell* 50:509, 1987.

46. FRIEND SH, BERNARDS R, ROGELJ S, WEINBERG RA, RAPAPORT JM, ALBERT DM, DRYJA TP: A human DNA segment with properties of the gene that predisposes to retinoblastoma and osteosarcoma. *Nature* 323:643, 1986.

47. GILLIAM TC, TANZI RE, HAINES JL, BONNER TI, FARYNIARZ AG, HOBBS WJ, MacDONALD ME, CHENG SV, FOLSTEIN SE, CONNEALLY PM, WEXLER NS, GUSELLA JF: Localization of the Huntington's disease gene to a small segment of chromosome 4 flanked by D4S10 and the telomere. *Cell* 50:565, 1987.

48. REEDERS ST, BREUNING MH, DAVIES KE, NICHOLLS RD, JARMAN AP, HIGGS DR, PEARSON PL, WEATHERALL DJ: A highly polymorphic DNA marker linked to adult polycystic kidney disease on chromosome 16. *Nature* 317:542, 1985.

49. SEIZINGER BR, ROULEAU GA, OZELIUS LJ, LANE AH, FARYNIARZ AG, CHAO MV, HUSON S, KORF BR, PARRY DM, PERICAK-VANCE MA, COLLINS FS, HOBBS WJ, FALCONE BG, IANNAZZI JA, ROY JC, ST. GEORGE-HYSLOP PH, TANZI RE, BOTHWELL MA, UPADHYAYA M, HARPER P, GOLDSTEIN AE, HOOVER DL, BADER JL, SPENCE MA, MULVIHILL JJ, AYLSWORTH AS, VANCE JM, ROSSENWASSER GOD, GASKELL PC, ROSEO AD, MARTUZA RL, BREAKEFIELD XO, GUSELLA JF: Genetic linkage of von Recklinghausen neurofibromatosis to the nerve growth factor receptor gene. *Cell* 49:589, 1987.

50. SEIZINGER BR, ROULEAU GA, OZELIUS LJ, LANE AH, FARMER GE, LAMIELL JM, HAINES J, YUEN JWM, COLLINS D, MAJOOR-KRAKAUER D, BONNER T, MATHEW C, RUBENSTEIN A, HALPERIN J, McCONKIE-ROSELL A, GREEN JS, TROFATTER JA, PONDER BA, EIERMAN L, BOWMER MI, SCHIMKE R, OOSTRA B, ARONIN N, SMITH DI, DRABKIN H, WAZIRI MH, HOBBS WJ, MARTUZA RL, CONNEALLY PM, HSIA YE, GUSELLA JF: Von Hippel-Lindau disease maps to the region of chromosome 3 associated with renal cell carcinoma. *Nature* 332:268, 1988.

51. BODMER WF, BAILEY CJ, BODMER J, BUSSEY HJR, ELLIS A, GORMAN P, LUCIBELLO FC, MURDAY VA, RIDER SH, SCAMBLER P, SHEER D, SOLOMON E, SPURR NK: Localization of the gene for familial adenomatous polyposis on chromosome 5. *Nature* 328:614, 1987.

52. HERRERA L, KAKATI S, GIBAS L, PIETRZAK E, SANDBERG AA: Brief clinical report: Gardner syndrome in a man with an interstitial deletion of 5q. *Am J Med Genet* 25:473, 1986.

53. MARX JL: Putting the human genome on the map. *Science* 229:150, 1985.

54. EIBERG H, MOHR J, SCHMIEGELOW K, NIELSEN LS, WILLIAMSON R: Linkage relationships of paraoxonase (PON) with other markers: Indication of PON-cystic fibrosis synteny. *Clin Genet* 28:265, 1985.

55. TSUI L-P, BUCHWALD M, BARKER D, BRAMAN JC, KNOWLTON R, SCHUMM JW, EIBERT H, MOHR J, KENNEDY D, PLAVSIC N, ZSIGA M, MARKIEWICZ D, AKOTS G, BROWN V, HELMS C, GRAVIUS T, PARKER C, REDIKER K, DONIS-KELLER H: Cystic fibrosis locus defined by a genetically linked polymorphic DNA marker. *Science* 230:1054, 1985.

56. WHITE R, WOODWARD C, LEPPERT M, O'CONNELL P, HOFF M, HERBST J, LALOUEL J-M, DEAN M, VANDE WOUDE G: A closely linked genetic marker for cystic fibrosis. *Nature* 318:382, 1985.

57. WAINWRIGHT BJ, SCAMBLER PG, SCHMIDTKE J, WATSON EA, LAW H-Y, FARRALL M, COOKE HJ, EIBERT H, WILLIAMSON R: Localization of cystic fibrosis locus to human chromosome 7cen-q22. *Nature* 318:384, 1985.

58. BEAUDET A, BOWCOCK A, BUCHWALD M, CAVALLI-SFORZA L, FARRALL M, KING M-C, KLINGER K, LALOUEL J-M, LATHROP G, NAYLOR S, OTT J, TSUI L-C, WAINWRIGHT B, WATKINS P, WHITE R, WILLIAMSON R: Linkage of cystic fibrosis to two tightly linked DNA markers: Joint report from a collaborative study. *Am J Hum Genet* 39:681, 1986.

59. GROSVELD F, van ASSENDELFT GB, GREAVES DR, KOLLIAS G: Position independent, high level expression of the human β-globin gene in transgenic mice. *Cell* 51:975, 1987.

60. JELINEK WR, SCHMID CW: Repetitive sequences in eukaryotic DNA and their expression. *Annu Rev Biochem* 51:813, 1982.

61. BIRD AP: CpG-rich islands and the function of DNA methylation. *Nature* 321:209, 1986.

62. ALBERTS B, BRAY D, LEWIS J, RAFF M, ROBERTS K, WATSON JD: *Molecular Biology of the Cell.* New York, Garland, 1983.

63. DARNELL J, LODISH H, BALTIMORE D: *Molecular Cell Biology.* New York, Scientific American Books, 1986.

64. WATSON JD, HOPKINS NH, ROBERTS JW, STEITZ JA, WEINER AM: *Molecular Biology of the Gene.* Menlo Park, Benjamin/Cummings, 1987.

65. KORNBERG A: *DNA Replication.* San Francisco, Freeman, 1980.

66. WATSON JD, CRICK FHC: Molecular structure of nucleic acids. *Nature* 171:737, 1953.

67. KORNBERG A: *Supplement to DNA Replication.* San Francisco, Freeman, 1982.

68. MCMACKEN R, KELLY TJ: *Replication and Recombination: UCLA Symposia on Molecular and Cellular Biology, New Series.* New York, AR Liss, 1987.

69. KORNBERG A: DNA replication. *J Biol Chem* 263:1, 1988.

70. STRYER L: *Biochemistry.* San Francisco, Freeman, 1981.

71. PTASHNE M: *A Genetic Switch: Gene Control and Phage λ.* Cambridge, Cell Press, 1986.

72. MANIATIS T, GOODBOURN S, FISCHER JA: Regulation of inducible and tissue-specific gene expression. *Science* 236:1237, 1987.

73. GUARENTE L: UASs and enhancers: Common mechanism of transcriptional activation in yeast and mammals. *Cell* 52:303, 1988.

74. BERG JM: Potential metal-binding domains in nucleic acid binding proteins. *Science* 232:485, 1986.

75. EVANS RM, HOLLENBERG SM: Zinc fingers: Gilt by association. *Cell* 52:1, 1988.

76. SCHEVITZ RW, OTWINOWSKI Z, JOACHIMIAK A, LAWSON CL, SIGLER PB: The three-dimensional structure of *trp* repressor. *Nature* 317:782, 1985.

77. LANDSCHULZ WH, JOHNSON PF, MCKNIGHT SL: Leucine zipper: A hypothetical structure common to a new class of DNA binding proteins. *Science* 240:1759, 1988.

78. SINGH H, LEBOWITZ JH, BALDWIN AS, SHARP PA: Molecular cloning of an enhancer binding protein: Isolation by screening of an expression library with a recognition site DNA. *Cell* 52:415, 1988.

79. HARRIS H: *The Principles of Human Biochemical Genetics,* 3d ed. Amsterdam, North-Holland, 1980.

80. ANTONARAKIS SE, KAZAZIAN HH, ORKIN SH: DNA polymorphism and molecular pathology of the human globin gene clusters. *Hum Genet* 69:1, 1985.

81. BARKER D, SCHAFER M, WHITE R: Restriction sites containing CpG show a higher frequency of polymorphism in human DNA. *Cell* 36:131, 1984.

82. HARRIS H: Enzyme polymorphisms in man. *Proc R Soc Lond (Biol)* 174:1, 1966.

83. LEWONTIN RC, HUBBY JL: A molecular approach to the study of genetic heterozygosity in natural populations. II. Amount of variation and degree of heterozygosity in natural population of *Drosophila pseudoobscura.* *Genetics* 54:595, 1966.

84. GIBLETT ER: Genetic polymorphisms in human blood. *Annu Rev Genet* 11:13, 1977.

85. WALTON KE, STYER D, GRUENSTEIN EI: Genetic polymorphism in normal human fibroblasts as analyzed by two-dimensional polyacrylamide gel electrophoresis. *J Biol Chem* 254:7951, 1979.

86. MCCONKEY EH, TAYLOR BJ, PHAN D: Human heterozygosity: A new estimate. *Proc Natl Acad Sci USA* 76:6500, 1979.

87. COOPER DN, SMITH BA, BOOKE HJ, NIEMANN S, SCHMIDTKE J: An estimate of unique DNA sequence heterozygosity in the human genome. *Hum Genet* 69:201, 1985.

88. EMBURY SH, DOZY AJ, MILLER J, DAVIS JR, KLEMAN KM, PRESILER H, VICHINSKY E, LANDE WN, LUBIN B, KAN YW, MENTZER WC: Concurrent sickle cell anemia and α-thalassemia. Effect on severity of anemia. *N Engl J Med* 306:270, 1982.

89. HIGGS DR, ALDRIDGE BE, LAMB J, CLEGG JB, WEATHERALL DJ, HAYES RJ, GRANDISON Y, LOWRIE Y, MAON KP, SERJEANT BE, SERJEANT GR: The interaction of α-thalassemia and homozygous sickle cell disease. *N Engl Med* 306:1441, 1982.

90. COSTA T, SCRIVER CR, CHILDS B: The effect of Mendelian disease on human health: A measurement. *Am J Med Genet* 21:231, 1985.

91. MORGAN TH: The relation of genetics to physiology and medicine, in Baltimore D (ed): *Nobel Lectures in Molecular Biology 1933–1975.* New York, Elsevier North-Holland, 1977, p 3.

92. MCKUSICK VA, RUDDLE FH: The status of the gene map of the human chromosomes. *Science* 196:390, 1977.

93. RUDDLE FH: A new era in mammalian gene mapping: Somatic cell genetics and recombinant DNA methodologies. *Nature* 294:115, 1981.

94. RUDDLE FH: The William Allan Memorial Award address: Reverse genetics and beyond. *Am J Hum Genet* 36:944, 1984.

95. VOGEL F, MOTULSKY AG: *Human Genetics: Problems and Approaches,* 2d ed. Berlin, Springer-Verlag, 1986.

96. FRANCKE U, OCHS HD, deMARTINVILLE B, GIACALONE J, LINDGREN V, DISTÈCHE C, PAGON RA, HOFKER MH, van OMMEN G-JB, PEARSON PL, WEDGWOOD RJ: Minor Xp21 chromosome deletion in a male associated with expression of Duchenne muscular dystrophy, chronic granulomatous disease, retinitis pigmentosa, and McLeod syndrome. *Am J Hum Genet* 37:250, 1985.

97. GALJAARD H: *Genetic Metabolic Diseases: Early Diagnosis and Prenatal Analysis.* Amsterdam, Elsevier North-Holland, 1980.

98. SCRIVER CR, NEAL JL, SAGINUR R, CLOW A: The frequency of genetic disease and congenital malformation among patients in a pediatric hospital. *Can Med Assoc J* 108:1111, 1973.

99. BAIRD PA, ANDERSON TW, NEWCOMBE HB, LOWRY RB: Genetic disorders in children and young adults: A population study. *Am J Hum Genet* 42:677, 1988.

100. UNSCEAR: Genetic and somatic effects of ionizing radiation. New York, United Nations, 1986.

101. SORENSEN TIA, NIELSEN GG, ANDERSEN PK, TEASDALE TW: Genetic and environmental influences on premature death in adult adoptees. *N Engl J Med* 318:727, 1988.

102. YUNIS JJ: The chromosomal basis of human neoplasia. *Science* 221:227, 1983.

103. LE BEAU MM, ROWLEY JD: Chromosomal abnormalities in leukemia and lymphoma: Clinical and biological significance. *Adv Hum Genet* 15:1, 1986.

104. HALUSKA FG, TSUJIMOTO Y, CROCE CM: Oncogene activation by chromosome translocation in human malignancy. *Annu Rev Genet* 21:321, 1987.

105. OKAMOTO M, SASAKI M, SUGIO K, SATO C, IWAMA T, IKEUCHI T, TONOMURA A, SASAZUKI T, MIYAKI M: Loss of constitutional heterozygosity in colon carcinoma from patients with familial polyposis coli. *Nature* 331:273, 1988.

106. SOLOMON E, VOSS R, HALL V, BODMER WF, JASS JR, JEFFREYS AJ, LUCIBELLO FC, PATEL I, RIDER SH: Chromosome 5 allele loss in human colorectal carcinomas. *Nature* 328:616, 1987.

107. KOVACS G, ERLANDSSON R, BOLDOG F, INGVARSSON S, MÜLLER-BRECHLIN R, KLEIN G, SÜMEGI J: Consistent chromosome 3p deletion and loss of heterozygosity in renal cell carcinoma. *Proc Natl Acad Sci USA* 85:1571, 1988.

108. DE GROUCHY J, TURLEAU C: *Clinical Atlas of Human Chromosomes,* 2d ed. New York, Wiley, 1984.

109. SCHINZEL A: *Catalogue of Unbalanced Chromosome Aberrations in Man.* New York, Walter de Gruyter, 1983.

110. CARTER CO: Monogenic disorders. *J Med Genet* 14:316, 1977.

111. MOTULSKY AG: Frequency of sickling disorders in US blacks. *N Engl J Med* 288:31, 1973.

112. WEXLER NS, YOUNG AB, TANZI RE, TRAVERS H, STAROSTA-RUBINSTEIN S, PENNEY JB, SNODGRASS SR, SHOULSON I, GOMEZ F, RAMOS ARROYO MA, PENCHASZADEH GK, MORNEO H, GIBBONS K, FARYNIARZ A, HOBBS W, ANDERSON MA, BONILLA E, CONNEALLY PM, GUSELLA JF: Homozygotes for Huntington's disease. *Nature* 326:194, 1987.

113. SWIFT M, REITNAUER PJ, MORRELL D, CHASE CL: Breast and other cancers in families with ataxia-telangiectasia. *N Engl J Med* 316:1289, 1987.

114. KACSER H, BURNS JA: The molecular basis of dominance. *Genetics* 97:639, 1981.

115. HERSKOWITZ I: Functional inactivation of genes by dominant negative mutations. *Nature* 329:219, 1987.

116. BUNDEY S, EVANS K: Tuberous sclerosis—A genetic study. *J Neurol Neurosurg Psychiatry* 32:591, 1969.

117. JONES KL, SMITH DW, HARVEY MAS, HALL BD, QUAN L: Older paternal age and fresh gene mutation: Data on additional disorders. *J Pediatr* 86:84, 1975.

118. MURDOCH JL, WALKER BA, MCKUSICK VA: Parental age effects on the occurrence of new mutations for the Marfan syndrome. *Ann Hum Genet* 35:331, 1972.

119. BALLARD HS, FRAME B, HARTSOCK RJ: Familial multiple endocrine adenoma-peptic ulcer complex. *Medicine* 43:481, 1964.

120. LARSSON C, SKOGSEID B, ÖBERG K, NAKAMURA Y, NORDENSKJÖLD M: Multiple endocrine neoplasia type 1 gene maps to chromosome 11 and is lost in insulinoma. *Nature* 332:85, 1988.

121. STACEY A, BATEMAN J, CHOI T, MASCARA T, COLE W, JAENISCH R: Perinatal lethal osteogenesis imperfecta in transgenic mice bearing an engineered mutant pro-α1 (I) collagen gene. *Nature* 332:131, 1988.

122. BROWN MS, GOLDSTEIN JL: New directions in human biochemical genetics: Understanding the manifestations of receptor deficiency disorders. *Prog Med Genet* 1 (new series):103, 1976.

123. HERS HG: Inborn lysosomal diseases. *Gastroenterology* 48:625, 1965.

124. NEUFELD EF, TIMPLE WL, SHAPIRO LJ: Inherited disorders of lysosomal metabolism. *Annu Rev Biochem* 44:357, 1975.

125. VON FIGURA K, HASILIK A: Lysosomal enzymes and their receptors. *Annu Rev Biochem* 55:167, 1986.

126. CAVALLI-SFORZA LL, BODMER WF: *The Genetics of Human Populations.* San Francisco, Freeman, 1971.

127. CHARLESWORTH B: Driving genes and chromosomes. *Nature* 332:394, 1988.

128. ESTIVILL X, FARRALL M, SCAMBLER PJ, BELL GM, HAWLEY KMF, LENCH NJ, BATES GP, KRUYER HC, FREDERICK PA, STANIER P, WATSON EK, WILLIAMSON R, WAINWRIGHT BJ: A candidate for the cystic fibrosis locus isolated by selection for methylation-free islands. *Nature* 326:840, 1987.

129. LYON MF: X-Chromosome inactivation and developmental patterns in mammals. *Biol Rev* 47:1, 1972.

130. GARTLER SM, RIGGS AD: Mammalian X-chromosome inactivation. *Annu Rev Genet* 17:155, 1983.

131. VOGEL F, RATHENBERG R: Spontaneous mutation in man. *Adv Hum Genet* 5:223, 1975.

132. CHILDS B, DER KALOUSTIAN VM: Genetic heterogeneity. *N Engl J Med* 279:1205, 1267, 1968.

133. HARRIS H: Genetic heterogeneity in inherited disease. *J Clin Pathol (Suppl)* 27:32, 1974.

134. LEDLEY FD, LEVY HL, SHIH VE, BENJAMIN R, MAHONEY MJ: Benign methylmalonic aciduria. *N Engl J Med* 311:1015, 1984.

135. CARTER CO: Genetics of common disorders. *Br Med Bull* 25:52, 1972.

136. CARTER CO: Principles of polygenic inheritance. *Birth Defects* 13:69, 1977.

137. CHILDS B, SCRIVER CR: Age at onset and causes of disease. *Perspect Biol Med* 29:437, 1986.

138. VESELL ES: Pharmacogenetics: Multiple interactions between genes and environment as determinants of drug response. *Am J Med* 66:183, 1979.

139. BURTON BK: Inborn errors of metabolism: The clinical diagnosis in early infancy. *Pediatrics* 79:359, 1987.

140. NEUFELD EF, FRATANTONI JC: Inborn errors of mucopolysaccharide metabolism. *Science* 169:141, 1970.

141. NUDEL U, ROBZYK K, YAFFE D: Expression of the putative Duchenne muscular dystrophy gene in differentiated myogenic cell cultures and in the brain. *Nature* 331:635, 1988.

142. HOOPER M, HARDY K, HANDYSIDE A, HUNTER S, MONK M: HPRT-deficient (Lesch-Nyhan) mouse embryos derived from germline colonization by cultured cells. *Nature* 326:292, 1987.

143. KUEHN MR, BRADLEY A, ROBERTSON EJ, EVANS MJ: A potential animal model for Lesch-Nyhan syndrome through introduction of HPRT mutations into mice. *Nature* 326:295, 1987.

144. BERG K: Inactivation of one of the X chromosomes in females is a biological phenomenon of clinical importance. *Acta Med Scand* 206:1, 1979.

145. FIALKOW PJ, LISKER R, GIBLETT ER, ZAVALA C: Xg locus: Failure to detect inactivation in females with chronic myelocytic leukaemia. *Nature* 226:367, 1970.

146. SHAPIRO LJ, MOHANDAS T, WEISS R: Non-inactivation of an X-chromosome locus in man. *Science* 204:1224, 1979.

147. GOODFELLOW P, PYM B, MOHANDAS T, SHAPIRO LJ: The *MIC2X* locus escapes X inactivation. *Am J Hum Genet* 36:777, 1984.

148. MIGEON BR, CHILDS B: Hybridization of mammalian somatic cells. *Prog Med Genet* 7 (old series):1, 1970.

149. SAUNDERS M, SWEETMAN L, ROBINSON B, ROTH K, COHN R, GRAVEL RA: Biotin-response organicaciduria: Multiple carboxylase defects and complementation studies with propionicacidemia in cultured fibroblasts. *J Clin Invest* 64:1695, 1979.

150. GRAVEL RA, LEUNG A, SAUNDERS M, HOSLI P: Analysis of genetic complementation by whole-cell microtechniques in fibroblast heterokaryons. *Proc Natl Acad Sci USA* 76:6520, 1979.

151. SAIKI RK, SCHARF S, FALOONA F, MULLIS KB, HORN GT, ERLICH HA, ARNHEIM M: Enzymatic amplification of β-globin genomic sequences and restriction site analysis for diagnosis of sickle cell anemia. *Science* 230:1350, 1985.

152. SCHARF SJ, HORN GT, ERLICH HA: Direct cloning and sequence analysis of enzymatically amplified genomic sequences. *Science* 233:1076, 1986.

153. EMBURY SH, SCHARF SJ, SAIKI RK, GHOLSON MA, GOLBUS M, ARNHEIM N, ERLICH HA: Rapid prenatal diagnosis of sickle cell anemia by a new method of DNA analysis. *N Engl J Med* 316:656, 1987.

154. MCCABE ERB, HUANG S-Z, SELTZER WK, LAW ML: DNA microextraction from dried blood spots on filter paper blotters: Potential applications to newborn screening. *Hum Genet* 75:213, 1987.

155. KOGAN SC, DOHERTY M, GITSCHIER J: An improved method for prenatal diagnosis of genetic diseases by analysis of amplified DNA sequences: Application to hemophilia A. *N Engl J Med* 317:985, 1987.

156. STOFLET ES, KOEBERL DD, SARKAR G, SOMMER SS: Genomic amplification with transcript sequencing. *Science* 239:491, 1988.

157. WONG C, DOWLING CE, SAIKI RK, HIGUCHI RG, ERLICH HA, KAZAZIAN HH JR: Characterization of β-thalassaemia mutations using direct genomic sequencing of amplified single copy DNA. *Nature* 330:384, 1987.

158. ENGELKE DR, HOENER PA, COLLINS FS: Direct sequencing of enzymatically amplified human genomic DNA. *Proc Natl Acad Sci USA* 85:544, 1988.

159. TODD JA, BELL JI, MCDEVITT HO: HLA-DQβ gene contributes to susceptibility and resistance to insulin-dependent diabetes mellitus. *Nature* 329:599, 1987.

160. CONNER BJ, REYES AA, MORIN C, ITAKURA K, TEPLITZ RL, WALLACE RB: Detection of sickle cell β⁵-globin allele by hybridization with synthetic oligonucleotides. *Proc Natl Acad Sci USA* 80:278, 1983.

161. CHANG JC, KAN YW: A sensitive new prenatal test for sickle-cell anemia. *N Engl J Med* 307:30, 1982.

162. LATT SA, KURNIT DM, BRUNS GP, SCHRECK RR, MORTON CC, KUNKEL LM, LALANDE M, ALDRIDGE J, NEVE R, TANTRAVAHI U, KANDA N, LINDNER G, MERYASH D: Molecular genetic approaches to human diseases involving mental retardation. *Am J Ment Defic* 88:561, 1984.

163. LEONARD CO, CHASE GA, CHILDS B: Genetic counseling: A consumers' view. *N Engl J Med* 287:433, 1972.

164. SCRIVER CR AND COMMITTEE: in Marois M, Bennett HS, Klingberg MS, Brent RL, Lauder J, Saxen L (eds): *Population Screening: Report of a Workshop in Prevention of Physical and Mental Congenital Defects: Part B: Epidemiology. Early Detection and Therapy, and Environmental Factors.* New York, AR Liss, 1985, p 89.

165. KABACK MM, RIMOIN DL, O'BRIEN JS: *Tay-Sachs Disease: Screening and Prevention.* New York, AR Liss, 1977.

166. MILUNSKY A: Prenatal diagnosis of genetic disorders. *N Engl J Med* 300:157, 1976.

167. EPSTEIN CJ, GOLBUS MS: Prenatal diagnosis of genetic diseases. *Am Sci* 65:703, 1977.

168. NICHD NATIONAL REGISTRY FOR AMNIOCENTESIS STUDY GROUP: Midtrimester amniocentesis for prenatal diagnosis. *JAMA* 236:1471, 1976.

169. TABOR A, MADSEN M, OBEL EB, PHILIP J, BANG J, NØRGAARD-PEDERSEN B: Randomised controlled trial of genetic amniocentesis in 4606 low risk women. *Lancet* 1:1287, 1986.

170. BROCK DJH: Biochemical and cytological methods in the diagnosis of neural tube defects. *Prog Med Genet* 2(new series):1, 1977.

171. BRAMBATI B, OLDRINI A, FERRAZZI E, LANZANI A: Chorionic villus sampling: An analysis of the obstetric experience of 1000 cases. *Prenat Diagn* 7:157, 1987.

172. HOGGE WA, SCHONBERG SA, GOLBUS MS: Chorionic villus sampling: Experience of the first 1000 cases. *Am J Obstet Gynecol* 154:1249, 1986.

173. SMIDT-JENSEN S, HAHNEMANN N: Transabdominal chorionic villus sampling for fetal genetic diagnosis. Technical and obstetrical evaluation of 100 cases. *Prenat Diagn* 8:7, 1988.

174. PESCIA G, NGUYEN THE H: *Chorionic Villi Sampling (CVS).* New York, Karger, 1988.

175. POENARU L: First trimester prenatal diagnosis of metabolic diseases: A survey in countries from the European community. *Prenat Diagn* 7:333, 1987.

176. *Genetic Screening: Programs, Principles and Research.* Washington, DC, National Academy of Sciences, 1975.

177. MACCREADY RA, HUSSEY MG: Newborn phenylketonuria detection program in Massachusetts. *Am J Public Health* 54:2075, 1964.

178. RUCKNAGEL DL: A decade of screening in the hemoglobinopathies: Is a national program to prevent sickle cell anemia possible? *Am J Pediatr Hematol Oncol* 5:373, 1983.

179. Annotation: The prenatal diagnosis of thalassaemia. *Br J Haematol* 63:215, 1986.

180. SCRIVER CR, BARDANIS M, CARTIER L, CLOW CL, LANCASTER GA, OSTROWSKY JT: β-Thalassemia disease prevention: Genetic medicine applied. *Am J Hum Genet* 36:1024, 1984.

181. SOKAL DC, BYRD JR, CHEN ATL, GOLDBERG MF, OAKLEY GP: Prenatal chromosomal diagnosis: Racial and geographic variation for older women in Georgia. *JAMA* 244;1355, 1980.

182. UK collaborative study on α-fetoprotein in relation to neural tube defects: Maternal serum α-fetoprotein measurement in antenatal screening for anencephaly and spina bifida in early pregnancy. *Lancet* 1:1323, 1977.

183. DiMAIO MS, BAUMGARTEN A, GREENSTEIN RM, SAAL HM, MAHONEY MJ: Screening for fetal Down's syndrome in pregnancy by measuring maternal serum α-fetoprotein levels. *N Engl J Med* 317:342, 1987.

184. ROMERO R, PILU G, JEANTY P, GHIDINI A, HOBBINS JC: *Prenatal Diagnosis of Congenital Anomalies.* Norwalk, Appleton & Lange, 1988.

185. KUHL DE: Imaging local brain function with emission computed tomograpy. *Radiology* 150:625, 1984.

186. CHANCE B: Application of ³¹P-NMR to clinical biochemistry. *Ann NY Acad Sci* 428:318, 1984.

187. VALLE D: Genetic disease: An overview of current therapy. *Hosp Pract* 22:167, 1987.

187a. SCRIVER CR: Treatment in medical genetics, in Crow JF, Neel JV (eds): *Proceedings of the Third International Congress on Human Genetics.* Baltimore, Johns Hopkins University Press, 1967, p 45.

188. HOLTZMAN NA, DRONMAL RA, VAN DOORNINCK W, AZEN C, KOCH R: Effect of age at loss of dietary control on intellectual performance and behavior on children with phenylketonuria. *N Engl J Med* 314:593, 1986.

189. KAUFMAN FR, DONNELL GN, ROE TF, KOGUT MD: Gonadal function in patients with galactosemia. *J Inherited Metab Dis* 9:140, 1986.

190. BRUSILOW SW, VALLE D, BATSHAW ML: New pathways of waste nitrogen excretion in inborn errors of urea synthesis. *Lancet* 2:452, 1979.

191. BRUSILOW SW: Inborn errors of urea synthesis, in Lloyd JK, Scriver CR (eds): *Genetic and Metabolic Disease in Pediatrics.* Borough Green, Butterworths, 1985, p 140.

192. HAVEL RJ, HUNNINHAKE DB, ILLINGWORTH DR, LEES RS, STEIN EA, TOBERT JA, BACON SR, BOLOGNESE JA, FROST PH, LAMKIN GE, LEES AM, LEON AS, GARDNER K, JOHNSON G, MELLIES MK, RHYMER PA, TUN P: Lovastatin (Mevinolin) in the treatment of heterozygous familial hypercholesterolemia. *Ann Intern Med* 107:609, 1987.

193. CHEN YT, CORNBLATH M, SIDBURY JB: Cornstarch therapy in type I glycogen storage disease. *N Engl J Med* 310:171, 1984.

194. WOLF B, GRIER RE, SECOR-MCVOY JR, HEARD GS: Biotinidase deficiency: A novel vitamin recycling defect. *J Inherited Metab Dis (Suppl)* 8:53, 1985.

195. HEARD GS, WOLF B, JEFFERSON LG, WEISSBECKER KA, NANCE WE, SECOR-MCVOY JR, NAPOLITANO A, MITCHELL PL, LAMBERT FW, LINYEAR AS: Neonatal screening for biotinidase deficiency: Results of a 1 year pilot study. *J Pediatr* 108:40, 1986.

196. WEWERS MD, CASOLARO MA, SELLERS SE, SWAYZE SC, MCPHAUL KM, WITTES JT, CRYSTAL RG: Replacement therapy for α_1-antitrypsin deficiency associated with emphysema. *N Engl J Med* 316:1055, 1987.

197. HERSHFIELD MS, BUCKLEY RH, GREENBERG ML, MELTON AL, SCHIFF R, HATEM C, KURTZBERG J, MARKERT ML, KOBAYASHI RH, KOBAYASHI AL, ABUCHOWSKI A: Treatment of adenosine deaminase deficiency with polyethylene glycol-modified adenosine deaminase. *N Engl J Med* 316:589, 1987.

198. KRIVIT W, WHITLEY CB: Bone marrow transplantation for genetic diseases. *N Engl J Med* 3165:1085, 1987.

199. LUCARELLI G, GALIMBERTI M, POLCHI P, GIARDINI C, POLITI P, BARONCIANI D, ANGELUCCI E, MANENTI F, DELFINI C, AURELLI G, MURETTO P: Marrow transplantation in patients with advanced thalassemia. *N Engl J Med* 316:1050, 1987.

200. MALATACK JJ, FINEGOLD DN, IWATSUKI S, SHAW BW, GARTNER JC, ZITELLI BJ, ROE T, STARZL TE: Liver transplantation for type I glycogen storage disease. *Lancet* 1:1073, 1983.

201. BILHEIMER DW, GOLDSTEIN JL, GRUNDY SM, STARZL TE, BROWN MS: Liver transplantation to provide low-density lipoprotein receptors and lower plasma cholesterol in a child with homozygous familial hypercholesterolemia. *N Engl J Med* 311:1658, 1984.

202. DOWTON SB: Presented at the annual meeting of the Society for Inherited Metabolic Disorders, March 1988.

203. STARZL TE: Changing concepts: Liver replacement for hereditary tyrosinemia and hepatoma. *J Pediatr* 106:604, 1985.

204. DEMETRIOUS AA, WHITING JF, FELDMAN D, LEVENSON SM, CHOWDHURY NR, MOSCIONI AD, KRAM M, CHOWDHURY JR: Replacement of liver function in rats by transplantation of microcarrier-attached hepatocytes. *Science* 233:1090, 1986.

205. SHULL RM, HASTINGS NE, SELCER RR, JONES JB, SMITH JR, CULLEN WC, CONSTANTOPOULOS G: Bone marrow transplantation in canine mucopolysaccharidosis. I: Effects with the central nervous system. *J Clin Invest* 79:435, 1987.

206. ANDERSON WF: Prospects for human gene therapy. *Science* 226:401, 1984.

207. WILLIAMS DA, ORKIN SH: Somatic gene therapy: Current status and future prospects. *J Clin Invest* 77:1053, 1986.

208. CLINE MJ: Gene therapy: Current status. *Am J Med* 83:291, 1987.

209. DZIERZAK EA, PAPAYANNOPOULOU T, MULLIGAN RC: Lineage-specific expression of a human β-globin gene in murine bone marrow transplant recipients reconstituted with retrovirus-transduced stem cells. *Nature* 331:35, 1988.

210. WILSON JM, JOHNSTON DE, JEFFERSON DM, MULLIGAN RC: Correction of the genetic defect in hepatocytes from the Watanabe heritable hyperlipidemic rabbit. *Proc Natl Acad Sci USA,* 85:4421, 1988.

211. ST. LOUIS D, VERMA IM: An alternative approach to somatic cell gene therapy. *Proc Natl Acad Sci USA* 85:3150, 1988.

212. Molecular biology of *Homo sapiens. Cold Spring Harbor Symp Quant Biol* 51:1, 1986.

213. DESNICK RJ, PATTERSON DF, SCARPELLI DG: Animal models of inherited metabolic diseases. *Prog Clin Biol Res* 94:1, 1982.

214. POPKO B, PUCKETT C, LAI E, SHINE HD, READHEAD C, TAKAHASHI N, HUNT SW, SIDMAN RL, HOOD L: Myelin deficient mice: Expression of myelin basic protein and generation of mice with varying levels of myelin. *Cell* 48:713, 1987.

215. LEVINE M, RUBIN G, TJIAN R: Human DNA sequences homologous to a protein coding region conserved between homeotic genes of *Drosophila. Cell* 38:667, 1984.

216. CHAPMAN VM, MILLER DR, ARMSTRONG D, CASKEY CT: Recovery of induced mutations for X chromosome-linked muscular dystrophy in mice. *Proc Natl Acad Sci USA,* in press.

217. BEAUDET AL: Molecular genetics and medicine, in Braunwald E, Isselbacher KJ, Petersdorf RG, Wilson JD, Martin JB, Fauci AS (eds): *Harrison's Principles of Internal Medicine.* New York, McGraw-Hill, 1987, p 296.

218. ROMMENS JM, IANNUZZI MC, KEREM B-S, DRUMM ML, MELMER G, DEAN M, ROZMAHEL R, COLE JL, KENNEDY D, HIDAKA N, ZSIGA M, BUCHWALD M, RIORDAN JR, TSUI L-C, COLLINS FS: Identification of the cystic fibrosis gene: Chromosome walking and jumping. *Science* 245:1059, 1989.

219. RIORDAN JR, ROMMENS JM, KEREM B-S, ALON N, ROZMAHEL R, GRZELCZAK Z, ZIELENSKI J, LOK S, PLAVSIC N, CHOU J-L, DRUMM ML, IANNUZZI MC, COLLINS FS, TSUI L-C: Identification of the cystic fibrosis gene: Cloning and characterization of complementary DNA. *Science* 245:1066, 1989.

220. KEREM B-S, ROMMENS JM, BUCHANAN JA, MARKIEWICZ D, COX TK, CHAKRAVARTI A, BUCHWALD M, TSUI L-C: Identification of the cystic fibrosis gene: Genetic analysis. *Science* 245:1073, 1989.

221. LEMNA WK, FELDMAN GL, KEREM B-S, FERNBACH SD, ZEVKOVICH EP, O'BRIEN WE, RIORDAN JR, COLLINS FS, TSUI L-C, BEAUDET AL: Mutation analysis for heterozygote detection and the prenatal diagnosis of cystic fibrosis. *N Engl J Med* 322:291, 1990.

SELECTED READINGS

ALBERTS B, BRAY D, LEWIS J, RAFF M, ROBERTS K, WATSON JD: *Molecular Biology of the Cell*, 2d ed. New York, Garland Publishing, 1989.
  A lengthy and thorough text providing the advanced college student or graduate student with an in-depth view of cellular and molecular biology.

CONNOR JM, FERGUSON-SMITH MA: *Essential Medical Genetics*, 2d ed. London, Blackwell Scientific Publications, 1987.
  A succinct, clearly presented overview of medical genetics.

DARNELL J, LODISH H, BALTIMORE D: *Molecular Cell Biology*. New York, W. H. Freeman & Co., 1986.
  A lengthy and thorough text providing the advanced college student or graduate student with an in-depth view of cellular and molecular biology.

deGROUCHY J, TURLEAU C: *Clinical Atlas of Human Chromosomes*, 2d ed. New York, John Wiley & Sons, 1984.
  Clearly presented, succinct atlas of human chromosome aberrations with excellent clinical photographs.

EMERY AEH, RIMOIN DL: *Principles and Practice of Medical Genetics*. Edinburgh, Churchill Livingston, 1983.
  A voluminous medical textbook for practioners of clinical genetics; hundreds of disorders are discussed with an emphasis on medical diagnosis and genetic counseling.

HARRIS H: *The Principles of Human Biochemical Genetics*, 3d ed. Elsevier/North-Holland Biomedical Press, Amsterdam, 1980.
  A classical text in human biochemical genetics emphasizing the extraordinary biochemical diversity as it relates to genetics, medicine, and human biology.

JONES KL: *Smith's Recognizable Patterns of Human Malformation*, 4th ed. Philadelphia, W. B. Saunders, 1988.
  Compendium of phenotypic features with clinical photographs of the recognized aberrations in human morphologic development.

LEWIN B: *Genes*, 3d ed. New York, John Wiley & Sons, 1987.
  Concise, clearly written view of the central dogma of molecular genetics, from gene to protein.

McKUSICK VA: *Mendelian Inheritance in Man*, 9th ed. Baltimore, Johns Hopkins Press, 1990.
  A catalog of human Mendelian disorders providing a paragraph of description and numerous references regarding each; genetic loci and map locations are also cataloged.

THOMPSON JS, THOMPSON MW: *Genetics in Medicine*, 4th ed. Philadelphia, W. B. Saunders, 1986.
  An introductory medical genetics text designed for medical students emphasizing the basic genetic principles.

VOGEL F, MOTULSKY AG: *Human Genetics: Problems and Approaches*, 2d ed. Berlin, Springer-Verlag, 1986.
  An in-depth text emphasizing the principles of human genetics with a strong medical orientation; excellent sections on principles of cytogenetics, Mendelian principles, polygenic disorders, and many other topics.

WATSON JD, TOOZE J, KURTZ DT: *Recombinant DNA: A Short Course*. New York, W. H. Freeman & Co., 1983.
  An excellent, concise introduction to recombinant DNA methodology.

WATSON JD, HOPKINS NH, ROBERTS JW, STEITZ JA, WEINER AM: *Molecular Biology of the Gene*, 4th ed. Menlo Park, Benjamin/Cummings Publishing Co., 1987.
  A classical text describing the central dogmas of molecular biology in prokaryotes and eukaryotes; a specialized second volume concentrates on development, immunogenetics, eukaryotic viruses, and cancer.

WEATHERALL DJ: *The New Genetics and Clinical Practice*, 2d ed. Oxford, Oxford University Press, 1985.
  A short text emphasizing the application of molecular biological techniques to clinical medicine drawing heavily from studies of hemoglobinopathies.

Genetic Map of the Human Genome Autosomes, and X, Y, and Mitochondrial Chromosomes

A new morbid anatomy map (Fig. 1-9) is located on pp. 14-17. Information shown there is complemented by this appendix, which gathers together extensive material about human loci. As you can see, a great many human genes have been mapped and a large proportion of those mapped genes occur in mutant form, leading in turn to a human genetic disorder. The analogous gene is often mapped in the mouse.

Loci are listed by chromosome. For example, lpter-p36.13, which is the first entry in the table, indicates that the adenovirus 12 chromosome modification site maps to chromosome 1 between the terminus of the short (p) arm and band 36.13 on the short (p) arm. *Location* indicates the chromosome localization. *Symbol* indicates the official symbol for each locus as assigned by the human gene mapping workshops. *Status* indicates the level of confidence regarding chromosome assignments: P = provisional, C = confirmed, and L = limbo (in-dicating that there is controversy regarding the assignment). *Title* indicates the name for the gene or locus in question. *MIM* number indicates the number of the entry in McKusick's *Mendelian Inheritance in Man*. This number can be used in the published book or in the on-line database to obtain a brief descriptive paragraph and numerous references concerning the locus. *Comments* provides some additional information where appropriate. *Disorders* indicates the name for a human pathological condition which is associated with mutation at this locus. *Mouse* indicates the mouse chromosome assignment with the mouse gene symbol in parenthesis.

This up-to-date information is from the on-line databases of *Mendelian Inheritance in Man* (OMIM) at The Johns Hopkins Hospital and the Howard Hughes Medical Institute's Human Gene Mapping Library (HGML) in New Haven (Yale University).

Gene Map of the Autosomes

More than 2300 loci are known with confidence to exist on autosomes, on the basis mainly of characteristic mendelian patterns of inheritance of alternative forms of particular traits. (Another 2000 loci have been less securely identified on autosomes.) As indicated by the following data, some mapping information is available concerning almost three-fourths of the well confirmed autosomal loci. In addition to the loci listed here, anonymous DNA segments (some expressed), antigens defined by monoclonal antibodies, surface antigens, some 'like' genes, and pseudogenes, and function-unknown electrophoretic (O'Farrell) protein spots have been assigned to individual autosomes. The number in parentheses after the name of each item in the disorder field indicates whether the mutation was positioned by mapping the 'wildtype' gene (1), by the mapping disease phenotype itself (2), or by both approaches (3). Multiple allelic disorders in the disorder column are separated by semicolons. Brackets indicate 'nondisease' and braces indicate susceptibilities.

Chromosome No. 1

Location	Symbol	Status	Title	MIM #	Comments	Disorder	Mouse
1pter-p36.13	A12M2	P	Adenovirus-12 chromosome modification site-1p	102920			
1pter-p36.13	ENO1, PPH	C	Enolase-1	172430		Enolase deficiency (1)	4(Eno-1)
1pter-p36.13	GDH	C	Glucose dehydrogenase	138090			
1pter-p36	HLM2	C	Oncogene HLM2	131190			
1pter-p32	GALE	C	UDP galactose-4-epimerase	230350		Galactose epimerase deficiency (1)	
1pter-p22.1	TFS1	P	Transformation suppressor-1	190190			
1pter-p21	GLUT5	P	Glucose transporter, kidney	138230			
1pter-q12	DRNT	P	Dioxin receptor, nuclear translocator	126110			3(Dmt)
1p36.33-p36.22	CA6	P	Carbonic anhydrase VI	114780			
1p36.3	RNU1	C	RNA, U1 small nuclear	180680	?same as A12M2		
1p36.2	ANP, ANF, PND	C	Atrial natriuretic peptide; pronatriodilatin	108780			4(Pnd)
1p36.2-p36.13	PGD	C	6-Phosphogluconate dehydrogenase	172200			4(Pgd)
1p36.2-p36.1	FGR, SRC2	P	Oncogene FGR	164940	same as SRC2		
1p36.2-p34	ALPL, HOPS	C	Alkaline phosphatase, liver/bone/kidney type	171760		Hypophosphatasia, infantile 241500 (3); ?Hypophosphatasia, adult 146300 (1)	?4(Akp-2); ?1(Akp-1)
1p36.2-p34	EL1	C	Elliptocytosis-1 (protein 4.1)	130500	linked to RH	Elliptocytosis-1 (3)	
1p36.2-p34	EKV	C	Erythrokeratodermia variabilis	133200	theta = 0.03 with RH	Erythrokeratodermia variabilis (2)	
1p36.2-p34	RD	C	Radin blood group	111620			
1p36.2-p34	RH	C	RHESUS BLOOD GROUP CLUSTER		Order: 1pter--D-C-E--cen	Erythroblastosis fetalis (1); ?Rh-null hemolytic anemia (1)	
1p36.2-p34	RHC	C	Rhesus system C polypeptide	111700			
1p36.2-p34	RHD	C	Rhesus system D polypeptide	111680			
1p36.2-p34	RHE	C	Rhesus system E polypeptide	111690			
1p36.2-p34	SC	C	Scianna blood group	111750			
1p36.1-p35	APNH	P	Antiporter, sodium-potassium ion, amiloride-sensitive	107310			
1p36.1	TRN	P	tRNA asparagine	189880			
1p36	BRCD2	P	Breast cancer, ductal	211420		Breast cancer, ductal (2)	
1p36	CMM, HCMM	P	Malignant melanoma, cutaneous	155600		Malignant melanoma, cutaneous (2)	
1p36	TRE, TRNE	P	tRNA glutamic acid	180640			

Location	Symbol		Title	MIM No.	Comments	Disorder	Mouse
1p35-p32	LCK	P	Lymphocyte-specific tyrosine kinase	153390			4(lck)
1p35-p31.3	GLUT1	C	Glucose transporter protein-1	138140	probably in 1p33		
1p34	AK2	C	Adenylate kinase-2, mitochondrial	103020			4(Ak-2)
1p34	FUCA1, FUCA	C	Alpha-L-fucosidase-1	230000		Fucosidosis (1)	4(Fuca)
1p34	FUCT	L	Alpha-L-fucosidase regulator	136830	?very close to FUCA1		
1p34	MPLV	P	Myeloproliferative leukemia virus, human homolog of	159530			
1p34	UROD	C	Uroporphyrinogen decarboxylase	176100		Porphyria cutanea tarda (1); Porphyria, hepatoerythropoietic (1)	
1p34-p12	HMG17	P	Nonhistone chromosomal protein HMG-17	163910			
1p33	SCL	P	Stem-cell leukemia	184750			
1p33-p32	LAR	P	Leukocyte antigen related tyrosine phosphorylase	179590			
1p32	BLYM1, BLYM	P	Oncogene BLYM1, chicken bursal lymphoma	164830			
1p32	MYCL1, LMYC	P	Oncogene MYC, lung carcinoma-derived	164850			Y(L-myc)
1p32	NB, NBS	C	Neuroblastoma (neuroblastoma suppressor)	256700		Neuroblastoma (2)	
1p32	TCL5	P	T-cell leukemia/lymphoma-5	187040	?same as SCL; proximal to MYCL1		
1p32	UMPK	C	Uridine monophosphate kinase	191710			
1p32-p31	RAB3B	P	Brain antigen RAB3B	179510			
1p32-p31	JUN	P	Oncogene JUN	165160			
1p31	ACADM, MCAD	P	Acyl-CoA dehydrogenase, medium chain	201450		Acyl-CoA dehydrogenase, medium chain, deficiency of (1)	
1p31	GST1	C	Glutathione-S-transferase-1	138350			
1p22.1-qter	SDH	P	Succinate dehydrogenase	185470	1 of 2 polypeptides		4(Pgm-2)
1p22.1	PGM1	C	Phosphoglucomutase-1	171900			
1p22.1-q21.1	CD3Z, TCRZ	P	Antigen CD3Z, zeta polypeptide	186780			1(Cd-3z)
1p22	C8A	P	C8, alpha polypeptide	120950	close to PGM1; alpha and gamma coded by separate genes	C8 deficiency, type I (2)	
1p22	C8B	P	C8, beta polypeptide	120960	close to PGM1	C8 deficiency, type II (2)	
1p22	NGFB	C	Nerve growth factor, beta	162030	same 310kb fragment as TSHB		3(Ngfb)
1p22	NRAS1	C	Oncogene NRAS1	164790	1p12-p11 by A; ?same as NGF		3(Nras)
1p22	TSHB	C	Thyroid stimulating hormone, beta subunit	188540	centromeric to NGFB	Hypothyroidism, nongoitrous (1)	3(Tshb)
1p22-p21	F3, TFA	C	Clotting factor III	134390			
1p22-q23	CMT1B	C	Charcot-Marie-Tooth disease, slow nerve conduction type Ib	118200	ca. 15cM from FY	Charcot-Marie-Tooth disease, slow nerve conduction type Ib (2)	
1p22-qter	EPHX, EPOX	P	Epoxide hydroxylase, microsomal (epoxide hydrolase)	132810		?Fetal hydantoin syndrome (1)	1(Eph-1)
1p21	AMY2A	C	Amylase, pancreatic, alpha 2A	104650			3(Amy-2)
1p21	AMY2B	C	Amylase, pancreatic, alpha 2B	104660			
1p21	AMY1	C	Amylase, salivary	104700	multiple amylase genes		3(Amy-1)
1p21	COL11A1	P	Collagen, type XI, alpha 1	120280			
1p21-p13	AMPD1	P	Adenosine monophosphate deaminase-1	102770			

Location	Symbol	Status	Title	MIM #	Comments	Disorder	Mouse
1p21-q23	APOA2	C	Apolipoprotein A-II	107670			1(Alp-2, Apoa-2)
1p21-qter	ACTA, ASMA	C	Actin, skeletal muscle alpha chains	102610	?near centromere suggested by mouse data		3(Acts)
1p13	ASG	L	Aspermiogenesis factor	108420			
1p13	CD2	C	T-cell surface CD2 antigen	186990	1q25 = conflicting localization		3(Cd-2)
1p13	CD58, LFA3	C	Antigen CD58, lymphocyte function-associated antigen 3	153420	?same as MSK1; gene cloned		
1p13	HSDB	P	3-beta-hydroxysteroid dehydrogenase/isomerase	201810		Adrenal hyperplasia II (1)	
1p13-p12	RAP1A, KREV1	P	RAS-related protein RAP1A	179520			
1p13-p11	ATP1A1	P	ATPase, sodium-potassium, alpha-1 polypeptide	182310			3(Atpa-1)
1p	C1QA	P	Complement component, C1q, A chain	120550		?C1q deficiency (1)	
1p	C1QB	C	Complement component C1q, B chain	120570		?C1q deficiency (1)	
1p	NBCCS, BCNS, NBCS	L	Nevoid basal cell carcinoma syndrome	109400		?Nevoid basal cell carcinoma syndrome (2)	
1cen-q32	ATP1A2	P	Sodium-potassium-ATPase, alpha-2 polypeptide	182340			1(Atpa-3)
1cen-q32	BCM1, BLAST1	P	B-cell activation marker	109530			
1cen-q32	NCF2	P	Neutrophil cytosolic factor-2	233710		Chronic granulomatous disease due to deficiency of NCF-2 (1)	
1cen-q32	OCT1, OTF1	P	Lymphoid octomer-binding transcription factor-1	153250			
1cen-q32	PFKM	P	Phosphofructokinase, muscle type	232800		Glycogen storage disease, type VII (1)	
1q	ATP1B	P	Sodium-potassium ATPase, beta polypeptide	182330			1(Atpb)
1q11	D1Z1	C	Satellite DNA II	126370	1qh		
1q12-q21	CAGRA, CFAG, CFA	P	Cystic fibrosis antigen (calgranulin A)	219710	probable cluster with CAGRB, CACY, CAPL; on mouse 3		
1q12-q22	TRNL	P	tRNA asparagine-like	189890			
1q12-q23	CRP	C	C-reactive protein	123260			
1q12-q23	APCS, SAP	C	Amyloid P component, serum	104770	probably close to CRP	{?Amyloidosis, secondary, susceptibility to} (2)	1(Sap)
1q2	CAE	C	Cataract, zonular pulverulent	116200	close to FY	Cataract, zonular pulverulent (2)	
1q2	EL2	L	Elliptocytosis-2	130600	?linked to FY; ?same locus as alpha-spectrin	?Elliptocytosis-2 (2)	
1q21	A12M3	P	Adenovirus-12 chromosome modification site-1q2	102940	class 1, U2 snRNA pseudogenes, 180690, at this site		
1q21	FLG	P	Filaggrin	135940		?Ichthyosis vulgaris, 146700 (1)	
1q21	GBA	C	Acid beta-glucosidase (glucocerebrosidase)	230800		Gaucher disease (1)	3(Gba)
1q21	H1F2	P	H1 histone, family 2	142710			
1q21	H3F2	P	H3 histone, family 2	142780			

Location	Symbol		Title	MIM #	Comments	Disorder	Mouse
1q21	H4F2, HCB	P	H4 histone, family 2	142750	100-200 histone genes; some on chromosome 6 and 12, as well as perhaps 7		
1q21	IVL	P	Involucrin	147360			
1q21	MUC1, PUM	C	Mucin, urinary, peanut lectin binding	158340	5cM proximal to SPTA1		
1q21	SPTA1	C	Spectrin, alpha, erythrocytic-1	182860	?same locus as EL2	Elliptocytosis-2 (2); Pyropoikilocytosis (1); Spherocytosis, recessive (1)	1(Spna-1)
1q21-q22	ADPRT	P	ADP ribosyltransferase	161010			
1q21-q22	FY	C	Duffy blood group	110700	distal to 1qh; 20cM from AMY1	[Vivax malaria, susceptibility to] (1)	1(Fce-1a)
1q21-q22	PKLR, PK1, PKR	C	Pyruvate kinase, liver and RBC type	266200		PK deficiency hemolytic anemia (1)	
1q21-q23	FCE1A	P	Fc IgE receptor, alpha polypeptide	147140			
1q21-q23	UGP1	C	Uridyl diphosphate glucose pyrophosphorylase-1	191750			
1q21-q24	GRMP	P	Granulocyte membrane protein	173610			
1q21-q25	CACY	P	Calcyclin	114110			3(Cacy)
1q22-q23	CD1A	P	Thymocyte antigen CD1A	188370	genes A, B, C, D in cluster		3(Ly-38)
1q22-q23	CD1B	P	Thymocyte antigen CD1B	188360			
1q22-q23	CD1C	P	Thymocyte antigen CD1C	188340			
1q22-q24	SKI, SK, D1S3	P	Oncogene Sloan-Kettering, chicken virus	164780			
1q23	F5	C	Clotting factor V	227400		Factor V deficiency (1)	
1q23	MS336	P	Minisatellite 33.6	157560			
1q23-q24	FCG2, IGFR2, CD32	C	Fc fragment of IgG, low affinity II, receptor for (CD32) (Immunoglobulin G Fc receptor II)	146790	FCG2 and FCG3 within 250kb		1(Ly-17, Cd32)
1q23-q24	FCG3, CD16, IGFR3	C	Fc fragment of IgG, low affinity III, receptor for (CD16) (Immunoglobulin G Fc receptor III)	146740	FCG2 and FCG3 within 250kb		
1q23-q25	LYAM1, LAM1	P	Lymphocyte adhesion molecule 1	153240			
1q23.1-q23.9	AT3	C	Antithrombin III	107300	ca. 10cM from FY	Antithrombin III deficiency (3)	1(At-3)
1q24-q25	ABLL, ARG	P	Oncogene ARG (or ABL-like)	164690			1(Abll)
1q24-q31	CHR39A	P	Cholesterol repressible protein 39A	118460			
1q24-q31	FPSL1	P	Farnesylpyrophosphate synthetase-like 1	134631			
1q24-q31.2	FRNS	L	Fryns syndrome	229850		?Fryns syndrome (2)	
1q31	CTSE	P	Cathepsin E	116890			
1q31	LAMB2	C	Laminin B2	150290	at least 3 genes, ?linked		1(Lamb-2)
1q31-q32	CD45, LCA, T200	C	Leukocyte common antigen (T200)	151460			1(Ly-5)
1q31-q32.1	F13B	C	Clotting factor XIII, B subunit	134580			
1q31-q32.1	MCT	L	Microcephaly, true	251200		?Microcephaly, true (2)	
1q31-q41	PIGR	P	Polymeric immunoglobulin receptor	173880			
1q31-q41	TRK	P	Oncogene TRK	164970	NA2 protein in TRK oncogene		
1q31-q41	TPM	P	Tropomyosin, nonmuscle	191030			
1q32	RCAC	C	REGULATOR OF COMPLEMENT ACTIVATION CLUSTER		MCP, CR1, CR2, DAF, C4BP in 750kb segment		

Location	Symbol	Status	Title	MIM #	Comments	Disorder	Mouse
1q32	C4BP, C4BR	C	Complement component-4 binding protein	120830			1(C4bp)
1q32	CR1, C3BR	C	Complement component-3b, C3b, receptor	120620		CR1 deficiency (1); ?SLE (1)	
1q32	CR2, C3DR	C	Complement component-3d, C3d, receptor	120650			
1q32	DAF	C	Decay-accelerating factor of complement	125240			
1q32	HF, CFH	C	Complement factor H	134370			1(Cfh)
1q32	LPS, PIT, VDWS	C	Lip pit syndrome (van der Woude syndrome)	119300	del (1q32-q41); linked to REN	van der Woude syndrome (2)	
1q32	MCP	P	Membrane cofactor protein	120920			
1q32	REN	C	Renin	179820	q32.3-q42.3 excluded by D; q42 = conflicting assignment		1(Ren-1)
1q32	SNRPE	C	Small nuclear ribonucleoprotein polypeptide E	128260			
1q32	US2	P	Usher syndrome, type 2	276900		Usher syndrome, type 2 (2)	
1q32.1-q42	GUK1	C	Guanylate kinase-1	139270			
1q32.1-q42	GUK2	C	Guanylate kinase-2	139280	genetic independence of GUK1 and GUK2 unproved		
1q32.3-q42.3	DH	L	Diaphragmatic hernia	222400		?Diaphragmatic hernia (2)	
1q41	TGFB2	P	Transforming growth factor beta-2	190220			1(Tgf-b2)
1q41-q42	PPOL, PARP	C	Poly-ADP-ribose polymerase (NAD(+) ADP-ribosyltransferase)	173870	?processed pseudogenes on 13, 14q22	?Fanconi anemia (1); ?Xeroderma pigmentosum (1)	
1q42	PEPC	C	Peptidase C	170000	1q25, 1q32 = conflicting localizations		1(Pep-3)
1q42-q43	A12M1	P	Adenovirus-12 chromosome modification site-1q1	102930			
1q42-q43	AGT	C	Angiotensinogen	106150	same site as A12M1		8(Agt)
1q42-q43	RN5S	C	5S ribosomal RNA genes	180420			
1q42-qter	XPAC, XPA	P	Fast kinetic complementation DNA repair in xeroderma pigmentosum, group A	278700	should be on 1p in light of mouse location	?Xeroderma pigmentosum A (1)	4(Xpa)
1q42.1	FH	C	Fumarate hydratase	136850		?Fumarase deficiency (1)	
1q43	NID	P	Nidogen	131390			
Chr.1	ADSS, ADEH	P	Adenylosuccinate synthetase (Ade(-)H-complementing)	103060			
Chr.1	CAGRB	P	Calgranulin B	219720			
Chr.1	CAPL	P	Calcium placental protein	114210			3(Capl)
Chr.1	CHC1, RCC1	P	Regulator of chromosome condensation	179710			
Chr.1	GNAI3	P	Guanine nucleotide binding protein, alpha inhibiting, polypeptide 3	139370			
Chr.1	GNAT2	P	Guanine nucleotide binding protein, alpha transducing, polypeptide 2	139340			17(Gnat-2)
Chr.1	GNB1	P	Guanine nucleotide binding protein, beta polypeptide 1	139380			19(Gnb-1)
Chr.1	HKR3	P	Oncogene HKR3	165270			
Chr.1	KRL3	P	Kruppel-like zinc finger protein-3	149430			

Chr.1	MTR	P	5-Methyltetrahydrofolate:L-homocysteine S-methyltransferase; tetrahydropteroyl-glutamate methyltransferase	156570	
Chr.1	MYF4	P	Myogenic factor-4	159980	
Chr.1	PFN2, PFL	P	Profilin-2	176590	
Chr.1	PLA2L	P	Pancreatic phospholipase A2-like	see 172410	
Chr.1	TPR	P	Tumor potentiating region (translocated promoter region)	189940	fused with MET in chemically induced tumor

In addition: 2 surface antigens defined by monoclonals, 4 O'Farrell protein spots, 13 'like' genes, 9 pseudogenes, and 10 fragile sites (HGM10). The order of closely linked loci (of ENO1 and 6PGD; of EL1, RH, and FUCA; of UMPK and SC; and of FY and CAE) is uncertain. ²However, the following order of loosely linked segments seems established':
6PGD--RH--UMPK--PGM1--AMY--1qh12--FY--PEPC. (From Rao et al., Am. J. Hum. Genet. 31: 680-696, 1979.)

Chromosome No. 2

Location	Symbol	Status	Title	MIM #	Comments	Disorder	Mouse
2pter-p25.1	COI	L	Coloboma of iris	120200		?Coloboma of iris (2)	
2pter-p12	RHOH6	P	Oncogene RHO H6	165370			
2pter-p12	TPO, TPX	C	Thyroid peroxidase	274500		Thyroid iodine peroxidase deficiency (1)	
2p25	ACP1	C	Acid phosphatase-1	171500	linked to ACP1		12(Acp-1)
2p25	AN1	P	Aniridia-1	106200	see 14q24	Aniridia-1 (2)	
2p25	CAP	L	Cataract, anterior polar	115650		?Cataract, anterior polar (2)	
2p25	ODC1	C	Ornithine decarboxylase-1	165640			12(Odc-1)
2p25	POMC	C	Proopiomelanocortin	176830	?close to ACP1	ACTH deficiency (1)	12(Pomc-1)
2p25-p24	RRM2	P	Ribonucleotide reductase, M2 subunit	180390	pseudogenes on 1p, 1q, Xp		4,7,12,13(Rrm-2)
2p24	APOB	C	Apolipoprotein B	107730	1 gene for liver apo-B100 and gut apo-B48; Ag linked	Hypobetalipoproteinemia (1); ?Abetalipoproteinemia (1); Hyperbetalipoproteinemia (1); Apolipoprotein B-100, defective (1)	12(Apob)
2p24	MYCN, NMYC	C	Oncogene NMYC	164840	proximal to APOB		12(N-myc)
2p23	MDH1	C	Malate dehydrogenase, soluble	154200	proximal to APOB		
2p23-qter	ERCC3, XPB	P	Excision-repair, complementing defective, in Chinese hamster, number 3	133510	same as XPB	Xeroderma pigmentosum, group B, 278710 (1)	
2p23-qter	IFNB3	C	Beta-3-interferon	147860			
2p22-p11	GLAT	P	Galactose enzyme activator	137030			
2p21	CAD	P	CAD trifunctional protein of pyrimidine biosynthesis	114010	proximal to 21.01		
2p21	HPEC	L	Holoprosencephaly	236100		?Holoprosencephaly (2)	
2p13	TGFA	C	Transforming (or tumor) growth factor, alpha type	190170			
2p13-cen	REL	P	Oncogene REL, avian reticuloendotheliosis	164910			11(Rel)
2p12	IGK, KM	C	IMMUNOGLOBULIN KAPPA LIGHT CHAIN GENE CLUSTER		2p11.2 by high resolution in situ mapping; order: pter-C-J-V-cen		6(Igk)
2p12	IGKV	C	Variable region of kappa light chain	146980	25+ genes in 4 classes		
2p12	IGKJ	C	J region of kappa light chain	146970	5 genes		
2p12	IGKC	C	Constant region of kappa light chain	147200	1 gene		
2p12	IGKDE	P	Immunoglobulin kappa polypeptide deleting element	146780			6(Rs)
2p12	CD8, T8, LEU2	C	Leu-2 T-cell antigen (T8 lymphocyte antigen)	186910	distal to IGK		6(Lyt-3; ?Ly-2)
2p11	FABP1, FABPL	C	Fatty acid binding protein, liver	134650			6(Fabp-l; ?lvp-1)
2p11-q11	PLGL	P	Plasminogen-like	173340			
2p	AKE	L	Acrokeratoelastoidosis	101850	?linked to ACP1, JK, IGKC	?Acrokeratoelastoidosis (2)	

Location	Symbol	Status	Name	Comments	Disorder	MIM	Mouse
2p	CPS1	P	Carbamoylphosphate synthetase I (mitochondrial CPS)	urea cycle enzyme	Carbamoylphosphate synthetase I deficiency (1)	237300	
2p	OAK	L	Optic atrophy, Kjer type	?linked to JK; lod = 2.15 at theta 0.14 male, 0.27 female	?Optic atrophy, Kjer type (2)	165500	
2cen-q13	INHBB	P	Inhibin, beta-2			147390	1(Inhbb)
2cen-q13	MAL	P	T-lymphocyte maturation-associated protein			188860	
2q	TUBA1	P	Tubulin, alpha, testis-specific			191110	
2q12-q21	DBI	P	Diazepam binding inhibitor			125950	
2q13-q14	PROC	C	Protein C		Protein C deficiency (1)	176860	
2q13-q21	IL1A	C	Interleukin-1, alpha	tight linkage to IL1B in mouse		147760	2(Il-1a)
2q13-q21	IL1B	P	Interleukin-1, beta form			147720	2(Il-1b)
2q14-q21	GYPC, GE, GPC	P	Blood group Gerbich (glycophorin C)			110750	
2q14-q21	LCO, LCA	P	Liver cancer oncogene (Oncogene LCA)			165320	
2q31	COL3A1	C	Collagen III, alpha-1 chain		Ehlers-Danlos syndrome, type IV (3); Familial aneurysm (2)	120180	1(Col3a1)
2q31	COL5A2	C	Collagen V, alpha-2 chain	very close to COL3A1		120190	
2q31-q32	NEB	C	Nebulin			161650	
2q31-q37	HOX4	C	Homeo box-4	linked to Km in mice ?Hox5		142980	2(Hox-4)
2q31-qter	ELN	P	Elastin			130160	
2q32-q33.3	RPE	C	Ribulose 5-phosphate 3-epimerase			180480	
2q32-q34	CHRND, ACHRD	P	Cholinergic receptor, nicotinic, delta polypeptide	linked to Idh-1 in mouse		100720	1(Achr-d)
2q32-q34	CHRNG, ACHRG	P	Cholinergic receptor, nicotinic, gamma polypeptide	tightly linked to CHRND?		100730	1(Acr-g)
2q32.1-qter	MYL1	C	Myosin light chain, skeletal fast			160780	1(Myl-1)
2q33	CTLA4	P	Cytotoxic T-lymphocyte-associated serine esterase-IV			123890	
2q33-q35	CHE2	I	Cholinesterase, serum, 2	see chr.16		177500	1(Len-2)
2q33-q35	CRYG, CCL	C	CRYSTALLIN, GAMMA POLYPEPTIDE CLUSTER		Cataract, Coppock-like (3)		
2q33-q35	CRYG1	C	Crystallin, gamma polypeptide 1			123660	
2q33-q35	CRYG2	C	Crystallin, gamma polypeptide 2			123670	
2q33-q35	CRYG3	C	Crystallin, gamma polypeptide 3			123680	
2q33-q35	CRYG4	C	Crystallin, gamma polypeptide 4			123690	
2q33-q35	CRYG5	C	Crystallin, gamma polypeptide-5			123710	
2q33-q35	CRYG6	P	Crystallin, gamma polypeptide 6			123720	
2q33-qter	INHA	P	Inhibin, alpha			147380	1(Inha)
2q33.3	IDH1	C	Isocitrate dehydrogenase, soluble			147700	1(Idh-1)
2q34	TCL4	P	T-cell leukemia/lymphoma-4			186860	
2q34-q35	MAP2	P	Microtubule-associated protein-2			157130	
2q34-q36	FN1	C	Fibronectin-1	structural gene; see chr. 8, 11	?Ehlers-Danlos syndrome, type X (3)	135600	1(Fn-1)
2q35	DES	P	Desmin			125660	
2q35-q36	VIL	P	Villin			193040	1(Vil)
2q36-q37	GCG	C	Glucagon		[?Hyperproglucagonemia] (1)	138030	2(Gcg)

Location	Symbol	Status	Title	MIM #	Comments	Disorder	Mouse
2q37	ALPI	C	Alkaline phosphatase, adult intestinal	171740	close to ALPP		2(Alp-3)
2q37	ALPP, PLAP	C	Alkaline phosphatase, placental	171800			4(Akp-2)
2q37	ALPPL	P	Alkaline phosphatase, placental-like	171810			
2q37	COL6A3	P	Collagen VI, alpha-3 chain	120250	close to CRBP1		1(Col6a3)
2q37	RMSA	C	Rhabdomyosarcoma, alveolar	268220	see 11p	Rhabdomyosarcoma, aveolar (2)	
2q37.3	WS1	C	Waardenburg syndrome, type I	193500	paracentric inversion; 2q37.3 = alternative location	Waardenburg syndrome, type I (2)	1(Spl)
Chr.2	ADCP2	C	Adenosine deaminase complexing protein-2	107720			
Chr.2	ADRA2CR	P	Alpha-2C-adrenergic receptor	104260			
Chr.2	CD8B	P	Antigen CD8B	186730			6(Ly-3)
Chr.2	EN1	P	Engrailed-1	131290			
Chr.2	GAD	P	Glutamate decarboxylase	266100		?Pyridoxine dependency with seizures (1)	
Chr.2	GLI2	P	Oncogene GLI2	165230			
Chr.2	GNT1	P	Phenol UDP-glucuronosyltransferase	191740			
Chr.2	LCT, LAC, LPH	C	Lactase (lactase-phlorizin hydrolase)	223000		?Lactase deficiency, congenital (1); ?Lactase deficiency, adult, 223100 (1)	
Chr.2	SCN2A, NAC2	P	Sodium channel, neuronal (type II)	182390	4 related genes on chr.2		
Chr.2	RACH	P	Acetylcholinesterase regulator, or derepressor	100680			
Chr.2	SFTP3	C	Pulmonary surfactant-associated protein-3, 18kD	178640	SFTP2 in previous listing		
Chr.2	SPTB2, SPTBN1	P	Nonerythroid spectrin, beta type	182790			
Chr.2	UGP2	P	Uridyl diphosphate glucose pyrophosphorylase-2	191760			
Chr.2	UV24	P	Ultraviolet damage, repair of, in UV24	192070			
Chr.2	VNRA	P	Vibronectin receptor, alpha polypeptide	193210			
Chr.2	ZNF2	P	Zinc finger protein 2	194500			

In addition: 1 surface antigen, defined by monoclonals, 1 O'Farrell protein spot, 6 'like' genes, 8 pseudogenes, and 8 fragile sites (HGM10).

Chromosome No. 3

Location	Symbol	Status	Title	MIM #	Comments	Disorder	Mouse
3pter-p21	CCK	C	Cholecystokinin	118440			9(Cck)
3p25	RAF1	C	Oncogene RAF1	164760	homologous sequences on 10q24-q25 linked to RAF1		6(Raf-1)
3p25-p24	TSP1	P	Testis-specific protein-1	187420			
3p25-p24	VHL	C	von Hippel-Lindau syndrome	193300		von Hippel-Lindau syndrome (2)	
3p24.3	THRB, THR1, ERBA2	C	Thyroid hormone receptor, beta (ERBA2)	190160		Thyroid hormone resistance, 274300, 188570 (3)	
3p24	RARB, RAR2, HAP	C	Retinoic acid receptor, beta polypeptide	180220	= HAP = HBV-activated protein		
3p23-p22	ACAA	P	Peroxisomal 3-oxoacyl-CoA thiolase	261510		Pseudo-Zellweger syndrome (1)	
3p23-p21	SCLC1, SCCL	C	Small-cell cancer of lung	182280	centromeric to ERBA2	Small-cell cancer of lung (2)	
3p21.2-p21.1	ITIH1	P	Inter-alpha-trypsin inhibitor, heavy chain-1	147270			
3p21.2-p21.1	ITIH3	P	Inter-alpha-trypsin inhibitor, heavy chain-3	146650			
3p21.1	ACY1	C	Aminoacylase-1	104620			9(Acy)
3p21	ALAS1	C	Delta-aminolevulinate synthase	125290			
3p21	RHOH12	P	Oncogene RHO H12	165390			
3p21-p14.2	GLB1	C	Beta-galactosidase-1	230500	3p14.2-p11 excluded	GM1-gangliosidosis (1); Mucopolysaccharidosis IVB (1)	9(Bgl)
3p14.2	RCC1, RCC	C	Renal cell carcinoma	144700	at site of FRA3B	Renal cell carcinoma (2)	
3p14.2-qter	APOD	P	Apolipoprotein D	107740			
3p13-q12	GPX1	C	Glutathione peroxidase-1	138320		Hemolytic anemia due to glutathione peroxidase deficiency (1)	
3p11.1-q11.2	PSA, PROS	C	Protein S, alpha polypeptide	176880		Protein S deficiency (1)	
3p11.2-q11.2	PSB, PROS2	P	Protein S, beta polypeptide	177030	2 protein S genes in primates		
3p	MYL3	P	Myosin light chain alkali, ventricular and skeletal slow	160790			9(Myl-3)
3cen-q22	MER6, RHN	P	Rh-null, regulator type	268150	monoclonal ID8	Rh-null disease (1)	
3q12-q13	MOX2	C	MRC OX-2 antigen	155970			
3q13	UMPS, OPRT	C	Orotate phosphoribosyltransferase/OMP decarboxylase (UMP synthase)	258900		Oroticaciduria (1)	
3q13.3-q22	PCCB	C	Propionyl CoA carboxylase, beta polypeptide	232050	pccB complementation group	Propionicacidemia, type II or pccB type (1)	
3q21	TF	C	Transferrin	190000		Atransferrinemia (1)	9(Trf)
3q21-q22	RBP1, CRBP1	C	Cellular retinol binding protein I	180260	close to CRBP2		9(Crbp-1)
3q21-q23	LTF	C	Lactotransferrin	150210			9(Ltf)
3q21-q23	RP1	P	Retinitis pigmentosa-1	180100		Retinitis pigmentosa-1 (2)	
3q21-q24	CP	C	Ceruloplasmin	117700	ca. 15cM from TF	[Hypoceruloplasminemia, hereditary] (1)	9(Cp)
3q21-q24	RHO	C	Rhodopsin	180380			
3q21-q27	MME, CD10, CALLA	P	Membrane metallo-endopeptidase (common acute lymphocytic leukemia antigen)	120520			

Location	Symbol	Status	Title	MIM #	Comments	Disorder	Mouse
3q21-qter	ACPP	P	Acid phosphatase, prostate-specific	171790			
3q21-qter	RBP2, CRBP2	P	Cellular retinol binding protein II	180280	close to CRBP1		9(Crbp-2)
3q25-q26	SI	P	Sucrase-isomaltase	222900		Sucrose intolerance (1)	
3q25.2	ACHE	L	Acetylcholinesterase	100740	coamplified with CHE1		
3q25.2	CHE1	C	Pseudocholinesterase-1	177400	distal to CP, TF	Postanesthetic apnea (1)	
3q26.1-q26.3	GLUT2	C	Glucose transporter protein-2	138160			
3q26.2	TFRC	C	Transferrin receptor	190010			
3q27	FIM3	P	Friend murine leukemia virus integration site 3, homolog of	136770			
3q27-q29	AHSG	C	Alpha-2HS-glycoprotein	138680	linked to TF, CHE1; ?order = cen-TF-CHE1-AHSG		
3q28	SST	C	Somatostatin	182450			16(Smst)
3q29	MAP97, MFJ1, MFI2	P	Melanoma-associated antigen p97	155750	identical to TFRC		
Chr.3	AF8T	P	Temperature sensitive, tsAF8, complement	116950			
Chr.3	CRYG8	P	Crystallin, gamma polypeptide 8	123730			
Chr.3	DHFRP4	C	Dihydrofolate reductase pseudogene-4	see 126060			
Chr.3	GAP43	P	Neuron growth-associated protein 43	162060			16(Gap43)
Chr.3	GNAI2B	P	Guanine nucleotide binding protein, alpha inhibiting, polypeptide 2	139360			9(Gnai-2)
Chr.3	GNAT1	P	Guanine nucleotide binding protein, alpha transducing, polypeptide 1	139330			9(Gnat-1)
Chr.3	GST1L, GSTM	P	Glutathione-S-transferase 1-like (mu-like)	138380			
Chr.3	HRG	P	Histidine-rich glycoprotein	142640		Thrombophilia due to elevated HRG (2)	
Chr.3	HV1S	I	Herpes virus sensitivity	142450	see chr. 11		
Chr.3	RPN1	P	Ribophorin I	180470			
Chr.3	TRV4	P	Truncated endogenous retroviral sequence-4	190970			6(Rpm-1)

In addition: 7 surface antigens, most defined by monoclonals, 4 'like' genes, 4 pseudogenes, and 4 fragile sites (HGM10).

Chromosome No. 4

Location	Symbol	Status	Title	MIM #	Comments	Disorder	Mouse
4pter-p15	RAF2	P	Oncogene RAF2	see 164760	processed pseudogene		6(Raf-2)
4pter-q21	PPAT	P	Phosphoribosylpyrophosphate amidotransferase	172450			
4p16.3	HD	C	Huntington disease	143100	distal to D4S10	Huntington disease (2)	
4p16.1	D4S10	C	G8 DNA segment	see 143100	theta .03–.05, vs. HD		
4p16.1	HOX7	P	Homeo box-7	142983		Wolf-Hirschorn syndrome (3)	
4p15.3	QDPR, DHPR	C	Quinoid dihydropteridine reductase	261630		Phenylketonuria due to dihydropteridine reductase deficiency (1)	5(Qdpr)
4p14-q12	PGM2	C	Phosphoglucomutase-2	172000			5(Pgm-1)
4p13-p12	GABRA2	P	Gamma-aminobutyric acid receptor, alpha-2 polypeptide	137140			
4p13-p12	GABRB1	P	Gamma-aminobutyric acid receptor, beta-1 polypeptide	137190			
4p11-q12	PEPS	C	Peptidase S	170250			5(Pep-7)
4cen-q21	MT2P1	C	Metallothionein II processed pseudogene	see 156360			
4q11-q12	KIT	C	Oncogene KIT	164920			5(Kit)
4q11-q13	AFP	C	Alpha-fetoprotein	104150	order: 5'-ALB-3'--5'-AFP-3'	AFP deficiency, congenital (1)	5(Afp)
4q11-q13	ALB	C	Albumin	103600	linked to GC	Analbuminemia (1); [Dysalbuminemic hyperthyroxinemia] (1); [Dysalbuminemic hyperzincemia] (1)	5(Alb-1)
4q11-q13	HPAFP	P	Hereditary persistence of alpha-fetoprotein	104140	?same locus as AFP	[Hereditary persistence of alpha-fetoprotein] (3)	
4q11-q13	JPD, JP	P	Periodontitis, juvenile	170650	linked to GC, which is probably between DGI1 and JP	Periodontitis, juvenile (2)	
4q11-q13	STATH, STR	P	Statherin	184470			
4q12	GC, DBP	C	Group-specific component (vitamin D binding protein)	139200	4q13-q21.1 by in situ hybridization		
4q12	PBT	L	Piebald trait	172800		?Piebaldism (2)	5(W)
4q12	PDGFRA, PDGFR2	C	Platelet-derived growth factor receptor alpha polypeptide	173490			
4q12-q21	PF4	P	Platelet factor 4	173460			
4q13-q21	AREG	P	Amphiregulin	104640			
4q13-q21	DGI1	C	Dentinogenesis imperfecta-1	125490	ca. 11cM from GC	Dentinogenesis imperfecta-1 (2)	
4q13-q21	GRO, MGSA	P	Melanoma growth stimulatory activity	155730			5(Mgsa)
4q13-q21	IL8	P	Interleukin-8	146930			
4q16.1	ADRA2BR	C	Alpha-2B-adrenergic receptor (renal type)	104250	linked to D4S10		
4q21	IGCJ, JCH	P	J region of immunoglobulin heavy chain	147790		?Leukemia, acute lymphocytic, with 4/11 translocation (3)	5(Igj)

69

Location	Symbol	Status	Title	MIM #	Comments	Disorder	Mouse
4q21	INP10, IP10	C	Interferon-inducible cytokine IP-10	147310	?involved in monocytic leukemia with t(4;11)(q21;q23)		
4q21-q23	GNPTA	P	N-acetyl-alpha-glucosaminylphosphotransferase	252500		Mucolipidosis II (1); Mucolipidosis III (1)	
4q21-q24	FDH	C	Formaldehyde dehydrogenase	136490	4q24-qter (M. Smith)		
4q21-q25	ADHX, ADH5	C	Alcohol dehydrogenase, class III	103710			
4q21-q31	LPC2A	P	Lipocortin IIa	151710			
4q21-qter	AGA	C	Aspartylglucosaminidase	208400		Aspartylglucosaminuria (1)	
4q22	ADHC1	C	ALCOHOL DEHYDROGENASE, CLASS I, CLUSTER	103700	ADH1,ADH2,ADH3 loci for alpha, beta, and gamma chains		3(Adh-1,3)
4q22	ADH1	C	Alcohol dehydrogenase, alpha polypeptide	103720			
4q22	ADH2	C	Alcohol dehydrogenase, beta polypeptide	103730			
4q22	ADH3	C	Alcohol dehydrogenase, gamma polypeptide	103740			
4q22	ADH4	P	Alcohol dehydrogenase, class II, pi polypeptide				
4q23-q27	RGS	P	Rieger syndrome	180500	chr.21 and others implicated in some cases; ?not in 4q26	Rieger syndrome (2)	
4q25	EGF	C	Epidermal growth factor	131530	linked to ADH3; cen-ADH3-EGF-IL2-qter		3(Egf)
4q25	IF	C	Complement component I (C3b inactivator)	217030	40kb distal to EGF	C3b inactivator deficiency (1)	
4q26-q27	IL2, TCGF	C	T-cell growth factor (interleukin-2)	147680			3(Il-2)
4q26-q28	FGC	C	FIBRINOGEN GENE CLUSTER		likely order: gamma-alpha-beta		
4q26-q28	FGB	C	Fibrinogen, beta chain	134830	4q31 by A; proximal to GYPB/GYPA	Dysfibrinogenemia, beta types (1)	
4q26-q28	FGA	C	Fibrinogen, alpha chain	134820		Dysfibrinogenemia, alpha types (1)	
4q26-q28	FGG	C	Fibrinogen, gamma chain	134850	linked to MN	Dysfibrinogenemia, gamma types (1); Hypofibrinogenemia, gamma types (1)	
4q28-q31	ASMD	P	Anterior segment mesenchymal dysgenesis	107250	linked to MN	Anterior segment mesenchymal dysgenesis (2)	
4q28-q31	ENX2	P	Endonexin II	131230			
4q28-q31	FABP2	P	Fatty acid binding protein, intestinal	134640	see unassigned linkage groups, Ib4		3(Fabp-i)
4q28-q31	HCL2, RHC	P	Red hair color	266300	male lod = 3.79 at theta 0.32 vs. GC		
4q28-q31	MN, GYPA	C	MN blood group (glycophorin A)	111300			
4q28-q31	SF	C	Stoltzfus blood group	111800	ca. 25cM from MNSs		
4q28-q31	SS, GYPB	C	Ss blood group (glycophorin B)	111740			
4q28-q31	TYS	C	Sclerotylosis	181600		Sclerotylosis (2)	
4q31-q32	TDO2, TPH2, TRPO	C	Tryptophan oxygenase	191070	tightly linked to MN		
4q31.1	MLR, MCR, MR	C	Mineralocorticoid receptor	264350		Pseudohypoaldosteronism (1)	

Location	Symbol		Gene name	MIM #	Comments	Disorder
4q32.1	HVBS6, HCC2	P	Hepatitis B virus integration site 6 (hepatocellular carcinoma-2)	142380		Hepatocellular carcinoma (3)
4q35	F11	P	Factor XI	264900	not closely linked to MNS	Factor XI deficiency (1)
Chr.4	ANT1	P	Adenine nucleotide translocator 1 (ADP/ATP translocator of skeletal muscle)	103220		
Chr.4	ATPBL1	P	Sodium-potassium-ATPase, beta-polypeptide-like	182370		
Chr.4	CD38	P	Antigen CD38 of acute lymphoblastic leukemia	107270		
Chr.4	FGFB	P	Fibroblast growth factor, basic	134920		
Chr.4	GTB	I	Galactosyltransferase, 4-beta	137060	many alternate names see chr.9	
Chr.4	LAG5	P	Leukocyte antigen group five	151450		
Chr.4	MNB	L	Mannosidase, beta-	248510	linked in mouse to Adl-3	3(Bmn)
Chr.4	OPN	P	Osteopontin	166490		
Chr.4	PDE1A	P	Phosphodiesterase-1A	171890		
Chr.4	TS13	P	Temperature sensitivity complementation, ts13	187320		

In addition: 1 antigen, 4 'like' genes, 1 pseudogene, and 4 fragile sites (HGM10). Possible order: CEN--GC--DGI1--SS--MN--FGG. FGB--FGA--FGG in this order in 50kb segment.

Chromosome No. 5

Location	Symbol	Status	Title	MIM #	Comments	Disorder	Mouse
5pter-q11	RARS	P	Arginyl-tRNA synthetase	107820	very close to LARS		
5p14	MLVI2	P	Maloney leukemia virus integration site-2	154330			
5p14-p13	HMGCS	C	3-hydroxy-3-methylglutaryl coenzyme A synthase; HMG CoA synthase	142940	like HMGCR, regulated transcriptionally by steroid; ?2 genes closely situated		
5p14-p13	ZNF4	P	Zinc finger protein-4	194520			
5p13	C9	P	Complement component-9	120940		C9 deficiency (1)	
5p13-p12	GHR, GHBP	C	Growth hormone receptor	262500		Laron dwarfism (1)	
5p13-p12	PRLR	P	Prolactin receptor	176761	related to GHR		
5p13-cen	TARS	P	Threonyl-tRNA synthetase	187790	linked to LARS		
5cen-q11	LARS, RNTLS	C	Leucyl-tRNA synthetase	151350			
5q	GAP	P	Guanine triphosphatase (GTPase) activating protein	139150	excluded from 5q13-q15		13(Gap)
5q11	MFD1	L	Treacher Collins mandibulofacial dysostosis	154500	t(5;13)(q11;p11)	?Treacher Collins mandibulofacial dysostosis (2)	
5q11-q13	ARSB	C	Arylsulfatase B	253200		Maroteaux-Lamy syndrome (1)	13(As-1)
5q11.1-q13.2	DHFR	C	Dihydrofolate reductase	126060	5q23 = conflicting localization; to other chrs. with amplification	?Megaloblastic anemia (1)	13(Dhfr)
5q11.2-q13	HTR1A	P	5-hydroxytryptamine-1A receptor	109760			
5q11.2-q13.3	SCZD1	P	Schizophrenia-1	181510	cosegregation with partial trisomy	Schizophrenia (2)	
5q12-q13	ZNF5	P	Zinc finger protein-5	194530			
5q12-q32	MAR	P	Macrocytic anemia, refractory	153550	resulting from 5q-	Macrocytic anemia of 5q- syndrome, refractory (2)	
5q13	HEXB	C	Beta-hexosaminidase, beta chain	268800		Sandhoff disease (1)	13(Hex-2)
5q13.3-q14	HMGCR	C	3-hydroxy-3-methylglutaryl coenzyme A reductase; HMG CoA reductase	142910			
5q21-q23	CAMK4	P	Ca(2+)-calmodulin-dependent protein kinase type IV of brain	114080			
5q22-q23	APC, GS, FPC	C	Adenomatous polyposis of the colon (Gardner syndrome; familial polyposis coli)	175100		Gardner syndrome (2); Polyposis coli, familial (2);?Familial colorectal cancer (2)	
5q23	DTS	C	Diphtheria toxin sensitivity	126150		[Diphtheria, susceptibility to] (1)	
5q23-q31	CD14	P	Monocyte differentiation antigen CD14	158120			
5q23-q31	EGR1	C	Early growth response-1	128990			18(Egr-1)
5q23-q31	IL3	P	Interleukin-3	147740			11(Il-3)
5q23-q32	CSF2, GMCSF	C	Granulocyte-macrophage colony-stimulating factor	138960	9kb from CSF2 order: cen-CSF2-CSF1-FMS-qter		11(Csfgm)
5q23.3-q31.1	IL5	C	Interleukin 5	147850			11(Il-5)

Location		Symbol	Name	MIM	Comments	Disorder	Mouse
5q31	C	GRL	Glucocorticoid receptor, lymphocyte	138040		Cortisol resistance (1)	18(Grl-1)
5q31	C	IL4	Interleukin-4	147780			11(Il-4)
5q31-q32	C	ADRB2R, BAR2	Beta-2-adrenergic receptor	109690			
5q31-q32	P	PDGFRB, PDGFR, PDGFR1	Platelet-derived growth factor receptor-1	173410	between GMCSF and FMS		18(Pdgfr)
5q31-q33	C	EMTB, RPS14	Emetine resistance (ribosomal protein S14)	130620			
5q31-q33	C	ON, SPARC	Osteonectin (secreted protein, acidin, cysteine-rich)	182120	see 180460		11(Sparc)
5q31.3-q33.2	C	ECGF	Endothelial cell growth factor	131220			
5q32	C	HLADG, DHLAG	Histocompatibility class II antigens, gamma chain	142790			18(Ii)
5q32-q34	P	CBP68	Calcium-binding protein p68	114070			
5q33-qter	C	F12, HAF	Clotting factor XII (Hageman factor)	234000		Factor XII deficiency (1)	
5q33-qter	P	RHOH9	Oncogene RHO H9	165380			
5q33.1	L	CMD1	Campomelic dysplasia with sex reversal	211970	?or 8q21.4; balanced translocation	?Campomelic dysplasia with sex reversal (2)	
5q33.1	P	CSF1, MCSF	Macrophage colony stimulating factor	120420			3(Csfm)
5q33.2-q33.3	C	CSF1R, FMS	Oncogene FMS (McDonough feline sarcoma)	164770	= receptor for CSF1; FMS2 is 5' end		18(Fms)
5q34	P	GLUT6	Glucose transporter-6	138240			
5q34-q35	P	GABRA1	Gamma-aminobutyric acid receptor, alpha-1 polypeptide	137160			
5q35	C	CHR	Chromate resistance (sulfate transport)	118840			
Chr.5	P	C6	Complement component-6	217050	linked to C7 in dog, marmoset	C6 deficiency (1); Combined C6/C7 deficiency (1)	
Chr.5	P	C7	Complement component-7	217070	linked to C6 in dog, marmoset	C7 deficiency (1)	
Chr.5	P	ERBAL3, EAR3	ERBA-related gene-3	132890			
Chr.5	P	FGFA	Fibroblast growth factor, acidic	134910	same locus as ECGF		
Chr.5	P	GM2A	GM2-activator protein	272750		GM2-gangliosidosis, AB variant (1)	
Chr.5	P	HARS	Histidyl-tRNA synthetase	142810			
Chr.5	P	HFSP	Hanukah factor serine protease	140050			
Chr.5	P	SPINK1, PSTI	Serine protease inhibitor, Kazal type I (pancreatic secretory trypsin inhibitor)	167790			
Chr.5	P	ZNF3	Zinc finger protein-3	194510	?relation to ZNF4, ZNF5		

In addition: 1 surface antigen, 1 O'Farrell protein spot, 5 'like' genes, 5 pseudogenes, and 6 fragile sites (HGM10). Critical segment in *cri du chat* syndrome near 5p15.3-p15.2 junction.

Chromosome No. 6

Location	Symbol	Status	Title	MIM #	Comments	Disorder	Mouse
6pter-p23	ME2	P	Malic enzyme, mitochondrial	154270	10cM distal to F13A		7(Mod-2)
6pter-p23	OFC, CL	P	Orofacial cleft (cleft lip with or without cleft palate; isolated cleft palate)	119530	linked to F13A	Orofacial cleft (2)	
6pter-p21	TUBB	P	Tubulin, beta, M40	191130			
6pter-q12	PIM1	P	Oncogene PIM1	164960			17(Pim-1)
6p25-p24	F13A1	C	Factor XIII, A1 polypeptide	134570	F13A1, F13A2, F13A3 may be clustered loci	Factor XIII, A component deficiency (1)	
6p25-q24	F13A2	P	Factor XIII, A2 polypeptide	134620			
6p25-p24	F13A3	P	Factor XIII, A3 polypeptide	134630			
6p23-p22.3	FIM1	P	Friend murine leukemia virus integration site 1, homolog of	136750			
6p23-q12	HYS, MEA	P	H-Y antigen, structural gene for	143170	male enhanced antigen		
6p23-q12	INSL	P	Insulin-like DNA sequence	147490			
6p23-q12	RNTMI, TRM1	P	Initiator methionine tRNA	180620	2 of 12+ RNTMI genes are on chr. 6		
6p22.2-q21.3	PRL	C	Prolactin	176760	?between 6cen and GLO1		
6p22-p21.3	HSPA1, HSP70	C	Heat shock proteins-70	140550	also 14q22-q24, chr.21, and at least 1 other chromosome		
6p21.3	ASD2	P	Atrial septal defect, secundum type	108800	lod = 3.612 at theta 0.0 with HLA	Atrial septal defect, secundum type (2)	
6p21.3	BAT1	P	HLA-B associated transcript-1	142560	5 BATs in 160kb segment including also TNFA, TNFB		
6p21.3	BAT2	P	HLA-B associated transcript-2	142580			
6p21.3	BAT3	P	HLA-B associated transcript-3	142590			
6p21.3	BAT4	P	HLA-B associated transcript-4	142610			
6p21.3	BAT5	P	HLA-B associated transcript-5	142620			
6p21.3	BF	C	Properdin factor B	138470	no crossover with C2; less than 1kb from C2, 30kb from C4; C2, BF, C4A, C4B = class III		17(Bf)
6p21.3	C2	C	Complement component-2	217000	no crossover with BF	C2 deficiency (3)	17(C2)
6p21.3	C4A, C4S	C	Complement component 4A, or C4S	120810	order: HLA-B, C2, BF, C4A, C4B, CYP21, DR	C4 deficiency (3)	17(C4)
6p21.3	C4B, C4F	C	Complement component 4B, or C4F	120820	10kb from C4S	C4 deficiency (3)	17(C4)
6p21.3	CYP21, CA21H, CAH1	C	Congenital adrenal hyperplasia due to 21-hydroxylase deficiency; P450C21	201910	linked to C2, C4, BF; 2 loci, A and B; only B active	Adrenal hyperplasia, congenital, due to 21-hydroxylase deficiency (3)	17(P450-21)

74

Location	Status	Symbol	Title	MIM	Comments	Disorder	Mouse
6p21.3	P	GLUR	Renal glucosuria	233100	closer to HLA-A than HLA-B	[Renal glucosuria] (2)	
6p21.3	C	HFE	Hemochromatosis	235200	close to HLA-A; ?between HLA-A and HLA-B or distal to HLA-A	Hemochromatosis (2)	
6p21.3	C	MHC	MAJOR HISTOCOMPATIBILITY COMPLEX		class I distal to class II		17(Mhc)
6p21.3	P	HLA60, TCA	HLA-6.0	186840			17(Qa)
6p21.3	C	HLAA	HLA-A tissue type	142800	HLA-A, -B, -C, -6.0 = class I		17(H-2D)
6p21.3	C	HLAB	HLA-B tissue type	142830			
6p21.3	C	HLAC	HLA-C tissue type	142840			
6p21.3	C	HLADP	HLA-DP tissue type	142880	2 different alpha, 2 different beta chains		17(H-2L)
6p21.3	C	HLADQ	HLA-DQ tissue type	146880	1 Dx alpha, 1 Dx beta; 1 DC alpha, 1 DC beta chains		
6p21.3	C	HLADR	HLA-DR tissue type	142860	1 alpha, 3 different beta chains		17(H-2I)
6p21.3	C	HLADZ	HLA-DZ tissue type	142930	1 alpha, 1 beta chain; DZ, DR, etc. = class II		
6p21.3	P	HLAE	HLA-E tissue type	143010			
6p21.3	P	HLAF	HLA-F tissue type	143110			
6p21.3	L	IDDM	Insulin dependent diabetes mellitus	222100	?linkage or association, with HLA	?Diabetes mellitus, insulin dependent (2)	
6p21.3	C	IGLP1	Immune response to synthetic polypeptides-1	147080			
6p21.3	C	IGLP2	Immune response to synthetic polypeptides-2	147090			
6p21.3	P	IHG, ITG	Blastogenic response to synthetic polypeptides	146950, 146960	in A/B segment		
6p21.3	P	IPHEG, IGAT	Blastogenic response to synthetic polypeptides	146810, 146820	in B/D segment		
6p21.3	P	IS, ISCW, ISSCW	Immune suppression to streptococcal antigen	146850	HLA-linked		
6p21.3	L	LQT	Long QT syndrome	192500	?ca. 5cM from MHC near HLA-A end	?Long QT syndrome (2)	
6p21.3	P	MLRW	Mixed lymphocyte reaction, weak	157860	?linkage disequilibrium with HLA-B12		
6p21.3	P	NDF	Neutrophil differentiation factor	202700	?linked to HLA; see chr. 10	?Kostmann agranulocytosis (2)	
6p21.3	I	NEU, NEU1	Neuraminidase-1; sialidosis	162050, 256550	?linkage or association, with HLA	?Sialidosis (2)	17(Neu-1)
6p21.3	L	PDB	Paget disease of bone	167250	?linkage or association, with HLA	?Paget disease of bone (2)	
6p21.3	C	PLT1	Primed lymphocyte test-1	176680	near HLA-D		
6p21.3	P	RDBP	RD RNA-binding protein	154040	between C4 and BF		
6p21.3	L	RWS	Ragweed sensitivity	179450	?linkage or association, with HLA	?Ragweed sensitivity (2)	17(Rd)

Location	Symbol	Status	Title	MIM #	Comments	Disorder	Mouse
6p21.3-p21.2	LAP	L	Laryngeal adductor paralysis	150270	?linkage to HLA and GLO1	?Laryngeal adductor paralysis (2)	
6p21.3-p21.2	HMAA	P	Human monocyte antigen A	143070	between HLADQ and GLO		
6p21.3-p21.2	HMAB	P	Human monocyte antigen B	143080			
6p21.3-p21.2	GLO1	C	Glyoxalase I	138750	ca. 3cM proximal to HLA		17(Glo-1)
6p21.3-p21.2	CP20	L	Lymphocyte cytosolic protein, molecular weight 20kD	153380			
6p21.3-p21.2	MLN	P	Motilin	158270			
6p21.3-p21.2	SCA1	C	Spinocerebellar ataxia-1	164400	telomeric to GLO1 and centromeric to HLA; other evidence puts it distal to HLA	Spinocerebellar ataxia-1 (2)	
6p21.3-p21.1	B144	P	B144 protein	109170	10kb 3' from TNFA		
6p21.3-p21.1	PGC	C	Preprogastricsin	169740	cen-PGG-GLO1-HLA		17(Upg-1)
6p21.3-p21.1	TNFA, TNF1	P	Tumor necrosis factor, alpha	191160	5'-TNFB--TNFA-3' in 7kb segment (pter-cen); 210kb from HLA-B		17(Tnfa)
6p21.3-p21.1	TNFB, TNF2	P	Tumor necrosis factor, beta	153440	cen-DR-210H-C4-BF-C2-TNFA-TNFB-HLA-B		17(Tnfb)
6p21.2	COL11A2	C	Collagen, type XI, alpha-2 polypeptide	120290	45kb centromeric of HLA-DPB2; 3'--5'-cen		
6p21.2-p12	MUT, MCM	C	Methylmalonyl CoA mutase	251000		Methylmalonicaciduria, mutase deficiency type (1)	17(Mut)
6p21.1-p12	PGK1P2	C	Phosphoglycerate kinase-1 pseudogene-2	172270	proximal to MHC		17(Pgk-2)
6p21	EJM, JME	C	Epilepsy, juvenile myoclonic	254770	linked to BF and HLA	Epilepsy, juvenile myoclonic (2)	
6p21	MAPT2	P	Microtubule-associated protein tau-2	see 157130	see 17q21		
6p21-qter	TPX1	P	Testis-specific protein TPX-1	187430			17(Tpx-1)
6p12	GST2	C	Glutathione S-transferase-2	138360			
6p12-p11	RASK1, KRAS1P	C	Oncogene, Kirsten rat sarcoma virus-1	190110	pseudogene		
6p	CSCI	L	Corticosterone side-chain isomerase	122550	?linked to MHC		
6q	IFNGR1	I	Immune interferon, receptor for	107470	both 6 and 18 required		10(Ifgr)
6q12	ME1	C	Malic enzyme, cytoplasmic	154250			9(Mod-1)
6q12	PGM3	C	Phosphoglucomutase-3	172100			9(Pgm-3)
6q13	COL9A1	P	Collagen, type IX, alpha-1 polypeptide	120210			
6q14-q21	NT5, NTE, E5NT	C	Ecto-5'-nucleotidase	129190			
6q16-q22	GJL	P	Gap junction protein, liver	137205			
6q21	BKMA1	P	Banded krait minor satellite DNA-1	see 109780	related to heterogametic sex		
6q21	SOD2	C	Superoxide dismutase-2, mitochondrial	147460			17(Sod-2)
6q21-qter	DMDL	P	Dystrophin-like protein	128240			
6q21-qter	TCP10A	P	T-complex locus TCP10A	187020			

Location	Symbol	Type	Title	MIM number	Method/Comments	Disorder	Mouse
6q21.1-q23	CGA	P	Chorionic gonadotropin, alpha chain	118850	shared with LH, FSH, TSH		4(Tsha)
6q22	MYB	C	Oncogene, avian myeloblastosis virus	189990			10(Myb)
6q22	ROS1, ROS, MCF3	C	Oncogene ROS (oncogene MCF3)	165020			
6q22-q27	CVL	P	Cytovillin	123900	coamplified with MYB		
6q23	ARG1	P	Arginase, liver	207800		Argininemia (1)	
6q24-q27	ESR, ER	C	Estrogen receptor	133430			
6q24-q27	MAS1	P	Oncogene MAS1	165180	?same as ESR		
6q25-q26	RCD1	L	Retinal cone dystrophy-1	180020		?Retinal cone dystrophy-1 (2)	
6q25-q27	IGF2R, MPRI	P	Insulin-like growth factor-2 receptor (mannose-6-phosphate receptor, cation-independent)	147280			
6q25-q27	TCP1	C	T-complex locus TCP-1	186980	tightly linked to PLG		
6q25-qter	FUCA2	C	Alpha-L-fucosidase-2	136820	linked to PLG		
6q25-qter	VMD2	L	Macular dystrophy, ?vitelline type	153700		Macular dystrophy, ?vitelline type (2)	
6q26-q27	PLG	C	Plasminogen	173350	20cM from TCP10A	Plasminogen Tochigi disease (1); Dysplasminogenemic thrombophilia (1); Plasminogen deficiency, types I and II (1)	17(Cp)
6q26-q27	VIP	C	Vasoactive intestinal peptide	192320			
6q27	LPA	C	Apolipoprotein Lp(a)	152200		{Coronary artery disease, susceptibility to} (1)	
Chr.6	ADCP1	I	Adenosine deaminase complexing protein-1	102710			
Chr.6	AMD	P	S-adenosylmethionine decarboxylase	180980	sequences on Xq22-q28		
Chr.6	ASSP2	P	Argininosuccinate synthetase pseudogene-2	107840	others on 8 or more other chromosomes including X and Y		
Chr.6	BEVI	C	Baboon M7 virus replication	109180			
Chr.6	DHFRP2	P	Dihydrofolate reductase pseudogene-2	see 126060			
Chr.6	EDN1	P	Endothelin-1	131240			
Chr.6	FEA	L	F9 embryonic antigen	137010			
Chr.6	G6PD2	P	Glucose-6-phosphate dehydrogenase, red cell locus-2	138080			
Chr.6	MRBC	P	Monkey RBC receptor	158050			
Chr.6	P	P	P blood group globoside	111400			
Chr.6	TS546	P	Temperature sensitivity complementation, cell cycle specific, ts546 cells	187330			

In addition: 2 surface antigens, most defined by monoclonals, 6 'like' genes, 6 pseudogenes, and 6 fragile sites (HGM10). Order: 6cen--DR--C2--BF--C4A--CA21HA--C4B--CA21HB--HLA-B--pter (Wilton and Charlton, 1986). Order of class II subregions: 6cen--DP--DZalpha--DObeta--DX--DQ--DRbeta--DRalpha (Hardy et al, 1986). Order in region of class I genes: 6cen--DR--HLA-B--0.01--HLA-C--0.7--HLA-A--pter. HLADP shows relatively high recombination with DQ but the physical distance by molecular studies is about same as DQ-to-DR. Recombinational hotspots probably exist within the DQ subregion and between HLA-A and HLA-C (which molecular data suggest are as close as B and C). Family data show HLA-A to HLA-C = 0.7cM; HLA-C to HLA-B = 0.1cM. Disease/MHC associations of various strengths are probably indicative of pleiotropic effects of specific alleles or haplotypes, not linkage. Two of the strongest are ankylosing spondylitis (106300) with HLA-B27 and narcolepsy (161400) with HLA-DR2.

Chromosome No. 7

Location	Symbol	Status	Title	MIM #	Comments	Disorder	Mouse
7pter-p14	GCTG	P	Gamma-glutamylcyclotransferase	137170			5(Actb)
7pter-q22	ACTB	P	Actin, cytoskeletal beta	102630	ca. 20 pseudogenes also		
7pter-q22	NPY	P	Neuropeptide Y	162640			
7p22-q21	PDGFA	C	Platelet-derived growth factor, A chain	173430			
7p22-p15	RAL	P	RAS-like protein	179550			
7p21.3-p21.2	CRS, CSO	C	Craniosynostosis	123100		Craniosynostosis (2)	
7p21	IFNB2, IL6, BSF2	C	Interferon, beta-2 (hepatocyte stimulating factor, interleukin-6)	147620	conflicting assignment = 7p31		
7p15.2-p15.1	PSP	C	Phosphoserine phosphatase	172480			5(Psph)
7p15	TCRG	C	T-cell antigen receptor, gamma subunit	186970	multiple V genes, two J-C duplexes		13(Tcrg)
7p15-p14	HOX1	C	Homeo box-1	142950			6(Hox-1)
7p15-p13	INHBA, INHB2	P	Inhibin, beta-1	147290			13(Inhba)
7p14-p12	ERBB	C	Oncogene ERBB	190140	?same as EGFR; similar sequences		11(Erbb)
7p14-p12	IBP1	C	Insulin-like growth factor, low molecular weight	146730			
7p14-cen	BLVR	C	Biliverdin reductase	109750			2(Blvr)
7p13	GCPS	C	Greig craniopolysyndactyly syndrome	175700	balanced translocation; same restriction fragment as TCRG	Greig craniopolysyndactyly syndrome (2)	13(Xt)
7p13-p12	PGAM2, PGAMM	C	Phosphoglycerate mutase, muscle form	261670		Myopathy due to phosphoglycerate mutase deficiency (1)	
7p13-q22	MDH2	C	Malate dehydrogenase, mitochondrial	154100			
7p13-qter	PRKAR1, PKR1	P	Protein kinase, cAMP-dependent, type I regulatory subunit	176890	not in 7q22-q31.3		5(Mor-1)
7p12.3-p12.1	EGFR	C	Epidermal growth factor receptor	131550			
7p11.4-q21	ARAF2	P	Oncogene ARAF2	164710			
7p11-q11.2	PKS1	P	Oncogene PKS1	165010			
7p	GHS	L	Goldenhar syndrome	141400		?Goldenhar syndrome (2)	
7cen-q11.2	ASL	C	Argininosuccinate lyase	207900		Argininosuccinicaciduria (1)	5(Asl)
7q11.12-q11.23	ZWS, ZS	P	Zellweger syndrome	214100		Zellweger syndrome (2)	
7q21	GNAI1	C	Guanine nucleotide binding protein, alpha inhibiting, polypeptide-1	139310			
7q21-q22	EPO	C	Erythropoietin	133170	close to COL1A2; no recombination	?Erythremia (1)	5(Epo)
7q21-q22	NKNA	P	Neurokinin A (substance P)	162320			
7q21-q31	ASNS, AS	C	Asparagine synthetase	108370	temperature sensitive G1 mutant		
7q21.1	PGY1, MDR1	C	P-glycoprotein-1 (multidrug resistance)	171050			5(Mdr-1)
7q21.1	PGY3, MDR3	P	P-glycoprotein-3 (multidrug resistance-3)	171060	within 500kb of MDR1		
7q21.1	SRL, SCN	P	Sorcin (class 4 gene)	182520			
7q21.1-q22	GUSB	C	Beta-glucuronidase	253220		Mucopolysaccharidosis VII (1)	5(Gus)

78

Location	Status	Gene/Description	Symbol	MIM No.	Comments	Disorder	Mouse
7q21.3-q22	C	Cytochrome P450C3 (nifedipine oxidase)	CYP3	124010			6(Cyp-3)
7q21.3-q22	C	Plasminogen activator inhibitor-1	PLANH1, PAI1	173360		?Thrombophilia due to excessive plasminogen activator inhibitor (1); Hemorrhagic diathesis due to PAI1 deficiency (1)	
7q21.3-q22.1	C	Collagen I, alpha-2 chain	COL1A2	120160	ca. 17cM from CF	Osteogenesis imperfecta, 2 or more clinical forms (3); Ehlers-Danlos syndrome, type VIIA2 (3); Marfan syndrome, atypical (1)	6(Cola-2)
7q22	C	Paraoxonase	PON, ESA	168820	Order: COL1A2-D7S15-PON-CF		
7q22	I	HISTONE CLUSTER A: H1, H2A, H2B	HCA	142710, 142720, 142760	7q32-q36 = conflicting localization; others find none on 7		13(Hist-1)
7q22-q31	P	Protein kinase, cAMP-dependent, type II regulatory subunit	PRKAR2, PKR2	176910			
7q22-q32	P	Kinase-like protein	G7P1	148750			
7q22-q34	P	2,3-bisphosphoglycerate mutase	BPGM	222800		Hemolytic anemia due to bisphosphoglycerate mutase deficiency (1)	
7q22-qter	P	Actin, cytoskeletal beta, pseudogene-5	ACTBP5	102640	ca. 20 in all; 1 on X chr; 2 on chr. 5; 3 on chr. 18; 4 on chr. 5, etc.		
7q22-qter	P	Blue cone pigment	BCP, CBT	190900		Colorblindness, tritan (2)	
7q22-qter	P	Carboxypeptidase A	CPA	114850	both CPA and TRY1 = serine proteases		6(Cpa)
7q22-qter	C	Neutrophil migration (granulocyte glycoprotein)	GP130, NM	162820	formerly neutrophil chemotactic response, NCR		
7q22-qter	P	Trypsin-1	TRY1, TRP1	276000		Trypsinogen deficiency (1)	6(Try-1)
7q31	P	INT1-related protein	IRP	147870	isolated by CMGT with MET		
7q31	C	Oncogene MET	MET	164860	ca. 1.2cM from CF		6(Met)
7q31-qter	C	Ornithine decarboxylase-2	ODC2	165650			
7q31.1-q31.3	C	Laminin B1	LAMB1	150240	7q22 = conflicting assignment		1(Lamb-1)
7q31.3-q32	C	Cystic fibrosis	CF	219700		Cystic fibrosis (2)	
7q32-q36	C	EPH tyrosine kinase/erythropoietin producing hepatoma amplified sequence (oncogene EPH)	EPHT	179610	distal and 5' to MET		
7q32-q36	P	Prolactin-inducible protein	PIP	176720			
7q34-qter	L	Smith-Lemli-Opitz syndrome	SLO	270400		?Smith-Lemli-Opitz syndrome (2)	
7q35	C	T-cell antigen receptor, beta subunit	TCRB	186930	7q32 by A; cluster of V, D, J, and C genes; many V, two D-J-C triplexes		6(Tcrb)
7q35-q36	P	Membrane protein band 3, nonerythroid	MPB3	109280			

Location	Symbol	Status	Title	MIM #	Comments	Disorder	Mouse
7q35-q36	MS3315	P	Minisatellite 33.15	157570			
7q36	EN2	P	Engrailed-2	131310			
Chr.7	DIA2	L	Diaphorase-2	125870			
Chr.7	DLD, LAD	P	Dihydrolipoamide dehydrogenase	246900		Lipoamide dehydrogenase deficiency (1)	
Chr.7	ERV3	P	Endogenous retrovirus-3	131170			
Chr.7	FPSL2	P	Farnesylpyrophosphate synthetase-2	134632			
Chr.7	GCF1	P	Growth rate controlling factor-1	139220			
Chr.7	GLI3	P	Oncogene GLI3	165240			
Chr.7	GNB2	P	Guanine nucleotide binding protein, beta-2	139390			
Chr.7	HADH, ACADL, LCAD	P	Hydroxyacyl-CoA dehydrogenase (acyl-CoA dehydrogenase, long chain)	143450		?Acyl-CoA dehydrogenase, long chain deficiency of (1)	
Chr.7	NCF1	P	Neutrophil cytosolic factor-1	233700		Chronic granulomatous disease due to deficiency of NCF-1 (1)	
Chr.7	NHCP2	P	Nonhistone chromosomal protein-2	118880			
Chr.7	PHKG	P	Phosphorylase kinase, muscle, gamma subunit	172470			
Chr.7	TTIM1, INM7	P	T-cell tumor invasion and metastasis-1 (invasion-metastasis of neoplasms, chromosome 7 determined)	147830			
Chr.7	UP	C	Uridine phosphorylase	191730	presumed pseudogene on 11		

In addition: 1 surface antigen, 2 O'Farrell protein spots, 5 'like' genes, 7 pseudogenes, and 9 fragile sites (HGM10).

80

Chromosome No. 8

Location	Symbol	Status	Title	MIM #	Comments	Disorder	Mouse
8p23.3-p23.1	F7E, F7R	C	Clotting factor VII expression, or regulator	134450			
8p23	DEF, HNP1	P	Defensin-1 (human neutrophil peptide-1)	125220			8(Defcr)
8p22	CTSB, CPSB	P	Cathepsin B	116810	13q14 by rat probe		
8p22	LPL, LIPD	P	Lipoprotein lipase (lipase D)	238600		Hyperlipoproteinemia I (1)	
8p21.1	GSR	C	Glutathione reductase	138300		Hemolytic anemia due to glutathione reductase deficiency (1)	8(Gr-1)
8p21	NEFL, NFL, NF68	C	Neurofilament, light polypeptide	162280	?NFI and NFH on 2 near cen, 7q		
8p21-q11.2	GNRH, LHRH	P	Luteinizing hormone releasing hormone (gonadotropin releasing hormone)	152760		?Hypogonadotropic hypogonadism due to GNRH deficiency, 227200 (1)	
8p12	PLAT, TPA	C	Plasminogen activator, tissue type	173370		Plasminogen activator deficiency (1)	8(Plat)
8p12-p11.2	FMSL, FLG	P	FMS-like gene	136350			
8p12-p11	POLB	C	Polymerase, DNA, beta	174760			
8p11	ANK, SPH2	C	Ankyrin (spherocytosis)	182900		Spherocytosis-2 (2)	
8q	GPB	C	Beta-glycerol phosphatase	109640			8(nb)
8q11-q12	MOS	C	Oncogene MOS, Moloney murine sarcoma virus	190060			4(Mos)
8q12	SGPA, PSA	P	Salivary gland pleomorphic adenoma	181030	12q13-q15 affected in subset	Salivary gland pleomorphic adenoma (2)	
8q12-q13	IL7	P	Interleukin 7	146660			
8q13	CRH	P	Corticotropin releasing hormone	122560			
8q13-qter	LYN	P	Oncogene Yamaguchi sarcoma viral related	165120			
8q13.3	BOS	L	Branchiootic syndrome	113650	?q21.13	?Branchiootic syndrome (2)	
8q21	BN51T, TSBN51	P	Temperature sensitive complementation, cell cycle specific, tsBN51	187280	block in progression through G1		
8q21	CYP11B1, P450C11	P	11-beta-hydroxylase; corticosteroid methyl oxidase II (CMO II)	202010	multifunctional enzyme	Adrenal hyperplasia, congenital, due to 11-beta-hydroxylase deficiency (1); CMO II deficiency (1)	
8q21	CYP11B2	P	Cytochrome P450 CYP11B2	124080			
8q21.1-q23	MRS	P	Myeloid-related sequence	159560		?ANLL-M2 (1)	
8q21.1-qter	GLYB	P	Glycine auxotroph B, complementation of hamster	138480	gly(-)B		
8q21.4	CMD1	L	Campomelic dysplasia with sex reversal	211970	?or 5q33.1; balanced translocation	?Campomelic dysplasia with sex reversal (2)	
8q22	CAC	C	CARBONIC ANHYDRASE CLUSTER				
8q22	CA1	C	Carbonic anhydrase I	114800		[Carbonic anhydrase I deficiency] (1)	3(Car-1)
8q22	CA2	C	Carbonic anhydrase II	259730	CA1, CA2 linked in monkey and mouse	Renal tubular acidosis-osteopetrosis syndrome (1)	3(Car-2)
8q22	CA3	C	Carbonic anhydrase III	114750			
8q22-q24	HSPG	P	Heparan sulfate proteoglycan, cell surface-associated	142460			

Location	Symbol	Status	Title	MIM #	Comments	Disorder	Mouse
8q23-q24	PENK	P	Proenkephalin	131330			
8q23-q24.1	EXT	L	Multiple exostoses	133700		?Multiple exostoses (2)	
8q24	EBS1	C	Epidermolysis bullosa, Ogna type	131950	closely linked to GPT	Epidermolysis bullosa, Ogna type (2)	15(Gpt-1)
8q24	GPT	C	Glutamate-pyruvate transaminase	138200			
8q24	PDS	L	Pendred syndrome	274600		?Pendred syndrome (2)	
8q24	PVT1	P	Oncogene PVT-1 (MYC activator)	165140			
8q24	VMD1	C	Macular dystrophy, atypical vitelliform	153840	5cm from GPT	Macular dystrophy, atypical vitelliform (2)	
8q24.1	MYC	C	Oncogene MYC, avian myelocytomatosis virus	190080	cen-5'-3'-ter	Burkitt lymphoma (3)	15(Myc)
8q24.11-q24.13	LGCR, LGS, TRPS2	C	Langer-Giedion syndrome	150230	?deletion of both EXT and TRP1 in LGS; ?critical segment = 8q24.11-q24.12	Langer-Giedion syndrome (2)	
8q24.12	TRPS1	P	Trichorhinophalangeal syndrome, type I	190350	?q24.11	Trichorhinophalangeal syndrome, type I (2)	
8q24.2-q24.3	TG	C	Thyroglobulin	188450	distal to MYC	Hypothyroidism, hereditary congenital, 1 or more types (1); ?Goiter, adolescent multinodular, 138800 (1)	?15(Tg)
Chr.8	CALB	P	Calbindin, 27kD	114050			
Chr.8	CYC1	P	Cytochrome c1	123980			
Chr.8	FNZ	L	Fibronectin	135600	?concerned with expression on cell surface		
Chr.8	FRV2	P	Full-length endogenous retroviral sequence-2	136870			
Chr.8	GLI4, HKR4	P	GLI-Kruppel family member GLI4 (Oncogene HKR4)	165280			
Chr.8	KRL4	P	Kruppel-like zinc finger protein 4	149440			
Chr.8	SFTP2	P	Pulmonary surfactant apoprotein-2	178620			
Chr.8	ZNF1	P	Zinc finger protein-1	194490			?8(Zfp-2)

In addition: 6 'like' genes, 5 pseudogenes, and 6 fragile sites (HGM10).

Chromosome No. 9

Location	Symbol	Status	Title	MIM #	Comments	Disorder	Mouse
9pter-p22	ZFY, TDFA	P	ZFY-related autosomal sequence	154230			
9pter-q12	RLXH1, RLN1	P	Relaxin, H1	179730			
9pter-q12	RLXH2, RLN2	P	Relaxin, H2	179740			
9pter-q34	LPC2B	P	Lipocortin IIb	151720			
9p24-p13	AK3	C	Adenylate kinase-3, mitochondrial	103030			
9p22	NKH1	L	Hyperglycinemia, isolated nonketotic, type I	238300		?Hyperglycinemia, isolated nonketotic, type I (2)	
9p22-p21	LALL	P	Lymphomatous acute lymphoblastic leukemia	247640		Acute lymphoblastic leukemia (2)	
9p22-p21	MTAP, MSAP	C	Methylthioadenosine phosphorylase	156540			
9p22-p13	ACO1	C	Aconitase, soluble	100880			4(Aco-1)
9p21	IFNB, IFNB1, IFF	C	Fibroblast interferon; beta-interferon	147640	distal to IFL, 9p23-p22 according to Rowley; IFF duplicate in some persons		4(Ifb)
9p21	IFNA, IFL, IFA	C	LEUKOCYTE INTERFERON GENE CLUSTER; ALPHA-INTERFERON	147660	very close to IFF by Fd, LD; 15-30 genes	Interferon, alpha, deficiency (1)	4(Ifa)
9p21-p12	RMRPR	P	Mitochondrial RNA-processing endoribonuclease	157660			4(Rmrpn)
9p13	GALT	C	Galactose-1-phosphate uridyltransferase	230400		Galactosemia (1)	4(Galt)
9p13	GT1	I	Galactosyltransferase-1	137060	?relation to GTB on chr.4		4(Ggt-1)
9cen-q34	FPGS	P	Folylpolyglutamate synthetase	136510			2(Fpgs)
9cen-qter	GRP78	P	Glucose-regulated protein	138120			
9q	C8G	P	Complement component 8, gamma polypeptide	120930	probably near C5, ORM1, ITIL		
9q11-q22	LPC1	P	Lipocortin I	151690			
9q12	DNCM	P	Cytoplasmic membrane DNA	126330			
9q13-q21.1	FRDA, FAT	C	Friedreich ataxia	229300	9qh	Friedreich ataxia (2)	
9q21	ALDH1	P	Aldehyde dehydrogenase-1	100640			19(Ahd-1,2)
9q21-q22	CTSL	P	Cathepsin L	116880			
9q22	ALDOB	C	Aldolase B; fructose-1-phosphate aldolase	229600		Fructose intolerance (1)	
9q31-qter	APPL1	P	Amyloid beta (A4) precursor protein-like-1	104740			
9q32-q33	ITIL, ITIL, HCP	C	Protein HC (alpha-1-microglobulin); inter-alpha-trypsin inhibitor, light chain	176870		?Familial Mediterranean fever, 249100 (1)	
9q32-q34	DYT1	C	Torsion dystonia, autosomal dominant	128100		Torsion dystonia (2)	
9q33-34	RPL7A, SURF3	P	Surfeit-3 (L7a ribosomal protein)	185640	in cluster with SURF1, SURF2, SURF4		
9q33-q34	SPTAN1, NEAS	C	Spectrin, alpha, nonerythrocytic 1 (alpha-fodrin)	182810			2(Spna-2)
9q33-q34	SURF1	P	Surfeit-1	185620			
9q33-q34	SURF2	P	Surfeit-2	185630			
9q33-q34	SURF4	P	Surfeit-4	185660			
9q33-q34	TSC1, TSC, TS	C	Tuberous sclerosis-1	191100	linked to ABO, ABL	Tuberous sclerosis-1 (2)	
9q33-qter	ITO	I	Hypomelanosis of Ito	146150	see chr.15	?Hypomelanosis of Ito (2)	

Location	Symbol	Status	Title	MIM #	Comments	Disorder	Mouse
9q34	ABO	C	ABO blood group	110300	linked to AK1		
9q34	ALAD	C	Delta-aminolevulinate dehydratase	125270	linked to ABO; ORM-13-ALAD-11-AK-13-ABO	Porphyria, acute hepatic (1); [Lead poisoning, susceptibility to] (1)	4(Lv)
9q34	ASS	C	Argininosuccinate synthetase	215700	14 pseudogenes on 11 chromosomes	Citrullinemia (1)	2(Ass)
9q34	DBH	C	Dopamine-beta-hydroxylase	223360	tightly linked to ABO		
9q34	GSN	P	Gelsolin	137350	40kb proximal to ABL		
9q34	NPS1	C	Nail-patella syndrome	161200	linked to AK1, ABO; no recombination with AK1	Nail-patella syndrome (2)	
9q34.1	ABL	C	Oncogene ABL (Abelson strain, murine leukemia virus)	189980	fusion hybrid gene with BCR1 in CML	Leukemia, chronic myeloid (3)	2(Abl)
9q34.1	AK1	C	Adenylate kinase-1, soluble	103000	proximal to Ph1 break, 9q34.1; AK1 to ORM =17cM	Hemolytic anemia due to adenylate kinase deficiency (1)	2(Ak-1)
9q34.1	C5	C	Complement component 5	120900		C5 deficiency (1)	2(Hc)
9q34.1-q34.3	ORM1, AGP1	C	Orosomucoid-1 (alpha-1-acid glycoprotein-1)	138600	linked to ABO, AK1, ALAD		4(Agp-1)
9q34.1-q34.3	ORM2	C	Orosomucoid-2	138610			4(Agp-2)
Chr.9	ALDH4	P	Aldehyde dehydrogenase-4	100670			
Chr.9	CPRO, CPO	P	Coproporphyrinogen oxidase	121300	?on 9p	Coproporphyria (1); Harderoporphyria (1)	
Chr.9	H142T	P	Temperature sensitivity complementation, H142	187290			
Chr.9	IGEP2	P	Immunoglobulin epsilon heavy chain pseudogene	147210			
Chr.9	IREBP	P	Iron-responsive element, binding protein for	147581			
Chr.9	VARS	P	Valyl-tRNA synthetase	192150			

In addition: 1 antigen, 3 O'Farrell protein spots, 5 'like' genes and 4 pseudogenes, and 6 fragile sites (HGM10).

Chromosome No. 10

Location	Symbol	Status	Title	MIM #	Comments	Disorder	Mouse
10pter-p11.1	PFKF, PFKP	C	Phosphofructokinase, platelet type	171840			
10p15	ITIH2	P	Inter-alpha-trypsin inhibitor, heavy chain-2	146640			
10p15-p14	IL2R, TAK	C	Interleukin-2 receptor; T-cell growth factor receptor	147730			
10p13	VIM	C	Vimentin	193060			
10p12-q23.2	GBM	C	Glioblastoma multiforme	137800		Glioblastoma multiforme	
10p11.2	FNRB, VLAB	C	Fibronectin receptor, beta subunit (common unit of very late activator proteins)	135630			
10p11.2	HK1	C	Hexokinase-1	142600		Hemolytic anemia due to hexokinase deficiency (1)	10(Hk-1)
10p11.2-q11.2	RBP3, IRBP	C	Interstitial retinol-binding protein	180290			
10q11	ERCC6	P	Excision repair cross complementing rodent repair deficiency, complementation group 6	133540			
10q11-q12	TST1, PTC, TPC	C	Thyroid papillary carcinoma oncogene	188550	?same as MEN2A	Thyroid papillary carcinoma (1)	
10q11-q24	ADK	C	Adenosine kinase	102750			14(Adk)
10q11-qter	ALDOBP	P	Aldolase B pseudogene	see 229600			
10q11.1-q24	PP	C	Inorganic pyrophosphatase	179030			10(Pyp)
10q21-q22	LPC2C	P	Lipocortin IIc	151730			
10q21-q22	SAP1, SAP2	C	Sphingolipid activator protein-1; sphingolipid activator protein-2	249900		Metachromatic leukodystrophy due to deficiency of SAP-1 (1)	
10q21-q24	SFTP1, PSAP	C	Pulmonary surfactant-associated protein, 35kD	178630			
10q21.1	MEN2A, MEN2	C	Multiple endocrine neoplasia, type II (or IIA); medullary thyroid carcinoma	171400	19cM from D10S5 at 10q21.1; ?allele for medullary thyroid carcinoma	Multiple endocrine neoplasia II (2); Medullary thyroid carcinoma (2)	
10q21.1	MEN3, MEN2B	C	Multiple endocrine neoplasia, type III (or IIB)	162300	?allelic to MEN2	Multiple endocrine neoplasia III(2)	
10q21.1-q22.1	KROX20, EGR2	P	KROX-20, Drosophila, homolog (early growth response-2)	129010			10(Krox-20; Egr-2)
10q21.1-q21.2	GLUD	C	Glutamate dehydrogenase	138130	?10q23-q24		14(Glud)
10q21.3-q23.1	P4HA, PO4HA	P	Prolyl 4-hydroxylase, alpha polypeptide	176710			
10q22	COL13A1	P	Collagen, type XIII, alpha-1 polypeptide	120350			
10q22.1	PRG	C	Proteoglycan, secretory granule (platelet proteoglycan protein core)	177040			
10q23-q24	DNTT, TDT	C	Terminal deoxynucleotidyltransferase	187410			19(Tdt)
10q23-q24	RBP4	C	Retinol binding protein, plasma	180250		Retinol binding protein, deficiency of (1)	
10q23-q25	ADRA2R	P	Alpha-2-adrenergic receptor	104210	same 250 kb segment as ADRA2R		
10q23-q25	ADRB1R	P	Beta-1-adrenergic receptor	109630	no recombination with ADRA2R		
10q24	TCL3	P	T-cell leukemia-3	186770		Leukemia, T-cell acute lymphocytic (2)	

Location	Symbol	Status	Title	MIM #	Comments	Disorder	Mouse
10q24-q25	LIPA	P	Lysosomal acid lipase-A	278000	?close to GOT	Wolman disease (1); Cholesterol ester storage disease (1)	19(Lip-1)
10q24-qter	PLAU, URK	C	Urokinase (plasminogen activator, urinary)	191840			9(Plau)
10q24.1-q24.3	CYP2C	C	Cytochrome P450, family II, subfamily C (mephenytoin 4-hydroxylase)	124020	multiple genes		19(P450-2c)
10q24.1-q25.1	GOT1	C	Glutamate oxaloacetate transaminase, soluble	138180	10q26.1 = conflicting localization		19(Got-1)
10q25-q26	IFNAI1, RNM561	P	Interferon-inducible mRNA 561	147690			
10q25.3	PGAMB, PGAM1	P	Phosphoglycerate mutase A, nonmuscle form	172250			19(Pgam-1)
10q26	OAT	C	Ornithine aminotransferase	258870	pseudogene at Xp11.2	Gyrate atrophy of choroid and retina (1)	7(Oat)
Chr.10	ATPM, OMR	P	Mitochondrial ATPase (oligomycin resistance)	164360			
Chr.10	CDC2	C	Cell cycle controller, CDC2	116940			
Chr.10	CHAT	P	Choline acetyltransferase	118490			
Chr.10	CYP2E	P	Cytochrome P450, family II, subfamily E	124040			15(Cyp2e)
Chr.10	CYP17, P450C17	P	Steroid 17-alpha-hydroxylase / 17,20 lyase	202110	at least 2 genes	Adrenal hyperplasia V (1)	
Chr.10	FUSE	P	Polykaryocytosis inducer	174750			
Chr.10	G10P2	P	Interferon, alpha-inducible protein (MW 54kD)	147040			
Chr.10	GSAS	P	Glutamate-gamma-semialdehyde synthetase	138250	GOT1 and GSAS in same pathway		
Chr.10	HEP10	P	Hepatic protein 10	142390			
Chr.10	M130	P	External membrane protein-130	133710			
Chr.10	NEU, NEUG	I	Glycoprotein neuraminidase; sialidosis	256550	see 6p	?Sialidosis (1)	
Chr.10	PROA	P	Proline(-) auxotroph, complementation of	176770			

In addition: 2 O'Farrell protein spots 4 'like' genes, and 1 pseudogene (HGM10).

Chromosome No. 11

Location	Symbol	Status	Title	MIM #	Comments	Disorder	Mouse
11pter-p15.5	RMS, RMSCR	P	Rhabdomyosarcoma, embryonal	268210	2q37 suggested by translocations	Rhabdomyosarcoma (2)	
11pter-p15.4	BWCR, BWS, WBS	C	Beckwith-Wiedemann syndrome	130650	partial trisomy	Beckwith-Wiedemann syndrome (2)	
11pter-p13	CD44, LHR	P	antigen CD44, (homing function), includes MDU2, MDU3, MIC4	153270			
11pter-p12	SAA	C	Serum amyloid A	104750	2 genes, ?closely linked	?Susceptibility to amyloid in FMF, 249100 (1)	7(Saa)
11pter-p11.2	CDw26, TP250	P	T-cell activation antigen CDw26	186710			
11p15.5	ADCR, ADCC	P	Adrenocortical carcinoma region	202300	11p12.08-p12.05 = conflicting localization;	Adrenocortical carcinoma (2)	
11p15.5	NAGC, HBBC	C	NON-ALPHA GLOBIN CLUSTER (HEMOGLOBIN BETA CLUSTER)				
11p15.5	HBB	C	Hemoglobin beta	141900		Sickle cell anemia (1); Thalassemias, beta- (1); Methemoglobinemias, beta- (1); Erythremias, beta- (1); Heinz body anemias, beta- (1); HPFH, deletion type (1)	7(Hbb)
11p15.5	HBD	C	Hemoglobin delta	142000			
11p15.5	HBGR	C	Hb gamma regulator	142270		?Hereditary persistence of fetal hemoglobin (3)	
11p15.5	HBG1	C	Hemoglobin gamma 136 alanine	142200		HPFH, nondeletion type A (1)	
11p15.5	HBG2	C	Hemoglobin gamma 136 glycine	142250		HPFH, nondeletion type G (1)	
11p15.5	HBE1	C	Hemoglobin epsilon	142100			
11p15.5	HRAS1, RASH1	C	Oncogene HRAS1, Harvey rat sarcoma-1	190020	pseudogene HRAS2 on X		7(Hras1)
11p15.5	IGF2	C	Insulin-like growth factor II, or somatomedin A	147470	separate gene for variant, 147410		
11p15.5	INS	C	Insulin	176730	5'--INS-12.6kb-IGF2--3'; cen-HBBC-10cM-INS-2cM-HRAS1-3cM-TH	Diabetes mellitus, rare form (1); MODY, one form, 125850 (3); Hyperproinsulinemia, familial (1)	6(Ins-1); 7(Ins-2)
11p15.5	MAFD1, MD1	L	Manic-depressive illness (major affective disorder 1)	125480		?Manic-depressive illness (2)	
11p15.5	TYH, TH	C	Tyrosine hydroxylase	191290	distal to HRAS1		7(Th)
11p15.5	WT2, WTCR2	P	Wilms tumor region-2	194090		Wilms tumor, type 2 (2)	
11p15.5-p15.4	HPX	C	Hemopexin	142290			
11p15.5-p15.3	LDHC	C	Lactate dehydrogenase C	150150	closely linked to LDHB in other species; in man syntenic with LDHA; ?close to LDHA		

Location	Symbol	Status	Title	MIM #	Comments	Disorder	Mouse
11p15.4	CALCA, CALC1	C	Calcitonin/calcitonin gene related peptide, alpha polypeptide	114130			7(Calc)
11p15.4-p15.1	MYF3, MYOD1	C	Myogenic factor-3	159970			
11p15	CTSD, CPSD	P	Cathepsin D	116840			
11p15	HPFH, FCP, HHPF	L	F-cell production	142470	ca.15cM from HBB; ?on Xq28	Heterocellular hereditary persistence of fetal hemoglobin (2)	
11p15	MER2	P	Red blood cell antigen MER2	179620			
11p15	MUC2	P	Mucin 2, intestinal	158370			
11p15	PTH	C	Parathyroid hormone	168450		?Hypoparathyroidism, familial (1)	7(Pth)
11p15	RRM1	P	Ribonucleotide reductase, M1 subunit	180410			
11p15-p14	LDHA	C	Lactate dehydrogenase A	150000	ca.9cM distal to CALC1	Exertional myoglobinuria due to deficiency of LDH-A (1)	7(Ldh-1)
11p15-p13	TPN, TRH1, TRPH	P	Tryptophan hydroxylase (tryptophan-5-monooxygenase)	191060			
11p14.3-p12	ST2	P	Suppressor of transformation/tumorigenicity-2	185440			
11p14.2-p12	CALCB, CALC2	C	Calcitonin gene related peptide beta	114160			
11p14-p13	CD59	P	Antigen CD59	107271			
11p14-p13	HVBS1, HBVS1	P	Hepatitis B virus integration site-1	114550		Liver cell carcinoma (1)	
11p13	AN2	C	Aniridia-2	106210	cen-CAT-WT-AN-pter distal to AN2	Aniridia-2 (2)	?2(Sey)
11p13	CAT	C	Catalase	115500		Acatalasemia (1)	2(Cas-1)
11p13	FSHB	C	Follicle stimulating hormone, beta polypeptide	136530		?Male infertility, familial (1)	2(Fshb)
11p13	TCL2	P	T-cell leukemia/lymphoma-2	151390	involved in t(11;14)(p15;q11.2); between HRAS1 and INS/IGF2	Leukemia, acute T-cell (2)	
11p13	WAGR, WTCR1	C	Wilms tumor/aniridia/gonadoblastoma/retardation complex	194070	actually clump of pter-FSHB-AN2-WT-CAT	Wilms tumor (2); Aniridia of WAGR syndrome (2); Gonadoblastoma (2); Mental retardation of WAGR (2)	
11p13-q13	ROM, ROSP1	P	Rod outer segment protein-1	180721			19(Rosp-1)
11p12-p11.22	SP1	P	Oncogene SP1	165170			
11p12-p11	ACP2	C	Acid phosphatase-2	171650		?Lysosomal acid phosphatase deficiency (1)	2(Acp-2)
11p11.2	TYRL	P	Tyrosinase-like	191270			
11p11-q12	F2	C	Prothrombin (clotting factor II)	176930		Hypoprothrombinemia (1); Dysprothrombinemia (1)	
11p	MDU3, INLU	P	Lutheran inhibitor, dominant (monoclonal antibody A3D8)	111150			
11q	NACAE, MDU1, M4F2	C	Sodium-calcium exchanger	158070			
11q	OSBP	P	Oxysterol binding protein	167040			19(Osbp)
11q	PC	P	Pyruvate carboxylase	266150		Pyruvate carboxylase deficiency (1)	
11q11-q13	C1NH, C1I, HANE	C	C1 inhibitor	106100		Angioedema, hereditary (1)	
11q11-q23	CLG, EBR1, CLGN	C	Collagenase (recessive epidermolysis bullosa dystrophica)	226600		Epidermolysis bullosa dystrophica, recessive (3)	

Location	Symbol		Title	MIM number	Comments	Disorder	Mouse
11q12-q13	APY, IGEL	P	Atopy (allergic asthma and rhinitis; immunoglobulin E level)	147050		Atopy (2)	
11q12-q13	CD20	P	Antigen CD20 (differentiation antigen B1)	112210			19(Cd20)
11q12-q13	COX8	P	Cytochrome c oxidase, subunit VIII	123870			
11q12.1-q13.5	FNL2	P	Fibronectin-like-2	135610			
11q12-qter	CD15	P	Myeloid-associated surface antigen CD15	159470			
11q13	CD5, LEU1	C	Lymphocyte antigen CD5	153340			19(Ly-1)
11q13	GST3	C	Glutathione-S-transferase-3	138370	formerly called GST1		9(Gsta)
11q13	HST, FGFR, HST1	C	Oncogene HST (fibroblast growth factor related)	164980	coamplified with INT2 in melanoma		
11q13	INT2	C	Oncogene INT2	164950	35kb 5' to HST1		7(Int-2)
11q13	MEN1	C	Multiple endocrine neoplasia I	131100	linked to PYGM	Multiple endocrine neoplasia I (1)	
11q13	PGA	C	PEPSINOGEN A CLUSTER	169700	about 20cM from CAT		
11q13	PGA3	C	Pepsinogen A3	169710			
11q13	PGA4	C	Pepsinogen A4	169720			
11q13	PGA5	C	Pepsinogen A5	169730	pter-5'HRAS--5'INS--cen		
11q13	PYGM, MGP	C	Muscle glycogen phosphorylase	232600		McArdle disease (1)	19(Pygm)
11q13	SEA	P	Oncogene SEA (S13 avian erythroblastosis)	165110	related to heterogametic sex		
11q13-q14	BKMA	P	BKM, banded krait minor satellite, DNA	see 109780			
11q13-q22	ESA4	C	Esterase-A4	133220			9(Es-17)
11q13-q23	TSHL	P	Tumor suppressor gene, HELA cell type	191181			
11q13-qter	GANAB	P	Neutral alpha-glucosidase AB	104160			
11q13-qter	MSK39	P	Antigen defined by monoclonal antibody 5.1H11	107240			
11q13.3	BCL1	C	B-cell leukemia-1; chronic lymphocytic leukemia	151400	t(11;14)--(q13.3;q32.3)	Leukemia/lymphoma, B-cell, 1 (2)	
11q14-q21	CPD3	L	Cerebellar ataxia	213200	?linked to ATN		
11q14-q21	TYR, ATN	C	Tyrosinase (albinism, tyrosinase negative)	203100	?linked to CPD3	Albinism (3)	7(c)
11q22	PGR	C	Progesterone receptor	264080	11q13 = earlier regionalization		9(Pgr)
11q22-q23	AT1	P	Ataxia-telangiectasia	208900		Ataxia-telangiectasia (2)	
11q22-qter	ANC	L	Anal canal carcinoma	105580	3p22 also deleted	Anal canal carcinoma (2)	
11q22.3	THY1	C	Thy-1 T-cell antigen	188230	11q23 = conflicting localization		9(Thy-1)
11q22.3-q23.1	CRYA2	P	Crystallin, alpha-B	123590			
11q23	CD3D, CD3, T3D	C	T3 T-cell antigen receptor, delta polypeptide	186790	3 CD3 genes in 50kb		9(T3d)
11q23	CD3E, TCRE, T3D	P	T3 T-cell antigen receptor, epsilon polypeptide	186830			9(T3e)
11q23	CD3G	C	T3 T-cell antigen receptor, gamma polypeptide	186740			9(T3g)
11q23	DRD2	P	Dopamine receptor, D2	126450	11q22-q23 juncture defective in "staggerer," a form of cerebellar ataxia in mice		
11q23	NCAM	C	Neural cell adhesion molecule	116930	?defect in NCAM		9(Ncam)
11q23	STMY	C	Stromelysin	185250			
11q23	TSC2	P	Tuberous sclerosis-2	191090		Tuberous sclerosis-2 (2)	

Location	Symbol	Status	Title	MIM #	Comments	Disorder	Mouse
11q23-qter	APOLP1	C	APOLIPOPROTEIN CLUSTER I		11q13 = earlier assignment		
11q23-qter	APOA1	C	Apolipoprotein A-I	107680		ApoA-I and apoC-III deficiency, combined (1); Hypertriglyceridemia, 1 form (1); Hypoalphalipoproteinemia (1); Amyloidosis, Iowa form 105100 (1)	9(Apl-1)
11q23-qter	APOC3	C	Apolipoprotein C-III	107720	2.6kb 3' to APOA1		
11q23-qter	APOA4	C	Apolipoprotein A-IV	107690	12 kb 3' to APOA1		9(Apoa-4)
11q23.1	EBVM1	P	Epstein-Barr virus modification site-1	132860			
11q23.2-qter	PBGD, UPS	C	Porphobilinogen deaminase (uroporphyrinogen I synthase)	176000		Porphyria, acute intermittent (1)	9(Ups)
11q23.3-qter	CBL2	P	Cas-Br-M ectropic retroviral transforming sequence (Oncogene CBL2)	165360			
11q24	ETS1	C	Oncogene ETS-1	164720	shown by HSR		9(Ets-1)
11q24-q25	SRPR	P	Signal recognition particle receptor	182180			
Chr.11	ADX	P	Adrenodoxin	103260	pseudogene on 20		
Chr.11	CD6, TP120	P	T-cell differentiation antigen CD6	186720			
Chr.11	FCT3A	P	Alpha-3-fucosyltransferase	104230			
Chr.11	FRV1	P	Full-length endogenous retroviral sequence-2	136840			
Chr.11	FTH	P	Ferritin, heavy chain	134770			
Chr.11	GLAU1	L	Congenital glaucoma-1	231300	see chr. 3	Glaucoma, congenital (2)	
Chr.11	HV1S	P	Herpes virus sensitivity	142450			
Chr.11	LEU7, HNK1	P	Leu-7 antigen of natural killer lymphocytes, HNK-1	151290			
Chr.11	NANTA3	P	Alpha-3-acetylneuraminyltransferase	104240			
Chr.11	TRV2	P	Truncated endogenous retroviral sequence-2	190950			

In addition: 19 surface antigens, most defined by monoclonals, 1 O'Farrell protein spot, 5 'like' genes, 6 pseudogenes and 8 fragile sites (HGM10). 11p physical map (HGM9): Cen--CAT--FSHB--LDHA--CALC1--PTH--HBBC--INS--HRAS1--pter. Genetic map (HGM9): Cen--CAT--18%--CALC1--8%--PTH--12%--HBBC--10%--INS--30%--HRAS1--pter; ?linkage heterogeneity (polymorphism) raised by some discrepant results. Map of apolipoprotein cluster I: ?11qter cen or 11qter 5'--APOA1-3'--(2.6kb)--3'--APOC3-5'--(4.5kb)--5'--APOA4-3'--?11cen or 11qter.

Chromosome No. 12

Location	Symbol	Status	Title	MIM #	Comments	Disorder	Mouse
12pter-p12	F8VWF, VWF	C	von Willebrand factor	193400		von Willebrand disease (1)	
12pter-p12	CD4, T4, LEU3	C	T-cell antigen CD4	186940	CD = 'cluster of differentiation' = nomenclature of leukocyte differentiation antigens		
12pter-q12	BCT1	C	Branched chain amino acid transaminase-1	113520		?Hyperleucinemia-isoleucinemia or hypervalinemia (1)	
12p13.31-p13.1	GAPD	C	Glyceraldehyde-3-phosphate dehydrogenase	138400			6(Gapd)
12p13.3	GLUT3	P	Glucose transporter-3	138170			
12p13.3-p12.3	A2M	P	Alpha-2-macroglobulin	103950			
12p13.2	SPC, PRP	P	SALIVARY PROLINE-RICH PROTEIN COMPLEX		cluster of genes		6(Prp)
12p13.2	G1, PRB3	C	Paroid salivary glycoprotein	168840	6 loci in 2 subfamilies; in 500 kb: PRH1, PRH2, PRB1, PRB2, = PRB3 in basic subfamily		
12p13.2	PE, PRB1	P	Salivary protein Pe	180970			
12p13.2	PM	C	Parotid middle band protein	168780	linked to PRH1, PRH2, G1		
12p13.2	PRH1	C	Proline-rich acidic protein, HaeIII type, 1	168730	PA, DB, PIF alleles		
12p13.2	PRH2, PR	C	Proline-rich acidic protein, HaeIII type, 2	168790			
12p13.2	PS	C	Parotid size variant	168810			
12p13.2	PB	C	Parotid basic protein	168750			
12p13.2	PPB	C	Post-parotid basic protein	168760			
12p13.2	CON1, PRB4	C	Salivary protein CON1	168870	close to PS; ?order: PS-PR-PM-G1-DB		
12p13.2	CON2	C	Salivary protein CON2	168880	close to PM		
12p13.2	PO	P	Salivary protein Po	180990	probably closely linked to CON2		
12p13.2	PCS, PC	P	Parotid proline-rich protein Pc	168710	linked to PS		
12p13	MPE, EMP	L	Eosinophils, malignant proliferation of	131440		?Eosinophilic myeloproliferative disorder (2)	
12p13	C1R	C	Complement component C1r	216950		C1r/C1s deficiency, combined (1)	
12p13	C1S	C	Complement component C1s	120580		C1r/C1s deficiency, combined (1)	
12p13	CD9, MIC3	C	Antigen CD9 identified by monoclonal antibodies 602-29, BA-2, et al.	143030			
12p13	GNB3	P	Guanine nucleotide binding protein, beta-3 polypeptide	139130			
12p13	TPI1, TPI	C	Triosephosphate isomerase	190450		Hemolytic anemia due to triosephosphate isomerase deficiency (1)	6(Tpi-1)

Location	Symbol	Status	Title	MIM #	Comments	Disorder	Mouse
12q13-p12.2	PZP	P	Pregnancy zone protein	176420			
12q13-q12	ATPSB, ATPMB	C	Adenosine triphosphate synthase, mitochondrial, beta polypeptide	102910			
12p12.2-p12.1	LDHB	C	Lactate dehydrogenase B	150100			6(Ldh-2)
12p12.1	KRAS2, RASK2	C	Oncogene Kras-2, Kirsten rat sarcoma virus	190070		Colorectal adenoma (1); ?Colorectal cancer (1)	6(Kras-2)
12p12.1-p11.2	PTHLH	P	Parathyroid hormone-like hormone	168470			6(Pthlh)
12p11.2-q11	KRT4, CYK4	C	Cytokeratin 4	123940			
12p11-qter	CS	C	Citrate synthase, mitochondrial	118950			10(Cs)
12p11-qter	ENO2	C	Enolase-2	131360	by A, pter-p13		
12p	KAR	L	Aromatic alpha-keto acid reductase	107920	?same as MDH1 on proximal 12p		
12p	ELA1	C	Elastase-1	130120	conflicting localization = 12p12.3		15(Ela-1)
12cen-q14	IAPP, IAP, DAP	C	Islet amyloid polypeptide (diabetes-associated peptide; amylin)	147940			
12cen-q14	MIP	P	Major intrinsic protein of lens fiber	154050			
12q	RARG	P	Retinoic acid receptor, gamma	180190			15(Rar-g)
12q11-q13	FNRA	P	Fibronectin receptor, alpha polypeptide	135620			
12q11-q21	KRTA	P	Keratin, acid or alpha-	139350	close to Hox-3 in mouse		15(Krta)
12q12-q13	INT1	C	Oncogene INT1, murine mammary cancer virus	164820			15(Int-1)
12q12-q13	MLA1	P	Melanoma-associated antigen ME491	155740			
12q12-q14	SHMT, GLYA	C	Serine hydroxymethyltransferase	138450	glycine A auxotroph probably 1 gene; 3 homeoboxes in 1 transcription unit		
12q13	HOX3	C	Homeo box-3	142970			15(Hox-3)
12q13	LALBA	P	Lactalbumin, alpha	149750			
12q13-q14	BABL, LIPO	C	Lipoma (breakpoint in benign lipoma); myxoid liposarcoma	151900	?recombination 12q13 and 16p11 for myxoid liposarcoma, 152410	Lipoma (2); Myxoid liposarcoma (2); ?Multiple lipomatosis (2)	
12q13-q21	NKNB	P	Neurokinin B	162330			
12q13.1-q13.3	COL2A1	C	Collagen II, alpha-1 chain	120140	conflicting: 12q14.3	Stickler syndrome (3); Spondyloepiphyseal dysplasia congenita (3); ?Kniest dysplasia (1); Langer-Saldino achondrogenesis-hypochondrogenesis (1); Osteoarthrosis, precocious (3)	
12q13.2-q13.3	GLI1	C	Oncogene GLI1	165220			
12q14	GNS, G6S	P	N-acetylglucosamine-6-sulfatase	252940		Sanfilippo syndrome D (1)	
12q14	RAP1B	P	RAS-related protein RAP1B	179530			
12q14	VDD1	C	Vitamin D dependency, type I	264700		Vitamin D dependency, type I (2)	
12q21	PEPB	C	Peptidase B	169900			10(Pep-2)
12q22-q23	HIS, HSTD	C	Histidase	235800		[Histidinemia] (1)	10(Hstd)
12q22-q24.1	IGF1	C	Insulin-like growth factor I, or somatomedin C	147440			
12q22-qter	ACADS	P	Acyl-CoA dehydrogenase, short chain	201470		Acyl-CoA dehydrogenase, short chain, deficiency of (1)	5(Bcd-1)
12q24.1	IFNG, IFI, IFG	C	Interferon, gamma or immune type	147570	3 introns; IFF, IFL none	Interferon, immune, deficiency (1)	10(Ifg)

Location	Symbol		Name	MIM no.	Disorder	Mouse
12q24.1	PAH, PKU1	C	Phenylalanine hydroxylase	261600	Phenylketonuria (3); [Hyperphenylalaninemia, mild] (3)	10(Pah)
12q24.2	ALDH2	C	Aldehyde dehydrogenase, mitochondrial	100650	Acute alcohol intolerance (1); ?Fetal alcohol syndrome (1)	4(Aldh-2)
Chr.12	ATP2B	P	ATPase, CA++ dependent, slow twitch/cardiac muscle	108740	?Brody myopathy (1)	
Chr.12	FRV3	P	Full-length endogenous retroviral sequence-3	136890		
Chr.12	GNAI2A, GNAIH	P	Guanine nucleotide binding protein, alpha inhibiting, polypeptide h (or polypeptide 2A)	139180		
Chr.12	GPD1	P	Alpha-glycerophosphate dehydrogenase; glycerol-3-phosphate dehydrogenase	138420		15(Gdc-1)
Chr.12	LYS, LYZ	P	Lysozyme	153450		
Chr.12	MPRD	P	Mannose-6-phosphate receptor, cation-dependent	154540		
Chr.12	MTRNS, MARS, METRS	P	Methioninyl-tRNA synthetase	156560		
Chr.12	MYF5	P	Myogenic factor-5	159990		
Chr.12	NTS	P	Neurotensin	162650		
Chr.12	OIAS	C	2',5'-oligoisoadenylate synthetase	164350		
Chr.12	PFKX	P	Phosphofructokinase X	171880		15(Pfkx)
Chr.12	PPLA2	P	Phospholipase A2, pancreatic	172410		
Chr.12	TRV3	P	Truncated endogenous retroviral sequence-3	190960		

In addition: 7 surface antigens, most defined by monoclonals, 3 O'Farrell protein spots, 3 'like' genes, 1 pseudogene and 5 fragile sites (HGM10). Probable order: 12pter--TPI1--GAPD--LDHB--ENO2--cen--SHMT--PEPB--12qter

93

Chromosome No. 13

Location	Symbol	Status	Title	MIM #	Comments	Disorder	Mouse
13p12	RNR1	C	Ribosomal RNA	180450			
13q12	FLT	P	Oncogene FLT (FMS-like tyrosine kinase)	165070			
13q14	XRS	L	X-ray sensitivity	194370			
13q14-q21	WND, WD	C	Wilson disease	277900	vs. ESD, max. lod = 5.49, theta = 0.03; distal to RB1	Wilson disease (2)	
13q14-q31	LSD	L	Letterer-Siwe disease	246400		?Letterer-Siwe disease (2)	
13q14.1	OSRC	P	Osteosarcoma	259500	probably same locus as retinoblastoma	Osteosarcoma, retinoblastoma-related (2)	
13q14.1-q14.2	RB1	C	Retinoblastoma-1	180200		Retinoblastoma (2)	14(Rb-1)
13q14.1-q14.3	LCP1	P	Lymphocyte cytosolic protein-1	153430			
13q14.11	ESD, FGH	C	Esterase D: S-formylglutathione hydrolase	133280	proximal to RB1, WND		14(Es-10)
13q21-q31	ATP1AL2	P	Sodium-potassium-ATPase, alpha-polypeptide-like	182360			
13q22-q34	ERCC5	C	Excision-repair, complementing defective, in Chinese hamster, number 5	133530			
13q22.1-q32.1	MGC	L	Megacolon (Hirschsprung disease)	249200	?linked to factors VII and X	?Megacolon (2)	
13q34	CBT1	L	Carotid body tumor-1	168000			
13q34	COL4A1	C	Collagen IV, alpha-1 chain	120130			
13q34	COL4A2	C	Collagen IV, alpha-2 chain	120090			
13q34	DJS	L	Dubin-Johnson syndrome	237500	with factor VII deficiency	?Dubin-Johnson syndrome (2)	
13q34	F7	C	Clotting factor VII	227500		Factor VII deficiency (1)	
13q34	F10	C	Clotting factor X	227600		Factor X deficiency (1)	
13q34	HHHS	L	Hyperornithinemia-hyperammonemia-homocitrullinemia syndrome	238970	associated with deficiency of factors VII and X in 3 unrelated cases	?HHH syndrome (2)	
13q34	RAP2	P	RAP2, member of RAS oncogene family (K-rev)	179540			
Chr.13	BRCD1, DBC, BCDS1	P	Breast cancer, ductal, suppressor-1	211410	evidence of 1p determinants	Breast cancer, ductal (2)	
Chr.13	PCCA	P	Propionyl CoA carboxylase, alpha subunit	232000		Propionicacidemia, type I or pccA type (1)	
Chr.13	TRV5	P	Truncated retroviral sequence-5	190980			
Chr.13	UVDR, ERCM2	P	UV-damage, excision repair of (XP complementation group I)	192060	also called UV-135	?Xeroderma pigmentosum, one type (1)	

In addition: 3 'like' genes, 4 pseudogenes and 3 fragile sites (HGM10).

Chromosome No. 14

Location	Symbol	Status	Title	MIM #	Comments	Disorder	Mouse
14p12	RNR2	C	Ribosomal RNA	180450			
14q11	TCRD	P	T-cell antigen receptor, delta subunit	186810			
14q11-q12	TRNP1, TRLPT	C	Transfer RNA cluster-1 (Pro-Leu-Pro-Thr)	189930			
14q11-q13	ANG	P	Angiogenin	105850			
14q11.2	CTLA1	P	Cytotoxic-T-lymphocyte-associated serine esterase-1	123910			14(Ctla-1)
14q11.2	CTSG	P	Cathepsin G	116830			
14q11.2	TCRA	C	T-cell antigen receptor, alpha subunit	186880	cen--V-C--ter	Leukemia/lymphoma, T-cell (3)	14(Tcra)
14q11.2-q13	MYH6, MYHCA	C	Myosin, heavy polypeptide 6, cardiac muscle, alpha	160710			?11(Myh)
14q11.2-q13	MYH7, MYHCB	P	Myosin, heavy polypeptide-7, cardiac muscle, beta	160760	5'-B-4.5kb-A-3'		
14q13.1	NP, NP1	C	Nucleoside phosphorylase	164050	centromeric to TCRA	Nucleoside phosphorylase deficiency, immunodeficiency due to (2)	14(Np-1,2)
14q21-q31	FOS	C	Oncogene FOS (FBJ murine osteosarcoma virus)	164810			12(Fos)
14q21-qter	WARS	C	Tryptophanyl-tRNA synthetase	191050			
14q22-q23.2	SPTB, SPH1	C	Beta-spectrin (spherocytosis-1)	182870		Elliptocytosis-3 (2); Spherocytosis-1 (3)	12(Spb)
14q22-qter	ADEB	P	Phosphoribosylformylglycinamidine synthetase (adenine (-)B auxotroph)	see 172460	?separate from ADEE locus		
14q23-q24.2	HOS	L	Holt-Oram syndrome	142900		?Holt-Oram syndrome (2)	
14q24	CAP	L	Cataract, anterior polar	115650	see 2p25	?Cataract, anterior polar (2)	
14q24	MTHFD, MTHFC, PGFT	C	5,10-methylenetetrahydrofolate dehydrogenase, 5,10-methenyltetrahydrofolatecyclohydrolase	172460	trifunctional protein		
14q24	TGFB3	P	Transforming growth factor beta-3	190230			12(Tgf-b3)
14q32	CHGA	C	Chromogranin A (parathyroid secretory protein 1)	118910			
14q32	CKBB	C	Creatine kinase, brain type	123280	distal to PI and AACT; closely linked to AKT1		
14q32	CKBE	P	Creatine kinase, brain type, ectopic expression of	123270	linked to IGH, PI; ?same locus as CKBB	[Creatine kinase, brain type, ectopic expression of] (2)	
14q32	VP, PPOX	P	Porphyria variegata (protoporphyrinogen oxidase)	176200		Porphyria variegata (2)	
14q32.1	AACT	C	Alpha-1-antichymotrypsin	107280	220kb from PI	Alpha-1-antichymotrypsin deficiency (1)	
14q32.1	PI, AAT	C	Protease inhibitor (alpha-1-antitrypsin)	107400		Emphysema-cirrhosis (1); Hemorrhagic diathesis due to 'antithrombin' Pittsburgh (1)	12(Aat)
14q32.1	TCL1	C	T-cell lymphoma-1	186960		Leukemia/lymphoma, T-cell (2)	

Location	Symbol	Status	Title	MIM #	Comments	Disorder	Mouse
14q32.3	AKT1	C	Oncogene AKT1	164730	proximal to IGH; ?identical to TCL1		12(Akt)
14q32.3	ELK2	P	Oncogene ELK-2	165350			
14q32.33	IGH	C	IMMUNOGLOBULIN HEAVY CHAIN GENE CLUSTER				12(Igh)
14q32.33	IGHR	L	Immunoglobulin heavy chain regulator	144120		?Combined variable hypogammaglobulinemia (1)	
14q32.33	IGHV	C	V (variable) region of heavy chains	147070	ca. 250 genes; orientation: cen-PI-D14S1-IGH-IGHV--qter; 3' centromeric, 5' telomeric; IgM telomeric to IgG	?Hyperimmunoglobulin G1 syndrome (2)	
14q32.33	IGD1	C	D (diversity) region of heavy chains	146910	many genes		
14q32.33	IGHJ	C	J (joining) region of heavy chains	147010	more than 4 genes		
14q32.33	IGHM, MU	C	Constant region of heavy chain of IgM	147020			
14q32.33	IGHD	C	Constant region of heavy chain of IgD	147170			
14q32.33	IGHG2	C	Constant region of heavy chain of IgG2	147110	5'-G2-17kb-G4-3'; closeness of IGG3 and IGG1 known from Lepore-like myeloma protein		
14q32.33	IGHG4	C	Constant region of heavy chain of IgG4	147130			
14q32.33	IGHG3	C	Constant region of heavy chain of IgG3	147120			
14q32.33	IGHG1	C	Constant region of heavy chain of IgG1	147100			
14q32.33	IGHE	C	Constant region of heavy chain of IgE	147180			
14q32.33	IGHEP1	C	Constant region of heavy chain of IgEP1	147160	IGEP2 on chr. 9; 147210		
14q32.33	IGHA1	C	Constant region of heavy chain of IgA1	146900			
14q32.33	IGHA2	C	Constant region of heavy chain of IgA2	147000			
Chr.14	CSPB	P	Serine protease B	182130			
Chr.14	ESAT	P	Esterase activator	133250			
Chr.14	FPSL3	P	Farnesylpyrophosphate synthetase-3	134633			
Chr.14	K12T	C	Temperature sensitivity complementation, K12	187310			
Chr.14	LCH	C	Lentil agglutinin binding	151020			
Chr.14	M195	P	External membrane protein-195	133740			
Chr.14	PYGL, PPYL	P	Liver glycogen phosphorylase	232700		Hers disease, or glycogen storage disease VI (1)	12(Pygl)
Chr.14	RIB1	L	Pancreatic ribonuclease	180440	?close to TCRA and NP		14(Rib-1)
Chr.14	TRV1	P	Truncated endogenous retroviral sequence-1	190940			

In addition: 1 antigen defined by monoclonal, 3 'like' genes, 4 pseudogenes and 2 fragile sites (HGM10). A Tunisian deletion indicates order: 5'--G3--G1--psi E1--A1--G2--G4--E--A2--3' (Lefranc et al., Nature 300: 760, 1982). Following information from M. J. Johnson and L. L. Cavalli-Sforza, Stanford Univ., Nov., 1983 and Hofker et al., PNAS 86: 5567, 1989: 5'(qter)--V--(7cM)--D--J--8kb--mu--5kb--delta--60kb--gamma-3--26kb--gamma-1--19kb--pseudo-epsilon-1 --13kb--alpha--1--80kb--gamma-2--18kb--gamma-4--23kb--epsilon--10kb--alpha-2--3'(centromere). Pseudo-gamma between alpha-1 and gamma-2 (Bech-Hansen et al., PNAS 80:6952, 1983; Migone et al., PNAS 81: 5811, 1984), about 35 kb from alpha-1. Comparable data in mouse for genes for kappa, lambda, and heavy chains of immunoglobulin and for T-cell alpha-, beta-, and gamma-genes are given in Figure 2 of Kronenberg et al., Ann Rev Immunol 4:529-591, 1986. See review in report of Keyeux et al., Genomics 5:431-441, 1989; they state the mu/delta interval as 8kb and refer to a gamma pseudogene between A1 and G2.

Chromosome No. 15

Location	Symbol	Status	Title	MIM #	Comments	Disorder	Mouse
15p12	RNR3	C	Ribosomal RNA	180450			
15p12-q21	SORD	C	Sorbitol dehydrogenase	182500			2(Sdh-1)
15q	NMB	P	Neuromedin B	162340			
15q11	DLX1	L	Dyslexia-1	127700	?near centromere; lod under 3.0 with HGM8 data	?Dyslexia-1 (2)	
15q11	PWCR, PWS	C	Prader-Willi syndrome	176270		Prader-Willi syndrome (2)	
15q11-q12	IGD2	P	Immunoglobulin heavy chain diversity region-2	146990	?functional		
15q11-q12	MIC7	P	Attached cell antigen 28.3.7	108990			
15q11-q13	ANCR, AGMS	P	Angelman syndrome	234400		Angelman syndrome (2)	
15q11-q13	ITO	L	Hypomelanosis of Ito	146150	see chr.9	?Hypomelanosis of Ito (2)	
15q11-q13	MANA	C	Alpha-mannosidase-A, cytoplasmic	154580			
15q11-q13	ACTC	P	Actin, cardiac alpha	102540			2(Actc-1)
15q11-qter	CVS, HCVS	P	Coronavirus 229E sensitivity	122460			
15q11-qter	P7B2	P	Pituitary polypeptide 7B2	173120			
15q13-q14	B2MR	C	Beta-2-microglobulin regulator	109710			
15q13-q15	IVD	P	Isovaleryl CoA dehydrogenase	243500		Isovalericacidemia (1)	
15q14-q15	FPSL4	P	Farnesylpyrophosphate synthetase-4	134634			
15q15-q21	CHR39B	P	Cholesterol repressible protein 39B	118480			
15q21-q22	B2M	C	Beta-2-microglobulin	109700	on 15q+ in APL	Hemodialysis-related amyloidosis (1)	2(B2m)
15q21-q22	LPC2D	P	Lipocortin IId	151740			
15q21-q23	LPC, LIPH, HL, HTGL	C	Hepatic triglyceride lipase	151670		?Hepatic lipase deficiency (1)	
15q21-qter	IDH2	C	Isocitrate dehydrogenase, mitochondrial	147650	close to CYP11 in mouse		7(Idh-2)
15q21.1	CYP19, ARO	C	Cytochrome P450 aromatization of androgen (aromatase)	107910		?Gynecomastia, familial, due to increased aromatase activity (1)	9(Cyp-19)
15q22	PK3, PKM2	C	Pyruvate kinase-3	179050			9(Pk-3)
15q22-q25.1	HEXA, TSD	C	Beta-hexosaminidase A, alpha chain	272800	on 15q+ in APL	Tay-Sachs disease (1); GM2-gangliosidosis, juvenile, adult (1); [Hex A pseudodeficiency] (1)	
15q22-q26	ACP5	P	Phosphatase, acid, type 5, tartrate-resistant	171640			
15q22-qter	CYP1A1, CYP1, P450C1	P	Dioxin-inducible P1-450 (TCDD-inducible P1-450)	108330	CYP2 = earlier symbol		9(P450-1)
15q22-qter	CYP1A2	P	Dioxin-inducible P3-450	124060	both CYP1 genes close to MPI in rodents		9(P450-1)
15q22-qter	MPI	C	Mannosephosphate isomerase	154550			9(Mpi-1)
15q23-q25	ETFA, GA2	P	Electron transfer flavoprotein, alpha subunit	231680		Glutaricaciduria, type II (1)	
15q23-q25	FAH	P	Fumarylacetoacetate	276700		Fumarylacetoacetate deficiency (1)	
15q24-q25	CTSH	P	Cathepsin H	116820		?Batten disease, 1 form, 204200 (1)	

Location	Symbol	Status	Title	MIM #	Comments	Disorder	Mouse
15q25-q26	FES	C	Oncogene FES, feline sarcoma virus	190030	?15q26; far from breakpoint in acute promyelocyte leukemia:t(15;17)(q22;q21)		7(Fes)
15q25-q26	FUR	C	Furin membrane associated receptor protein	136950	less than 1.1kb 5' to FES		
15q25-q26	IGF1R	P	Insulin-like growth factor-1 receptor	147370	?relation to FES		
15q25-q26	PEPN, CD13	C	Aminopeptidase N (antigen CD13, p150)	151530			
Chr.15	CHRNA, ACHRA	L	Cholinergic receptor, nicotinic, alpha polypeptide	100690	linked to Actc in mouse		17(?Achr-?)
Chr.15	CKMT	P	Creatine kinase, mitochondrial	123290			
Chr.15	COL1AR, COLR	P	Collagen, type 1, alpha, receptor	120340			
Chr.15	CSPG1	P	Chondroitin sulfate proteoglycan core protein	155760			
Chr.15	CYP11A, P450SCC, P450C11A1	P	P450 side chain cleavage enzyme (20,22 desmolase)	201710	?15q21.1 close to CYP11	Lipoid adrenal hyperplasia, congenital (1)	9(Cyp-11a)
Chr.15	GANC	P	Neutral alpha-glucosidase C	104180			
Chr.15	XPF	P	Xeroderma pigmentosum, group F	278760		Xeroderma pigmentosum, group F (2)	

In addition: 5 surface antigens, most defined by monoclonals, 2 O'Farrell protein spots, 2 pseudogenes and 1 fragile site (HGM10). Hemodialysis-related amyloidosis is presumably not genetic in a specific sense.

Chromosome No. 16

Location	Symbol	Status	Title	MIM #	Comments	Disorder	Mouse
16pter-p13.3	HBAC, ABC	C	ALPHA GLOBIN GENE CLUSTER		order: cen-APKD-HBZ1--HBA1-3'HVR-pter; distal to PGP		
16pter-p13.3	HBA1	C	Hemoglobin alpha-1	141800	1, 2, or 3 loci; 5'-zeta-pseudozeta-pseudoalpha-alpha-2-alpha-1-3'	Thalassemias, alpha- (1); Methemoglobinemias, alpha- (1); Erythremias, alpha- (1); Heinz body anemias, alpha- (1)	11(Hba)
16pter-p13.3	HBA2	C	Hemoglobin alpha-2	141850			11(Hba)
16pter-p13.3	HBQ1	P	Hemoglobin theta-1	142240			
16pter-p13.3	HBZ1	C	Hemoglobin zeta pseudogene (formerly zeta-1)	see 142310			
16pter-p13.3	HBZ2	C	Hemoglobin zeta (formerly zeta-2)	142310			
16pter-p13.3	HBHR	L	Hb H mental retardation syndrome	141750		Hb H mental retardation syndrome (2)	
16pter-p11	PDE1B	P	Phosphodiesterase-1B	171891			
16p13.31-p13.12	PGP	C	Phosphoglycolate phosphatase	172280	no recombination with PKD1		
16p13.31-p13.12	PKD1, APKD	C	Adult polycystic kidney disease	173900	rare form unlinked	Polycystic kidney disease (2)	
16p13.3-p13.13	ERCC4	P	Excision-repair, complementing defective, in Chinese hamster, number 4	133520			
16p13.1-p11	LAAC	C	LEUKOCYTE ADHESION, ALPHA, CLUSTER				
16q13.1-p11	CD11A, LFA1A	C	Lymphocyte function associated antigen-1, alpha subunit	153370			
16p13.1-p11	CD11C	P	Leukocyte surface antigen p150,95, alpha subunit	151510			
16p13.1-p11	CR3A, CD11B, MAC1A, MO1A	P	Complement component receptor-3 (Macrophage antigen-1, Mac-1, alpha subunit)	120980	?in same restriction fragment as LFA1A		
16p13	HAGH, GLO2	C	Glyoxalase II; hydroxyacyl glutathione hydrolase	138760		[Glyoxalase II deficiency] (1)	
16p11.2	PRKCB, PKCB	P	Protein kinase C, beta polypeptide	176970			
16p11.2	SPN, LSN, CD43	C	Sialophorin (leukosialin)	182160			
16p11-q23	CHE2	I	Cholinesterase, serum, 2	177500			
16p11-q24	UVO	P	Uvomorulin	192090	see chr. 2		8(Um)
16q12-q13.1	PHKB	P	Phosphorylase kinase, beta polypeptide	172490		?Phosphorylase kinase deficiency of liver and muscle, 261750 (2)	
16q12-q22	DIA4	C	Diaphorase-4	125860			
16q21	CETP	P	Cholesterol ester transfer protein, plasma	118470		CETP deficiency (1)	
16q21	CLG4	P	Collagenase, type IV	120360			
16q21	GOT2	C	Glutamate oxaloacetic transaminase, mitochondrial	138150	?pseudogenes on 12 and 1		8(Got-2)
16q21	PRM1	P	Sperm protamine P1	182880			16(Prm-1)
16q21	PRM2	L	Sperm protamine P2	182890			16(Prm-2)

99

Location	Symbol	Status	Title	MIM #	Comments	Disorder	Mouse
16q21-q23	CA7	P	Carbonic anhydrase VII	114770			
16q22	MT1	C	METALLOTHIONEIN I CLUSTER	156350			8(Mt-1)
16q22	MT2	C	METALLOTHIONEIN II CLUSTER	156360			8(Mt-2)
16q22	NCL, BD	C	Neuronal ceroid-lipofuscinosis (Batten disease)	204200	linked to HP	Batten disease (2)	
16q22-q24	ALDOA, ALDA	C	Aldolase A	103850		?Aldolase A deficiency (1)	
16q22.1	CA4	P	Carbonic anhydrase IV	114760	not proved to be expressed		
16q22.1	CPM, CAM	C	Cataract, Marner type	116800		Cataract, Marner type (2)	8(Hp)
16q22.1	HP	C	Haptoglobin	140100	just distal to fra16q22.1		
16q22.1	HPR	C	Haptoglobin-related locus	140210	2.2kb 3' to HP; multiple tandem genes in blacks		
16q22.1	LCAT	C	Lecithin-cholesterol acyltransferase	245900	very close to HP	Norum disease (3)	8(Lcat)
16q22.1-q22.3	TAT	C	Tyrosine aminotransferase, cytosolic	276600		Tyrosinemia, type II (1)	8(Tat-1)
16q22.3	CTRB	C	Chymotrypsinogen B	118890	HP-7cM-TAT-9cM-CTRB		8(Ctrb)
16q24	APRT	C	Adenine phosphoribosyltransferase	102600	distal to GOT2, DIA4; earlier mapped to 16q22.2-q22.3	Urolithiasis, 2,8-dihydroxyadenine (1)	8(Aprt)
Chr.16	ATP2A	P	ATPase, Ca++ transporting, fast-twitch, muscle	108730			
Chr.16	CTH	P	Cystathionase	219500		[Cystathioninuria] (1)	
Chr.16	DIP1, VDI	P	Vesicular stomatitis virus defective interfering particle repressor	125260			
Chr.16	ESB3	P	Esterase-B3	133290			
Chr.16	GCF2	P	Growth rate controlling factor-2	139230			
Chr.16	GRLL	P	Glucocorticoid receptor, lymphocyte, like	138060			
Chr.16	LIPB	P	Lysosomal acid lipase-B	247980			
Chr.16	NHCP1	P	Nonhistone chromosomal protein-1	118870			
Chr.16	TK2	P	Thymidine kinase, mitochondrial	188250			

In addition: 3 'like' genes, 3 pseudogenes and 5 fragile sites (HGM10). Order: pter--PGP--0.25--16qh--0.17--GOT2--0.08--HP--qter [Jeremiah et al., Ann. Hum. Genet. 46: 145, 1982).

Chromosome No. 17

Location	Symbol	Status	Title	MIM #	Comments	Disorder	Mouse
17pter-p21	TRNP2	P	Transfer RNA cluster-2 (Leu-Gln-Lys)	189920			11(Zfp-1)
17pter-p12	ZFP3	P	Zinc finger protein-3	194480			11(Mds)
17pter-p11	ENO3	P	Enolase-3, beta, muscle	131370			
17p13.3	MDCR, MDLS, MDS	C	Miller-Dieker lissencephaly syndrome	247200		Miller-Dieker lissencephaly syndrome (2)	
17p13.105-p12	POLR2, RPOL2, RNP2	C	RNA polymerase II, large subunit	180660			11(Rpol-2)
17p13.105-p12	TP53	C	Tumor protein p53	191170		Colorectal carcinoma, 114500 (1)	11(Trp53)
17p13	GLUT4	P	Glucose transporter, insulin-responsive	138190			11(Myh)
17p13	MYH1	C	MYOSIN, HEAVY CHAIN CLUSTER		a myosin gene cluster also on 7		
17p13	MYH1, MYHSA1	C	Myosin heavy chain, skeletal, adult-1	160730			
17p13	MYH2, MYHSA2	C	Myosin heavy chain, skeletal, adult-2	160740	17p13.105-p12		
17p13	MYH3, MYHSE1	C	Myosin heavy chain, embryonic-1	160720			
17p12	CRCR2, CRC17	P	Colorectal caarcinoma 2 (colorectal cancer-related sequence-17)	120460	?same as TP53	Colorectal cancer, 114500 (2)	
17p12-p11	CHRNB, ACHRB	C	Cholinergic receptor, nicotinic, beta polypeptide	100710	linked to Myh on mouse 11		11(?Achr-?)
17p11.2	SMCR	C	Smith-Magenis syndrome chromosome region	182290			
17p11.2-q23	CMT1A	C	Charcot-Marie-Tooth disease, slow nerve conduction type Ia	118220	?on proximal 17p	Charcot-Marie-Tooth disease, slow nerve conduction type Ia (2)	
17p11.1-qter	PNP, PPY	P	Pancreatic polypeptide	167780			
17p11-qter	ACTG	P	Cytoskeletal gamma-actin	102560			
17cen-q12	ALDOC, ALDC	C	Aldolase C	103870			
17cen-q25	ADXR	P	Adrenodoxin reductase	103270			
17cen-qter	GAS	C	Gastrin	137250			
17cen-qter	HTLVR	P	Receptor for HTLV-1 and HTLV-2	143090			
17q11-q12	EDHB17	P	Estradiol 17-beta-dehydrogenase	264300		Pseudohermaphroditism, male, with gynecomastia (1); Polycystic ovarian disease (1)	
17q11-q23	KRTB, CYK15	C	Keratin, basic or beta- (cytokeratin 15)	148030	tightly linked to Hox-2 in mouse; probable cluster of CYK genes		11(Krb)
17q11-q21	TCP228	P	T-cell specific protein p288	180710	?related gene at 5q31-q34		
17q11.1-q12	CRYB1	C	Crystallin, beta-B1	123610			
17q11.2	ERBA1, THRA	C	Oncogene ERB-A1 (avian erythroblastic leukemia virus)	190120	centromeric to NF1		11(Erba)
17q11.2	EVI2	P	Murine myeloid leukemia associated gene, human homolog of	158380			
17q11.2	NF1, VRNF	C	Neurofibromatosis, von Recklinghausen type	162200	?linked to GALK	Neurofibromatosis, von Recklinghausen (2)	

Location	Symbol	Status	Title	MIM #	Comments	Disorder	Mouse
17q11.2	WSS	L	Watson syndrome	193520	?allele at NF1 locus	?Watson syndrome (2)	
17q11.2-q12	CSF3, GCSF	C	Granulocyte colony-stimulating factor-3	138970			
17q12-q21.32	ERBB2	C	Oncogene ERB-B2	190150			
17q12-q22	PTMS	P	Parathymosin	168440			
17q21	ACC	P	Acetyl-CoA carboxylase	200350	proximal to q21.33	Acetyl-CoA carboxylase deficiency (1)	
17q21	MTBT1, MAPT1	P	Microtubule, beta, associated protein tau	157140	see 6p21		
17q21-q22	A12M4	C	Adenovirus-12 chromosome modification site-17	102970	in RNU2		
17q21-q22	EPB3, EMPB3	C	Erythroid membrane protein band 3	109270		[Acanthocytosis, 1 form] (1)	
17q21-q22	GALK	C	Galactokinase	230200	by CMGT, order = cen-GALK-TK1-COL1A1	Galactokinase deficiency (1)	11(Glk)
17q21-q22	HOX2, HU2	C	Homeo box-2	142960	5 or 6 genes, e.g., HOX2.1, HOX2.2		11(Hox-2)
17q21-q22	INT4	P	Oncogene INT-4 (murine mammary tumor virus integration site, v-int-4, oncogene homologue)	165330			11(Int-4)
17q21-q22	NGFR	C	Nerve growth factor receptor	162010	distal to APL breakpoint, q21; < 0.5mb from HOX2		
17q21-q22	NGL, NEU	C	Oncogene NGL (oncogene NEU, neuro- or glioblastoma derived; HER2; TKR1)	164870			
17q21-q22	RNU2	C	U2 snRNA GENE CLUSTER	180690			
17q21-q22	TOP2	P	DNA topoisomerase II	126430			
17q21.1	RARA	P	Retinoic acid receptor, alpha type	180240			
17q21.1-q21.3	GP3A	C	Platelet glycoprotein IIIa	173470	in same 260kb fragment as GP2B; PL(A) platelet antigen	Glanzmann thrombasthenia (1)	
17q21.3-q22	GIP	P	Gastric inhibitory polypeptide	137240			
17q21.3-q23	MPO	C	Myeloperoxidase	254600	translocated in t(15;17)(q22;q11.2)	Myeloperoxidase deficiency (1)	
17q21.31-q22.05	COL1A1	C	Collagen I, alpha-1 chain	120150	?proximal to GH1	Osteogenesis imperfecta, 2 or more clinical forms (3); Ehlers-Danlos syndrome, type VIIA1 (3); ?Marfan syndrome, atypical, 154700(1)	11(Cola-1)
17q21.32	GP2B	C	Platelet glycoprotein IIb	273800	3' to GP3A; BAK platelet antigen	Glanzmann thrombasthenia (1)	
17q22-q24	GHC	C	GROWTH HORMONE/PLACENTAL LACTOGEN GENE CLUSTER				
17q22-q24	CSHP1, CSL	C	Chorionic somatomammotropin pseudogene	see 150200			
17q22-q24	CSA, PL, CSH1	C	Chorionic somatomammotropin A	150200			
17q22-q24	CSB, CSH2	C	Chorionic somatomammotropin B	118820	at 3' end	[Placental lactogen deficiency] (1)	
17q22-q24	GH1, GHN	C	Growth hormone, normal	139250	5'-GH1-CSHP1-CSH1-GH2-CSH2-3'	Isolated growth hormone deficiency, Illig type with absent GH and Kowarski type with bioinactive GH (3)	11(Gh)
17q22-q24	GH2, GHV	C	Growth hormone, variant	139240			

Location	Symbol	Status	Title	MIM number	Comments	Disorder	Mouse
17q22-q24	PRKCA, PKCA	P	Protein kinase C, alpha form	176960	cen-COL1A1-PKCA-GH1		11(Pkca)
17q23	DCP, ACE1	P	Dipeptidylcarboxypeptidase-1 (angiotensin I converting enzyme)	106180			
17q23	GAA	C	Acid alpha-glucosidase	232300		Pompe disease (1); Acid-maltase deficiency, adult (1)	11(Umph-2)
17q23-q24	UMPH2	C	Uridine 5'-monophosphate phosphohydrolase-2; uridine monophosphatase-2	191720	between GAA and GHC		
17q23-q25	HLR1, G17P1	P	Helicase, RNA, nuclear 1, p68 (RNA-dependent ATPase)	180630			
17q23-qter	PEPE	C	Peptidase E	170200			
17q23.2-q25.3	TK1	C	Thymidine kinase-1	188300	to chromosome 15 in APL		11(Tk-1)
17q25	P4HB, PROHB	P	Prolyl-4-hydroxylase, beta subunit; disulfide isomerase; cellular thyroid hormone-binding protein p55	176790			
Chr.17	ALDH3	P	Aldehyde dehydrogenase-3	100660			
Chr.17	ALPPL	P	Placental alkaline phosphatase-like gene	see 171800			
Chr.17	APOH	P	Apolipoprotein H (beta-2-glycoprotein I)	138700		[Apolipoprotein H deficiency] (1)	
Chr.17	CD7	C	T-cell antigen CD7	186820			
Chr.17	G6PDL	P	Glucose-6 phosphate dehydrogenase-like	138110			
Chr.17	GALC	P	Galactocerebrosidase	245200		Krabbe disease (1)	?11(tw)
Chr.17	MYL4	C	Myosin light polypeptide-4, alkali; atrial, embryonic	160770			11(Myl-4)
Chr.17	PENT, PNMT	P	Phenylethanolamine N-methyltransferase	171190			
Chr.17	PFN1	P	Profilin-1	176610			
Chr.17	SMPD1, NPD	P	Sphingomyelinase (Niemann-Pick disease)	257200		Niemann-Pick disease (1)	
Chr.17	TSE1	P	Tissue-specific extinguisher-1	188830			11(Tse-1)

In addition: 3 surface antigens, most defined by monoclonals, 5 'like' genes, 3 pseudogenes and 1 fragile site (HGM10). Order by CMGT (Xu et al, 1988): pter--(TP53--POLR2--D17S1)--(MYHSA2--MYHSA1)--D17Z1--CRYB1--acute promyelocytic leukemia breakpoint--RNU2--HOX2--(NGFR--COL1A1--MPO)--GAA--UMPH2--GHC--TK1--GALK--qter.

103

Chromosome No. 18

Location	Symbol	Status	Title	MIM #	Comments	Disorder	Mouse
18p11.32	MCL	L	Multiple hereditary cutaneous leiomyomata	150800		?Leiomyomata, multiple hereditary cutaneous (2)	
18p11.31	LAMA	P	Laminin A	150320			
18p11.1-q11.2	PLI	P	Alpha-2-plasmin inhibitor	262850		Plasmin inhibitor deficiency (1)	
18q11-q12	JK	P	Kidd blood group	111000	previous suggestion of chr.7 or chr.2		
18q11-q12	LCFS2	L	Lynch cancer family syndrome II	114400	?linked to JK	?Lynch cancer family syndrome II (2)	
18q11.2-q12.1	PALB, TTR, TBPA	C	Thyroxine-binding prealbumin (transthyretin)	176300		Amyloid neuropathy, familial, several allelic types (3); [Dystransthyretinemic hyperthyroxinemia](1)	
18q21	GRP	C	Gastrin releasing peptide	137260	mammalian equivalent of bombesin		
18q21	SSAV1	P	Simian sarcoma-associated virus-1/Gibbon ape leukemia virus	182090			
18q21-q22.2	RCRD1	L	Retinal cone-rod dystrophy-1	120970		?Retinal cone-rod dystrophy (2)	
18q21.2-q22	PLANH2, PAI2	C	Plasminogen activator inhibitor, type II	173390			
18q21.3	BCL2, BCL3	C	B-cell CLL/lymphoma-2	151430	most frequent hematologic malignancy t(14;18)(q22;q21)	Leukemia/lymphoma, B-cell, 2 (2)	1(bcl-2)
18q21.3	YES1	C	Oncogene YES-1	164880			
18q21.31-qter	TS, TMS	C	Thymidylate synthase	188350	?on 18p or proximal 18q		
18q22-q23	ERV1	C	Oncogene ERV1; endogenous retrovirus-1	131150			
18q22-qter	MBP	C	Myelin basic protein	159430	defective in "shiverer," neurologic mutant in mouse		18(Mbp)
18q22.1	GTS	L	Gilles de la Tourette syndrome	137580	t(7;18)(q22;q22.1)	?Tourette syndrome (2)	
18q23	PEPA	C	Peptidase A	169800			18(Pep-1)
18q23.3	CRC18	P	Colorectal cancer-related sequence-18	120470		Colorectal cancer (1)	
Chr.18	DD	L	Diastrophic dysplasia	222600		?Diastrophic dysplasia (2)	
Chr.18	DHFRP1	P	Dihydrofolate reductase pseudogene-1	see 126060	shows +/- polymorphism		
Chr.18	IFNGR2	P	Interferon, gamma, receptor for	107470	both 6 and 18 required		
Chr.18	NARS, ASNRS	P	Asparaginyl-tRNA synthetase	108410			

In addition: 1 'like' gene, 4 pseudogenes and 2 fragile sites (HGM10). Subband critical to trisomy 18 phenotype = 18q12.2.

Chromosome No. 19

Location	Symbol	Status	Title	MIM #	Comments	Disorder	Mouse
19pter-p13.2	OK	P	Blood group OK	111380			
19pter-q13	CXB3S	P	Coxsackie virus B3 sensitivity	120050			
19pter-q12	EF2	C	Elongation factor-2	130610			
19p13.3-p13.2	AMH, MIF	P	Anti-Mullerian hormone	261550		Persistent Mullerian duct syndrome (1)	
19p13.3-p13.2	C3	C	Complement component-3	120700	LE ca. 7cM in males vs. C3 RFLP	C3 deficiency (1)	17(C3)
19p13.3-p13.2	E2A	P	Immunoglobulin enhancer binding factors E12/E47	147141			
19p13.3-p13.2	INSR	C	Insulin receptor	147670	1 gene for alpha and beta subunits	Leprechaunism (1); Diabetes mellitus, insulin-resistant, with acanthosis nigricans (1); ?Rabson-Mendenhall syndrome (1)	8(Insr)
19p13.2	RAB3A	P	RAS-associated protein RAB3A	179490			
19p13.2-p13.1	LDLR, FHC	C	Familial hypercholesterolemia (LDL receptor)	143890	ca. 20cM distal to C3	Hypercholesterolemia, familial (3)	9(Ldlr)
19p13.2-q12	MANB	C	Lysosomal alpha-D-mannosidase-B	248500		Mannosidosis (1)	
19p13.2-q13.4	DNL	P	Lysosomal DNA-ase	126350			
19p13.1-cen	LW	C	LW (Landsteiner-Weiner) blood group	111250	close to C3, LU		
19p13.1-q13.11	LE, LES	C	Lewis blood group	111100	linked to C3; order:FHC-C3-LE-DM-SE-LU		
19p13.1-q13.11	FUT1, H, HH	P	Fucosyltransferase-1 (Bombay phenotype)	211100	SE tightly linked		
19p13.1-q13.11	HCL1, BRHC	P	Brown hair color	113750			
19p13.1-q13.11	GEY	P	Green/blue eye color	227240	different locus for brown/blue		
19p13	LYL1	P	Leukemia, lymphoid, 1	151440			
19p13	RFX	P	HLA class II regulatory factor RF-X	209920		Severe combined immunodeficiency (SCID), HLA class II-negative type (1)	
19cen-q12	GPI	C	Glucosephosphate isomerase; neuroleukin	172400		Hemolytic anemia due to glucosephosphate isomerase deficiency (1); Hydrops fetalis (1)	7(Gpi-1)
19cen-q13.11	FUT2, SE	C	Fucosyltransferase-2 (secretor)	182100	H, SE = alpha-L-fucosyltransferases; from common ancestral genes		
19cen-q13.11	LU	C	Lutheran blood group	111200	linked to SE		
19cen-q13.11	PEPD	C	Peptidase D (prolidase)	170100	closely linked to APOC2	?Prolidase deficiency, 264130 (1)	7(Pep-4)
19cen-q13.2	MEL	C	Oncogene MEL	165040			
19cen-q13.3	LIPE, LHS	P	Lipase, hormone-sensitive	151750			

Location	Symbol	Status	Title	MIM #	Comments	Disorder	Mouse
19q12-q13.2	ATP1A3	C	Sodium-potassium-ATPase, alpha-3 polypeptide	182350			7(Atpa-2)
19q12-q13.2	MAG, GMA	C	Myelin-associated glycoprotein	159460			7(Gma)
19q12-q13.2	PVS	C	Polio virus sensitivity	173850		{Polio, susceptibility to} (2)	
19q13	APS	C	Prostate-specific antigen	176820	probably with cluster KLK1, KLK2		7(Aps)
19q13	BCL3	P	B-cell CLL/lymphoma-3	109560			
19q13	CKMM, CKM	C	Creatine kinase, muscle type	123310	distal to APOLP2		
19q13	DM	C	Myotonic dystrophy	160900	distal to APOLP2; ?proximal to CKM	Myotonic dystrophy (2)	
19q13	KLK2	P	Kallikrein, glandular	147960	12kb from APS		
19q13	NCA	P	Normal cross-reacting antigen	163980	closely related to CEA		
19q13.1	APOLP2	C	APOLIPOPROTEIN CLUSTER II		5'--APOE-4.3kb-APOC1-6kb-APOC1 pseudogene-22kb-APOC2--3'		
19q13.1	APOE	C	Apolipoprotein E	207760		Hyperlipoproteinemia, type III (1)	7(Apoe)
19q13.1	APOC1	C	Apolipoprotein C-I	107710			
19q13.1	APOC2	C	Apolipoprotein C-II	207750		Hyperlipoproteinemia, type Ib (1)	7(Pkcc)
19q13.1	PSBG1, B1G1, SP1	C	Pregnancy-specific beta-1-glycoprotein-1	176390			
19q13.1	RYR1, RYDR	P	Ryanodine receptor (sarcoplasmic reticulum calcium release channel)	180901			
19q13.1-q13.3	CEA	C	Carcinoembryonic antigen	114890	inconsistent regionalization = q31-q32		
19q13.1-q13.3	CYP2A, P450C2A	C	Cytochrome P-450, family II, subfamily A, phenobarbital inducible	123960	CYP1 = earlier symbol		
19q13.1-q13.3	CYP2B	C	Cytochrome P-450, family II, subfamily B, phenobarbital inducible	123930	same NoI fragment as CYP2A		7(Coh)
19q13.1-q13.3	CYP2F	P	Cytochrome P-450, family II, subfamily F	124070			
19q13.1-q13.3	MHS	P	Malignant hyperthermia, susceptibility to	145600		Malignant hyperthermia (2)	
19q13.1-q13.3	TGFB1	P	Transforming (or tumor) growth factor, beta form	190180	close to CYP2A		7(Tgfb)
19q13.1-qter	E11S	C	Echo 11 sensitivity	129150			
19q13.1-qter	RDRC, M7V1, M7VS1	C	RD114 virus receptor (Baboon M7 virus receptor)	109190			
19q13.2-q13.3	ERCC1, UV20	C	Complementation of CHO DNA-repair defect UV20	126380		?Xeroderma pigmentosum, 1 form (1)	
19q13.2-q13.3	ERCC2, EM9	P	Complementation of CHO DNA-repair defect EM9	126340			
19q13.2-q13.3	XRCC1	P	*X-ray-repair, complementing defective, in Chinese hamster	194360			
19q13.2-q13.4	KLK1, KLKR	P	Kallikrein, renal/pancreas/salivary	147910			7(Klk-1)
19q13.2-q13.4	PKCC, PKCG	C	Protein kinase C, gamma form	176980			
19q13.3	CD33	P	Myeloid differentiation antigen	159590			
19q13.3-q13.4	FTL	C	Ferritin, light chain	134790			

Location	Symbol	Title	MIM #	Comments	Disorder	Mouse
19q13.32	CGB	C	CHORIONIC GONADOTROPIN, BETA CHAIN	118860	at least 5 genes		
19q13.32	LHB	C	Luteinizing hormone, beta chain	152780	beta chains of FSH, TSH on 11p, 1p, respectively	?Male pseudohermaphroditism due to defective LH (1); ?Hypergonadotropic hypogonadism (1)	7(Lhb)
Chr.19	BCT2	P	Branched chain amino acid transaminase-2	113530		?Hypervalinemia or hyperleucine-isoleucinemia (1)	
Chr.19	BCKDHA, MSUD1	C	Branched chain ketoacid dehydrogenase, E1-alpha subunit	248600		Maple syrup urine disease (1)	
Chr.19	ERBAL2, EAR2	P	ERBA-related gene-2	132880			
Chr.19	G19P1, PKCSH	P	Protein kinase C substrate, H form	177060			
Chr.19	GUSM	P	Beta-glucuronidase, mouse, modifier of	231610			
Chr.19	HKR1	P	Oncogene HKR1	165250			
Chr.19	HKR2	P	Oncogene HKR2	165260			
Chr.19	KRL1	P	Kruppel-like zinc finger protein-1	149410			
Chr.19	KRL2	P	Kruppel-like zinc finger protein-2	149420			
Chr.19	OTF2, OCT2	P	Lymphoid-specific octamer-binding transcription factor-2	153260			
Chr.19	PGK2	C	Phosphoglycerate kinase-2 (testicular PGK)	172270			
Chr.19	RRAS	P	Oncogene RRAS	165090			7(Rras)
Chr.19	TRSP	P	Opal suppressor phosphoserine tRNA	165060	pseudogene on 22		
Chr.19	U1RNP, RNPU1Z, RPU1	P	U1 small nuclear ribonucleoprotein 70kD	180740			

In addition: 3 surface antigens, most defined by monoclonals, 1 O'Farrell protein spot, 2 'like' genes, 2 pseudogenes and 2 fragile sites (HGM10). Map (HGM9): pter--LDLR--(C3--LE)--LW--(PEPD--DM)--(SE--APOC2)--APOE--LU--qter. LDLR, distal 19p; C3, mid 19p; APOE, 19q. Order (Eiberg et al, 1983): LE--C3--DM--(SE--PEPD)--LU. Order (Breslow, 1984):FHC--C3--APOE/APOC2. APOC1 6kb 3' to APOE. Location 19p13.1-q13.11 for LE, HH, LW, PEPD, SE, GEY, LU is estimated from collation of physical and meiotic data.

107

Chromosome No. 20

Location	Symbol	Status	Title	MIM #	Comments	Disorder	Mouse
20pter-p12	SCG1, CHGB	P	Chromogranin B (secretogranin B)	118920			
20pter-p12	PDYN	P	Prodynorphin	131340			
20pter-p12	PRIP, PRNP	C	Prion protein	176640		?Creutzfeld-Jacob disease, 123400 (2); Gerstmann-Straussler disease, 137440 (2)	2(Prn-p)
20p12-cen	THBD, THRM	C	Thrombomodulin	188040			
20p11.23-qter	GHRF	C	Growth hormone releasing factor; somatocrinin	139190		?Isolated growth hormone deficiency due to defect in GHRF (1)	
20p11.2	AGS, AHD	C	Arteriohepatic dysplasia (Alagille syndrome)	118450		Arteriohepatic dysplasia (2)	
20p	ITPA	C	Inosine triphosphatase-A	147520		[Inosine triphosphatase deficiency] (1)	2(Itp)
20cen-q13.1	SAHH, AHCY	C	S-adenosylhomocysteine hydrolase	180960	~13cM from ADA		
20q11-q12	HCK	P	Hemopoietic cell kinase	142370			
20q12-q13	SRC, ASV, SRC1	C	Protooncogene SRC, Rous sarcoma	190090	?20q11.2		2(Src)
20q12-q13.1	PLC1	P	Phospholipase C-148	172420			
20q12-q13.2	TOP1	P	DNA topoisomerase I	126420			
20q13.11	ADA	C	Adenosine deaminase	102700		Severe combined immunodeficiency due to ADA deficiency (1); Hemolytic anemia due to ADA excess (1)	2(Ada)
Chr.20	ARVP, VP	P	Arginine vasopressin-neurophysin II	192340		?Diabetes insipidus, neurohypophyseal, 125700 (1)	
Chr.20	EBN, BNS	P	Seizures, benign neonatal	121200		Seizures, benign neonatal (2)	
Chr.20	DCE	P	Desmosterol-to-cholesterol enzyme	125650			
Chr.20	GNAS1, GNAS, GPSA	P	G-protein, stimulatory, alpha subunit (Gs-alpha)	139320		Pseudohypoparathyroidism, type Ia (1)	2(Gs-a)
Chr.20	GSL, NGBE	P	Neuraminidase/beta-galactosidase expression (galactosialidosis)	256540		Galactosialidosis (1)	
Chr.20	LEUT, HTL, HLT	P	Leucine transport, high	151310			
Chr.20	OT	P	Oxytocin-neurophysin I	167050	separated from VP by 12kb		
Chr.20	PYGB	P	Glycogen phosphorylase, brain	138550			2(Pygb)
Chr.20	RPN2	P	Ribophorin II	180490			2(Rpn-2)

In addition: 1 antigen, 2 'like' genes and 2 fragile sites (HGM10).

Chromosome No. 21

Location	Symbol	Status	Title	MIM #	Comments	Disorder	Mouse
21p12	RNR4	C	Ribosomal RNA	180450			
21q11.2-q21	AD1	C	Alzheimer disease-1	104300	near centromere	Alzheimer disease (2)	
21q21-qter	IFNAR	C	Antiviral protein; alpha-interferon receptor	107450			16(Ifrc)
21q21-qter	IFNBR	C	Antiviral protein; beta-interferon receptor	107460			
21q21.3-q22.05	APP, AAA, CVAP	C	Amyloid beta A4 precursor protein	104760	proximal to SOD; very distal q21 or boundary with q22	?Amyloidosis, cerebroarterial, Dutch type, 105160 (1)	16(Cvap)
21q22	S100B	P	S100 protein, beta polypeptide	176990			10(S100b)
21q22.1	PGFT, PAIS, GART	C	Phosphoribosylaminoimidazole synthetase; phosphoribosylglycineamide synthetase; phosphoribosylglycineamide formyltransferase	138440	multifunctional protein: Ade(-)C, Ade(-)G, GART		16(Prgs)
21q22.1	SOD1	C	Superoxide dismutase-1, soluble	147450	mid q22.1		16(Sod-1)
21q22.1-q22.3	ETS2	C	Oncogene ETS-2	164740	proximal q22.3		16(Ets-2)
21q22.1-qter	CD18, LCAMB, LAD	C	Cell adhesion molecule, leukocyte, beta subunit	116920	common subunit for CR3, LFA1, and P150,95	Leukocyte adhesion deficiency (2)	7(Ly-15)
21q22.3	BCEI	C	Breast cancer estrogen-inducible sequence	113710			
21q22.3	CBS	C	Cystathionine beta-synthase	236200	subtelomeric	Homocystinuria, B6-responsive and nonresponsive types (1)	17(Cbs)
21q22.3	COL6A1	P	Collagen VI, alpha-1 chain	120220			10(Col6a1)
21q22.3	COL6A2	P	Collagen VI, alpha-2 chain	120240			10(Col6a2)
21q22.3	CRYA1	C	Crystallin, alpha A	123580	alpha B on another chr., ?chr. 16		17(Crya-1)
21q22.3	ERG	C	Oncogene ERG	165080	related to ETS2; proximal to ETS2		
21q22.3	HMG14	C	Nonhistone chromosomal protein HMG-14	163920			
21q22.3	PFKL	C	Phosphofructokinase, liver type	171860		Hemolytic anemia due to phosphofructokinase deficiency (1)	17(Pfkl)
Chr.21	AABT	L	Beta-amino acids, renal transport of	109660			
Chr.21	BAS	L	Beta-adrenergic stimulation, response to	109670			
Chr.21	HTOR	L	5-hydroxytryptamine oxygenase regulator	143460			
Chr.21	MX1, MX, IFI78	P	Myxovirus (influenza) resistance-1 (interferon induced protein p78)	147150			16(Mx-1)
Chr.21	MX2	L	Myxovirus (influenza) resistance-2	147890			16(Mx-2)

In addition: 1 surface antigen, 5 O'Farrell protein spots, 1 'like' gene and 1 pseudogene (HGM10). Hyperuricemia, leukemia, Alzheimer disease, and cataract of Down syndrome may be explained by the presence of specific genes on chromosome 21. DSCR, Down syndrome chromosome region = proximal 21q22.3.

Chromosome No. 22

Location	Symbol	Status	Title	MIM #	Comments	Disorder	Mouse
22pter-q11.2	PVALB	P	Parvalbumin	168890	?role in DiGeorge syndrome		
22p12	RNR5	C	Ribosomal RNA	180450			
22q11	IDUA, IDA	P	Alpha-L-iduronidase	252800	on Ph1 chr.	Hurler syndrome (1); Mucopolysaccharidosis I (1); Hurler-Scheie syndrome (1); Scheie syndrome (1)	
22q11	CECR, CES	C	Cat eye syndrome	115470	partial tetrasomy of 22q11	Cat eye syndrome (2)	
22q11	DGCR, DGS	C	DiGeorge syndrome	188400		DiGeorge syndrome (2)	
22q11	NAGA	C	N-acetyl-alpha-D-galactosaminidase (alpha-galactosidase B)	104170	proximal to Ph1 break	Alpha-NAGA deficiency (1)	
22q11-q13	TSHR	C	Thyroid stimulating hormone receptor	275200	tight linkage to CYP2D	Hypothyroidism, nongoitrous, due to TSH resistance (1)	
22q11.1-q11.2	GGT, GTG	C	Gamma-glutamyl transpeptidase	231950	minor peak, q13.1 on Ph1 chr.; order 5' to 3':cen-V-C-ter	Glutathioninuria (1)	
22q11.12	IGL	C	IMMUNOGLOBULIN LAMBDA LIGHT CHAIN GENE CLUSTER				16(Igl)
22q11.12	IGLV	C	Variable region of lambda light chains	147240	many genes		
22q11.12	IGLJ	C	J region of lambda light chains	147230	nine J-C duplexes		
22q11.12	IGLC	C	Constant region of lambda light chains	147220	several genes		
22q11.2-q12.2	CRYB2	P	Crystallin, beta-B2	123620			
22q11.2-q12.2	CRYB3	P	Crystallin, beta-B3	123630			
22q11.2-q12.2	CYP2D, P450C2D	C	Cytochrome P450, family II, subfamily D	124030	debrisoquine 4-hydroxylase	{?Parkinsonism, susceptibility to} (1)	10(Cyp2d)
22q11.2-q13	MB	C	Myoglobin	160000			
22q11.2-qter	P1	P	P1 blood group	111410	?linked to DIA1 and SIS		
22q11.2-qter	SGLT1, NAGT	P	Sodium-glucose transporter-1	182380	linked to P1	Glucose/galactose malabsorption (1)	
22q11.2-qter	TCN2, TC2	C	Transcobalamin II	275350	distal to IGL;	Transcobalamin II deficiency (1)	11(Tcn-2)
22q11.21	BCR, CML, PHL	C	Chronic myeloid leukemia; breakpoint cluster region-1	151410	Ph1=t(9;22)(q34.1;q11.21); fusion gene with ABL in CML; cluster of 4 loci: cen-BCR2, BCR4, IGL-BCR1-BCR3-SIS	Leukemia, chronic myeloid (3)	
22q11.21	VPREB	P	Pre-B lymphocyte-specific protein	146770	between BCR2 and BCR4		
22q11.21-q13.1	NF2, ACN	C	Acoustic neuroma	101000	deletion of chr.22 markers	Acoustic neuroma (2)	
22q11.21-q13.31	ACO2	C	Aconitase, mitochondrial	100850	distal to Ph1 break		
22q12	ES	P	Ewing sarcoma	133450	(11;22)(q24;q12)	Ewing sarcoma (2)	
22q12.1-q12.2	LIF	P	Leukemia inhibitory factor	159540			

Location	Symbol	P/C	Gene name	MIM No.	Mouse homolog	Disorder
22q12.1-q13.1	NEFH	P	Neurofilament, heavy polypeptide	162230		
22q12.3-q13.1	SIS, PDGFB	C	Oncogene SIS (platelet derived growth factor, B chain)	190040	15(Sis)	
22q12.3-qter	MGCR, MGM	C	Meningioma	156100		Meningioma (2)
22q13-qter	ACR, ACRS	P	Acrosin (proacrosin)	102480		
22q13-qter	GLB2, PPGB	C	Beta-galactosidase-2 (GLB protective protein)	109680		
22q13.31-qter	ARSA	C	Arylsulfatase A	250100	15(As-2)	Metachromatic leukodystrophy (1)
22q13.31-qter	DIA1	C	NADH-diaphorase-1 (cytochrome b5 reductase)	250800	15(Dia-1)	Methemoglobinemia, enzymopathic (1)
Chr.22	ADSL, ADS	P	Adenylosuccinase (adenylosuccinate lyase)	103050	ade(-)I	Adenylosuccinase deficiency (1)
Chr.22	ASLP	P	Argininosuccinate lyase pseudogene	see 207900		
Chr.22	COMT	P	Catechol-O-methyltransferase	116790		
Chr.22	CST3	P	Cystatin C	105150		Cerebral amyloid angiopathy (1)
Chr.22	GNAZ	P	Guanine nucleotide-binding protein, alpha Z polypeptide	139160		
Chr.22	HCF2, HC2	P	Heparin cofactor II	142360		Thrombophilia due to heparin cofactor II deficiency (1)
Chr.22	MSK41	P	Antigen MSK41 identified by monoclonal antibody E3	107260		

In addition: 3 surface antigens, 3 'like' genes, 4 pseudogenes and 2 fragile sites (HGM10).

111

Gene Map of the X Chromosome

About 160 separate expressed genetic loci have been assigned to the X chromosome; for about an equal number of loci, X-chromosomal location has been suggested but not proved. Most of these loci have been placed on the X chromosome because of pedigree patterns and other characteristics of X-linked traits in families. Some have been assigned to the X chromosome by the same methods used in autosomal mapping: interspecies somatic cell hybridization (S, REa), or small, microscopically visible deletions (Ch). Some methods unique to the X chromosome have corroborated X-linkage or in some instances have given the first information on X-linkage or regional mapping: lyonization (L), Ohno's law of the evolutionary conservatism of the X chromosome in mammals (H), and X-autosome translocations in females affected by X-linked recessive disorders (X/A). The 'status' information in this case refers to certainty of regional assignment.

In addition: 3 surface antigens, 7 O'Farrell protein spots, 10 'like' genes, 9 pseudogenes and 2 fragile sites (HGM10).

Location	Symbol	Status	Title	MIM #	Comments	Disorder	Mouse
Xpter-p22.32	ARSC	P	Arylsulfatase C	301780			
Xpter-p22.32	KAL, KMS	C	Kallmann syndrome	308700	with ichthyosis in probable microdeletion syndrome	Kallmann syndrome (2)	
Xpter-p22.32	MIC2, MIC2X	C	MIC2 (monoclonal antibody 12E7)	313470	distal to STS		
Xpter-p22.32	STS, SSDD	C	Steroid sulfatase	308100	in nonlyonizing segment	Ichthyosis, X-linked (3); Placental steroid sulfatase deficiency (3)	X,Y(Sts)
Xpter-p22.32	XG	C	Xg blood group	314700	nonlyonizing		
Xpter-p22.32	CPXR	P	Chondrodysplasia punctata, X-linked recessive	302950		Chondrodysplasia punctata, X-linked recessive (2)	
Xpter-q21	PRPS2	P	Phosphoribosylpyrophosphate synthetase II	311860			
Xp22.31	DHOF, FODH	P	Focal dermal hypoplasia	305600		Focal dermal hypoplasia (2)	
Xp22.3	OA1	C	Ocular albinism, Nettleship-Falls type	300500	linked to XG	Ocular albinism, Nettleship-Falls type (2)	
Xp22	AGMX2, XLA2, IMD6	P	X-linked agammaglobulinemia, type 2	300310		Agammaglobulinemia, type 2, X-linked (2)	X(xid)
Xp22	AIC	C	Aicardi syndrome	304050		Aicardi syndrome (2)	
Xp22	GY	L	Hereditary hypophosphatemia II (gyro equivalent)	307810	close to hyp in mouse	?Hypophosphatemia with deafness (2)	
Xp22	HOMG, HSH, HMGX	C	Hypomagnesemia, X-linked primary	307600		Hypomagnesemia, X-linked primary (2)	
Xp22	HYP, HPDR1	C	Hereditary hypophosphatemia	307800	linked to DXS41	Hypophosphatemia, hereditary (2)	X(Hyp)
Xp22	MRX1	P	Mental retardation, X-linked nonspecific, I	309530	?11cM from XG	Mental retardation, X-linked nonspecific, I (2)	
Xp22	RS	C	Retinoschisis	312700	25cM from XG	Retinoschisis (2)	
Xp22	SEDL, SEDT	C	Spondyloepiphyseal dysplasia tarda	313400		Spondyloepiphyseal dysplasia tarda (2)	
Xp22-p21	GDXY, TDFX	P	Gonadal dysgenesis, XY female type	306100	?same as ZFX	Gonadal dysgenesis, XY female type (2)	
Xp22.3	HYR	P	H-Y regulator, or repressor	306970	structural HY locus on chr.6, 143170	?also Y	
Xp22.3-p22.1	AMGS, AMG, ALGN, AIH1	C	Amelogenin (amelogenesis imperfecta, hypoplastic type I)	301200		Amelogenesis imperfecta (1)	X(Amel)

Location	Symbol	Status	Title	MIM	Comments	Disorder	Mouse
Xp22.3-p21.1	NHS	P	Nance-Horan cataract-dental syndrome	302350		Nance-Horan syndrome (2)	
Xp22.3-p21.1	POLA	C	Polymerase, DNA, alpha	312040			
Xp22.2-p21.2	ZFX	P	Zinc finger protein, X-linked	314980		46,XY female (2)	X(Xfx)
Xp22.2-p22.1	CLS	P	Coffin-Lowry syndrome	303600	distal to DMD	Coffin-Lowry syndrome (2)	
Xp22.2-p22.1	CND	L	Corneal dermoids	304730	linked to DXS43		
Xp22.2-p22.1	PDHA1, PHE1A	P	Pyruvate dehydrogenase, E1-alpha polypeptide	312170		Pyruvate dehydrogenase deficiency (1)	X(Phe-1a)
Xp22.1-p21.2	GLR	P	Glycine receptor	305990			
Xp21.3-p21.2	AHC, AHX	C	Primary adrenal hypoplasia	300200	distal to GK	Adrenal hypoplasia, primary (2)	
Xp21.3-p21.2	GK	C	Glycerol kinase	307030	2Mb distal to DMD	Glycerol kinase deficiency (2)	
Xp21.3-p21.1	OA2	C	Ocular albinism, Forsius-Eriksson type	300600	?linked to XG	Ocular albinism, Forsius-Eriksson type (2)	
Xp21.2	DMD, BMD	C	Duchenne muscular dystrophy; Becker muscular dystrophy	310200	dystrophin gene; cen-5'-3'-pter; 2Mb; ?Xp21.13	Duchenne muscular dystrophy (3); Becker muscular dystrophy (3)	X(mdx)
Xp21.2-q21.1	LUS, XS	L	Lutheran suppressor, X-linked	309050			
Xp21.2-p21.1	XK	C	Xk	314850	~500kb distal to CGD	[McLeod phenotype] (2)	
Xp21.1	CYBB, CGD	C	Chronic granulomatous disease	306400	proximal to DMD	Granulomatous disease, chronic, X-linked (3)	X(Cybb)
Xp21.1	OTC	C	Ornithine transcarbamylase	311250	proximal to DMD, CGD	Ornithine transcarbamylase deficiency (3)	X(spf; Otc)
Xp21.1-p11.3	COD1, PCDX	P	Progressive cone dystrophy, X-linked	304020		Progressive cone dystrophy (2)	
Xp21	GTD	L	Gonadotropin deficiency	306190	distal to AHC	?Gonadotropin deficiency (2); ?Cryptorchidism (2)	
Xp21	RP3	C	Retinitis pigmentosa 3 (RP with metallic sheen in heterozygotes)	312610	probably between OTC and CGD	Retinitis pigmentosa 3 (2)	
Xp21-p11	GAPDP1	C	Glyceraldehyde-3-phosphate dehydrogenase pseudogene-1	305980			
Xp13-p11	ARAF1, RAFA1	P	Oncogene ARAF1	311010	close to DXS7		X(Araf)
Xp11.4	NDP, ND	C	Norrie disease	310600		Norrie disease (2)	
Xp11.4	PKS2	P	Oncogene PKS2	311020			
Xp11.4	PFC, PFD	C	Properdin P factor, complement (properdin P deficiency)	312060		Properdin deficiency, X-linked (3)	X(Prop)
Xp11.4-p11.23	A1S9T, A1S9	C	Temperature-sensitive mutation, mouse, complementation of (ts A1S9)	313660	escapes inactivation		
Xp11.4-p11.23	EPA, TIMP	C	Erythroid-potentiating activity (tissue inhibitor of metalloproteinases)	305370		?Menkes disease (1)	X(Timp)
Xp11.3	CSNB1	I	Congenital stationary nightblindness	310500		Nightblindness, congenital stationary, type I (2)	
Xp11.3	RP2	C	Retinitis pigmentosa 2	312600		Retinitis pigmentosa 2 (2)	
Xp11.3-p11	WAS, IMD2	C	Wiskott-Aldrich syndrome	301000	t(18;X)(q11.2;p11.2)	Wiskott-Aldrich syndrome (2)	
Xp11.23	MAOA	C	Monoamine oxidase A	309850	NDP, MAOA, MAOB closely linked		
Xp11.23	MAOB	C	Monoamine oxidase B	309860			
Xp11.2	SSRC	P	Sarcoma, synovial	312820		Sarcoma, synovial (2)	

Location	Symbol	Status	Title	MIM #	Comments	Disorder	Mouse
Xp11.2	IP1, IP	C	Incontinentia pigmenti-1, sporadic	308300	Xq21 = conflicting localization; both excluded by Fd	Incontinentia pigmenti (2)	
Xp11	SYN1	P	Synapsin I	313440			X(Syn-1)
Xp	CCT	L	Cataracts, congenital total	302200	?Cataracts, congenital total (2)		
Xq	A11	P	A-11 gene	300010			
Xcen-q13	AR, DHTR, TFM	C	Testicular feminization (androgen receptor)	313700		Testicular feminization (1); Reifenstein syndrome (1); Infertile male syndrome (1)	X(Tfm)
Xq11-q12	MRX2	L	Mental retardation, X-linked nonspecific, II	309540		Mental retardation, X-linked nonspecific, II (2)	
Xq11-q13	PGK1P1	C	Phosphoglycerate kinase-1 pseudogene-1	311810	probably Xq13.1		
Xq12-q13	MNK, MK	C	Menkes disease	309400	?proximal and close to PGKA	Menkes disease (2)	X(Mo)
Xq12-q13	PHKA	P	Phosphorylase kinase, alpha subunit	306000		Glycogen storage disease VIII (1)	X(Phka)
Xq12.2-13.1	EDA, HED	C	Anhidrotic ectodermal dysplasia	305100	~10cM distal to DXS1, proximal to DXYS1	Anhidrotic ectodermal dysplasia (2)	X(Ta)
Xq13	ALAS2, ASB, ANH1	P	Aminolevulinate, delta, synthase (sideroblastic anemia)	301300	somatic cell chromosome rearrangement	Anemia, sideroblastic/hypochromic (3)	
Xq13	CMTX, CMT2	C	Charcot-Marie-Tooth disease, X-linked	302800	5cM to DXYS1; very close to PGK	Charcot-Marie-Tooth disease, X-linked (2)	
Xq13	FGDY, AAS	P	Aarskog-Scott syndrome (faciogenital dysplasia)	305400		Aarskog-Scott syndrome (2)	
Xq13	PGKA, PGK1	C	Phosphoglycerate kinase-1	311800		Hemolytic anemia due to PGK deficiency (1)	X(Pgk-1)
Xq13	XCE, XIC	P	X chromosome controlling element (X-inactivation center)	314670	q13-q21; metaphase bend, or fold, at q13.3-q21.1		X(Xce)
Xq13-q13.3	SCAR	P	Single copy abundant mRNA	312880			
Xq13-q21	CHR39C	P	Cholesterol repressible protein 39C	302920			
Xq13-q21	SDYS, DGSX, GDS	L	Simpson dysmorphia syndrome (dysplasia-gigantism syndrome, X-linked)	312870	?linked to DXYS1	Dysplasia-gigantism syndrome, X-linked (2)	
Xq13-q21	WWS	P	Wieacker-Wolff syndrome	314580	linked to DXYS1	Wieacker-Wolff syndrome (2)	
Xq13-q21.1	DFN3	C	Conductive deafness with stapes fixation	304400	linked to DXS51	Conductive deafness with stapes fixation (2)	
Xq13-q21.1	ZNF6	P	Zinc finger protein-6	314990			
Xq13-q27	CCG1, BA2R, C1HR	C	Temperature sensitivity, mouse and hamster, complement	313650	?near HPRT		X(Ccg1)
Xq13.1-q21.1	SCIDX1, SCIDX, IMD4	C	Severe combined immunodeficiency, X-linked	300400	linked to DXS159	SCID, X-linked (2)	
Xq21	CPX	C	Cleft palate, X-linked	303400		Cleft palate, X-linked (2)	
Xq21-q22	FPSL5	P	Farnesylpyrophosphate synthetase	305425			
Xq21-q22	SPG2, SPPX2	P	Spastic paraplegia, X-linked, uncomplicated	312920		Spastic paraplegia, X-linked, uncomplicated (2)	

Location	Symbol	Status	Gene name	Comment	MIM	Disorder	Mouse
Xq21-q22	TBG	P	Thyroxine-binding globulin		314200	[Euthyroidal hyper- and hypothyroxinemia] (1)	
Xq21.2	TCD	C	Choroideremia		303100	Choroideremia (2)	
Xq21.3-q22	AGMX1, IMD1, XLA	C	X-linked agammaglobulinemia	0.0 recombination with DXYS1, DXYS12; ?Ig V-D-J recombinase	300300	Agammaglobulinemia, X-linked (2)	
Xq21.3-q22	GHDX	L	Growth hormone deficiency, X-linked	?contiguous gene syndrome with XLA	312000	?Growth hormone deficiency, X-linked (2)	
Xq21.3-q22	MGCN	P	Megalocornea, X-linked		309300	Megalocornea, X-linked (2)	
Xq21.3-q22	SBMA, KD, SMAX1	C	Kennedy spinal muscular atrophy	with DXYS1, lod=3.63, theta .05	313200	Kennedy disease (2)	
Xq22	GLA	C	Alpha-galactosidase A		301500	Fabry disease (3)	X(Ags)
Xq22	PLP, PMD	C	Myelin proteolipid protein		312080	Pelizaeus-Merzbacher disease (3)	X(Plp(jp))
Xq22-q24	ATS, ASLN	C	Alport syndrome	distal to DXS3	301050	Alport syndrome (2)	
Xq22-q26	PRPS1	C	Phosphoribosylpyrophosphate synthetase		311850	Phosphoribosylpyrophosphate synthetase-related gout (1)	
Xq22-q28	MYCL2	P	MYCL-related processed gene		310310		
Xq24-q27	HIGM1, IMD3	P	X-linked immunodeficiency with hyper-IgM		308230	Immunodeficiency, X-linked, with hyper-IgM (2)	
Xq25	OCRL, LOCR	C	Lowe oculocerebrorenal syndrome		309000	Lowe syndrome (2)	
Xq25-q26	LYP, IMD5, XLP, XLPD	C	Lymphoproliferative syndrome, X-linked	1cM from DXS42; no recombination with DXS37	308240	Lymphoproliferative syndrome, X-linked (2)	
Xq26-q27	HPTX, HYPX	P	Hypoparathyroidism, X-linked	?distal to F9	307700	Hypoparathyroidism, X-linked (2)	
Xq26-q27	POF	L	Premature ovarian failure		311360	Ovarian failure, premature (2)	
Xq26-q27.2	CDR	C	Cerebellar degeneration-related autoantigen	between HPRT and F9	302650		
Xq26-q27.2	HPRT	C	Hypoxanthine-guanine phosphoribosyltransferase		308000	Lesch-Nyhan syndrome (3); HPRT-related gout (1)	X(Hprt)
Xq26-q28	GLUDP1	C	Glutamate dehydrogenase pseudogene-1		305910		
Xq26.3-q27.1	ALDS, ADFN	P	Albinism-deafness syndrome	5cM proximal to F9	300700	Albinism-deafness syndrome (2)	
Xq27	DBL	P	Oncogene DBL	?same as MCF2	310970		
Xq27	MCF2	P	Oncogene MCF2	<270kb from F9 and telomeric	311030		
Xq27-q28	IP2	P	Incontinentia pigmenti-2 (familial, male-lethal type)		308310	Incontinentia pigmenti, familial (2)	X?streaked)
Xq27.1-q27.2	HEMB, F9	C	Hemophilia B; clotting factor IX	distal to HPRT; proximal part of Xq27	306900	Hemophilia B (3)	X(Cf-9)
Xq27.3	FRAXA	C	Fragile site Xq27.3		309550	Martin-Bell syndrome (2)	
Xq27.3	IDS, MPS2, SIDS	C	Hunter syndrome (sulfoiduronate sulfatase deficiency)		309900	Mucopolysaccharidosis II (2)	
Xq28	ALD	C	Adrenoleukodystrophy	cone pigment gene deleted in some ALD males	300100	Adrenoleukodystrophy (2)	
Xq28	CBBM, BCM	C	Blue-monochromatic colorblindness (blue cone monochromacy)		303700	Colorblindness, blue-monochromatic (3)	

Location	Symbol	Status	Title	MIM #	Comments	Disorder	Mouse
Xq28	CDPX2, CPXD, CPX	L	Chondrodysplasia punctata, X-linked dominant	302960	in mouse Bpa, bare-patches, close to G6pd and mdx	Chondrodysplasia punctata, X-linked dominant (2)	X(?Bpa)
Xq28	DIR, DI1	C	Nephrogenic diabetes insipidus	304800		Diabetes insipidus, nephrogenic (2)	
Xq28	DKC	P	Dyskeratosis congenita	305000		Dyskeratosis congenita (2)	
Xq28	EMD	C	Emery-Dreifuss muscular dystrophy	310300	combined with ALD in some cases; distal to DXS15	Emery-Dreifuss muscular dystrophy (2)	
Xq28	FCPX	L	F-cell production	305430		?Heterocellular hereditary persistence of fetal hemoglobin (2)	
Xq28	G6PD1	C	Glucose-6-phosphate dehydrogenase	305900	telomeric to GDX; proximal to F8, in same .29mb PFGE fragment	G6PD deficiency (3); Favism (1); Hemolytic anemia due to G6PD deficiency (1)	X(G6pd)
Xq28	GABRA3	C	Gamma-aminobutyric acid receptor, alpha-3 polypeptide	305660			
Xq28	GCP, CBD	C	Deutan colorblindness (green cone pigment)	303800	linked to G6PD; multiple genes	Colorblindness, deutan (2)	
Xq28	GDX	P	Protein GDX	312070	40kb 3' to G6PD		
Xq28	HEMA, F8C	C	Hemophilia A (clotting factor VIII)	306700	linked to G6PD, CB; proximal q28; DX13 and St14 distal	Hemophilia A (3)	X(Cf-8)
Xq28	HYCX	P	Hydrocephalus, X-linked	307000	linked to F8 and DXS52		
Xq28	L1CAM, CAML1	P	L1 cell adhesion molecule	308840	between RCP/GCP cluster and G6PD		X(Cam-L1)
Xq28	MAFD2, MDX	P	Manic-depressive illness, X-linked	309200	linkage to G6PD,CB in non-Ashkenazi Jews	Manic-depressive illness, X-linked (2)	
Xq28	MASA	P	MASA syndrome	309250		MASA syndrome (2)	
Xq28	MRSD, CHRS	P	Mental retardation-skeletal dysplasia	309620		Mental retardation-skeletal dysplasia (2)	
Xq28	MTM1, MTMX	P	Myotubular myopathy, X-linked	310400		Myotubular myopathy, X-linked (2)	
Xq28	P3	P	Protein P3	312090	order: G6PD-3'-(7kb)-5'-P3-3'-(0.5kb)-5'-GDX		
Xq28	RCP, CBP	C	Protan colorblindness (red cone pigment)	303900	5' to CBD	Colorblindness, protan (2)	X(Rsvp)
Xq28	TKCR	C	Goeminne TKCR syndrome	314300	distal to G6PD	Goeminne TKCR syndrome (2)	
Xq28	XM	P	Xm	314900	linked to DCB, PCB		

GENE MAP OF THE Y CHROMOSOME

1. According to the classical model (using the term of Good-fellow et al., J. Med. Genet. 22: 329-344, 1985), the Y chromosome has been thought to have several subregions: (1) an X-Y homologous, meiotic-pairing region occupying most of Yp and perhaps including a pseudoautosomal region of X-Y exchange; (2) a pericentric region containing the sex determining gene(s); and (3) a long arm heterochromatic, genetically inert region. Some recent findings support the classical model, whereas others refute it. Molecular studies indicate that Yp contains many sequences not homologous to Xp but with homology to Yq, Xq, or an autosome.

2. From the study of normal males and females, of persons with abnormal numbers of sex chromosomes, and of those carrying variant Y chromosomes, a factor (or factors) that determines the differentiation of the indifferent gonads into testes is known to be located on the Y chromosome, probably on the short arm; this may be called testis determining factor (TDF). (*See Mendelian Inheritance in Man*, 4th edition, figure 1, p.lix, 1975.) Translocation of this locus to Xp as the cause of XX males was suggested by Ferguson-Smith (Lancet 2: 475, 1966) and found confirmation in several observations (e.g., Evans et al., Hum. Genet. 49: 11, 1979). Location of TDF near the centromere was suggested by Davis (J. Med. Genet. 18: 161-195, 1981) and others; translocation to an X in XX males indicates a somewhat more distal location, at the junction of pseudoautosomal and Y-specific segments of Yp. Deletion of TDF in XY females was suggested by the observation of Disteche et al. (PNAS 83: 7841, 1986). Page et al. (Cell 51: 1091-1104, 1987) cloned part or all of what they thought to be the TDF gene, found that some sequences were highly conserved in mammals and even birds, and showed that the nucleotide sequence of the conserved DNA on the human Y chromosome corresponds to a protein with multiple 'finger' domains. The product probably binds to nucleic acids in a sequence-specific manner and may regulate transcription. TDF is probably located in band Yp11.2. ZFY (zinc finger protein, Y-linked) is the designation approved by HGM workshop committee, with ZFX (314980) being the X-linked counterpart. At this writing, evidence is accumulating that ZFY is not TDF.

3. A pseudoautosomal segment (PAS) of distal Yp and distal Xp (between which crossing-over occurs) has been suspected from microscopic observations and has been confirmed by studies using polymorphic DNA markers. (See Fig. 1 of Polani, Hum. Genet. 60: 207, 1982, and of Burgoyne, Hum. Genet. 61: 95, 1982, for a suggested homologous segment of X and Y.) DNA polymorphisms in a homologous segment of X and Y show 'pseudoautosomal' inheritance (Cooke et al., Nature 317:687, 1985; Simmler et al., Nature 317: 692, 1985). It appears that TDF is just proximal to PAS and that in PAS there is one, but only one, obligatory crossingover. The following order has been observed with regard to recombination with sex: Ypter--DXYS14--(50% recombination with sex)--DXYS15--(35.5%)--DXYS17--(11.5%)--MIC2--(2.7%)--TDF. These values are strictly additive indicating no double crossovers. Thus, the sequence can be written: Ypter

--DXYS14--14.5%--DXYS15--24%--DXYS17--8.8%--MIC2--2.7%--nonexchanging segment of Yp containing TDF.

4. The specific structural gene first to be identified confidently on the Y chromosome was that homologous to the X-linked gene for surface antigen MIC2 (Goodfellow et al., Nature 298: 346, 1983). Called MYC2Y, it was not only the first Y chromosome gene for which a gene product was identified, but also the first gene proved to have pseudoautosomal inheritance and the first gene proved to escape lyonization. The locus is in the Ypter-Yq11.2 segment. MIC2X (see 313470), a homologous locus, is at Xp22.32 (Buckle et al., Nature 317: 739, 1985).

5. Histocompatibility antigens determined by the Y chromosome were first found in the mouse (Eichwald, E. J. and Silmser, C. R., Transplant Bull. 2: 148-149, 1955; see review by Gasser, D. L. and Silver, W. K., Adv. Immun. 15:215-217, 1972) and later in the rat, guinea pig, and many other species. Their existence in man was first shown by the fact that mouse antisera react with human male lymphocytes but not with female lymphocytes (Wachtel et al., PNAS 71:1215-1218, 1974). The possibility that the locus that determines heterogametic sex determination and that for the H-Y antigen are one and the same was suggested by Wachtel et al. (New Engl. J. Med. 293:1070-1072, 1975). Subsequent evidence ruled out this possibility, however. (At the 1986 Cold Spring Harbor Symposium, 6 speakers discussed the Y chromosome at length, but H-Y was not once mentioned.) From the study of XX males and XY females, it can be concluded that the H-Y determinant on the Y (whatever its nature) and TDF was separate entities and not closely situated (Simpson, E., Cell 44: 813, 1986; Simpson et al., Nature 326: 876-878, 1987). H-Y (structural gene or regulator) is coded near the centromere, possibly on Yq, and cloning of the true TDF is in progress.

6. The existence of factors controlling spermatogenesis on the nonfluorescent part of the long arm of Y (distal part of Yq11) was suggested by study of 6 men with deletion of this segment and azoospermia (Tiepolo, L. and Zuffardi, O., Hum. Genet. 34: 110-124, 1976). This has been called azoospermia third factor (symbolized Sp-3), or more recently (HGM9), AZF (for azoospermia factor). This might be identical to H-Y because it maps to the same region. In mice, H-Y or a closely linked gene has been implicated in spermatogenesis (Burgoyne et al., Nature 320: 170, 1986).

7. That one or more genes concerned with stature are on the Y chromosome is suggested by the comparative heights of the XX, XY and XYY genotypes; that the effect of the Y chromosome on stature is mediated through a mechanism other than androgen is suggested by the tall stature of persons with XY gonadal dysgenesis (306100). See also the argument, from XO and XXY cases, that genes determining slower maturation must be on the Y (Tanner et al., Lancet II: 141-144, 1959). The postulated locus is symbolized STA (for 'stature'). Yamada et al. (Hum. Genet. 58:268-270, 1981) found a correlation between the length of heterochromatic band Yq12 and height; yet complete or almost complete lack of the heterochromatic segment in Amish males of the surname Byler had no effect on stature (or fertility) (Borgaonkar et al., Ann. Genet. 12:

262, 1969). The STA locus may be identical to the TSY (or GCY) locus (see later).

8. Alvesalo and de la Chapelle (Ann. Hum. Genet. 43:97-102, 1979; HGM5, Edinburgh, 1979) suggested, on the basis of tooth size in males of various Y chromosome constitutions, that a Y-chromosomal gene controlling tooth size is independent of the testis-determining gene and is carried by Yq11 (symbolized TS for 'tooth size,' or, more recently, in HGM8, GCY for 'growth control Y'. See Alvesalo and Portin, Am. J. Hum. Genet. 32:955-959, 1980; Alvesalo and de la Chapelle, Ann. Hum. Genet. 54:49-54, 1981. The dental growth factors are thought to coincide with determinants of stature.

9. An argininosuccinate synthetase pseudogene is on the Y (Daiger et al., Nature 298: 682, 1982), as is also an actin pseudogene (Heilig et al., EMBO J. 3:1803, 1984).

10. The Howard Hughes Medical Institute's Human Gene Mapping Library (HGML) has cataloged more than 100 seemingly low copy number anonymous DNA segments mapped exclusively to specific regions of the Y chromosome, as well as at least 60 DNA segments that map to both the Y and the X. Some segments map to both the Y and an autosome, and some repetitive DNA segments map to the Y exclusively or to both the Y and the X.

11. Repetitive sequences located exclusively or predominantly to the Y chromosome (e.g., Kunkel, Smith and Boyer, Biochemistry 18:3343-3353, 1979) map to the heterochromatic portion of Yq and are presumably genetically inert because persons lacking these are phenotypically normal and normally fertile.

THE MITOCHONDRIAL CHROMOSOME (CHROMOSOME M OR CHROMOSOME 25)

Each mitochondrion contains several circular chromosomes. The most important function of the mitochondria is synthesis of ATP by the process of oxidative phosphorylation (OXPHOS). OXPHOS involves 5 multi-polypeptide enzyme complexes in the mitochondrial inner membrane. The biogenesis of 4 of these 5 complexes is under the combined control of nuclear DNA and mitochondrial DNA (mtDNA). At least 69 separate polypeptides are known to be required for OXPHOS; only 13 of them are coded by mtDNA.

The 16,569 basepairs of the mitochondrial chromosome are the equivalent of 5,523 codons. Most of the mtDNA serves a coding function. The genes contain no intervening sequences, and little in the way of flanking sequences is present. The ribosomal and transfer RNAs are those involved in the synthesis of protein in the mitochondrion. Of the 22 tRNAs, 14 are coded on the L (light) strand. For all 13 reading frames, the function of the specific protein coded is known. The mtDNA code differs from that of the nuclear DNA and the genetic code of any presentday prokaryote. UGA codes for tryptophan (not termination), AUA codes for methionine (not isoleucine), and AGA and AGG code for termination (not arginine). The mitochondrial genome is transcribed as a single mRNA transcript which is subsequently cleaved into its several component genes.

Mitochondrial inheritance ('cytoplasmic inheritance' the old terminology) is exclusively matrilineal. Restriction fragment length polymorphisms (RFLPs) are known in mitochondrial DNA as in nuclear DNA. Mitochondrial restriction patterns can be used to construct a biological history of the human species.

Whereas each nuclear chromosome is present in only 2 copies per cell at the most, the mitochondrial chromosome is present in thousands of copies. The behavior of a mitochondrial mutation in inheritance might be expected, therefore, to be galtonian rather than mendelian.

In cultured cells, chloramphenicol resistance is demonstrably the result of mutation in the mtDNA gene for 16S rRNA (see 21465). Indeed, the specific nucleotide changes have been identified. A point mutation (substitution of nucleotide 1178) has been identified as a cause of Leber optic atrophy (Wallace et al., Science 242: 1427-1430, 1988). Deletions (which always avoid the origins of replication) have been observed in many patients with progressive external ophthalmoplegia alone or as part of Kearns-Sayre syndrome (Moraes et al., New Eng. J. Med. 320: 1293-1299, 1989). Deletion in the mitochondrial chromosome has also been found in mitochondrial myopathy (e.g., Holt et al., Nature 221: 717-719, 1988), in the Pearson marrow-pancreas syndrome (Rotig et al., Lancet 1: 902-903, 1989), the benign neoplasia called oncocytoma (Welter et al., Genes Chrom. Cancer 1: 79, 1989), and even a relation to aging has been suggested.

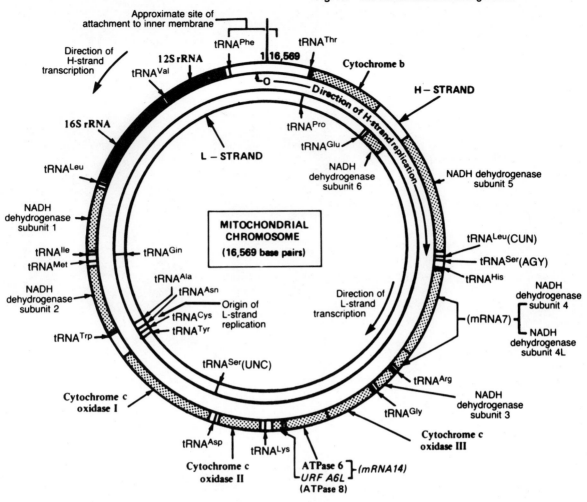

Fig. A1 The human mitochondrial genome.

Gene	Location (nucleotide pair)	Gene	Location (nucleotide pair)
(L-strand promoter	about 392-435)	tRNA asparagine	7518-7585
(major H-strand promoter	about 545-567)	cytochrome c oxidase subunit II	7586-8262
(minor L-strand start site	561)	tRNA lysine	8295-8364
tRNA phenylalanine	577-647	ATPase subunit 8 (URF A-L)	8366-8572
(minor H-strand start site	about 645)	ATPase subunit 6	8527-9207
12S rRNA	648-1601	cytochrome c oxidase subunit III	9207-9990
tRNA valine	1602-1670	tRNA glycine	9991-10058
16S rRNA	1671-3229	NADH dehydrogenase subunit 3	10059-10404
tRNA leucine (UUR)	3230-3304	tRNA arginine	10405-10469
NADH dehydrogenase subunit 1	3307-4262	NADH dehydrogenase subunit 4L	10470-10766
tRNA isoleucine	4263-4331	NADH dehydrogenase subunit 4	10760-12137
tRNA glutamine	4329-4400	tRNA histidine	12138-12206
tRNA methionine (including fMET)	4402-4469	tRNA serine (AGY)	12207-12265
NADH dehydrogenase subunit 2	4470-5511	tRNA leucine (CUN)	12266-12336
tRNA tryptophan	5512-5576	NADH dehydrogenase subunit 5	12337-14148
tRNA alanine	5587-5655	NADH dehydrogenase subunit 6 (on L)	14149-14673
tRNA asparagine	5657-5729	tRNA glutamic acid (L-strand)	14674-14742
(origin of L-strand replication	5729-5805)	cytochrome b	14747-15887
tRNA cysteine	5761-5826	tRNA threonine	15888-15953
tRNA tyrosine	5826-5891	tRNA proline (L-strand)	15955-16023
cytochrome c oxidase subunit I	5904-7444	(membrane attachment site	about 15925-499)
tRNA serine	7445-7516		

MAP SITES BY DISORDER (The Morbid Anatomy of the Human Genome)—see Figure 1-9

The following is an alphabetized list of disorders for which the mutation has been mapped to a specific site. In some instances, the disease phenotype was mapped by finding of linkage to a marker (e.g., Huntington disease) or by finding a specific chromosome change (e.g., Prader-Willi syndrome). In other instances, the disorder was located by virtue of mapping the 'wildtype' gene, combined with the presumption or proof that the given disorder represents a mutation in that structural gene (e.g., Tay-Sachs disease and hexosaminidase A). Cancers, which represent a form of somatic cell genetic disease, are, in selected instances, included here when a specific chromosomal change and/or relation to an oncogene indicates a specific localization of determinant(s). Malformations which are related to specific localized chromosomal change and again represent a form of somatic cell genetic disease are also included (e.g., Langer-Giedion syndrome). Certain 'nondiseases,' mainly genetic variations that lead to apparently abnormal laboratory test values (e.g., dysalbuminemic euthyroidal hyperthyroxinemia) are included in **brackets**. For some loci, multiple quite dissimilar disorders are caused by different mutations in the same gene; examples of allelic disorders are placed in **boxes** in the figure. **Braces** indicate examples of mutations which lead to universal susceptibility to a specific infection (diphtheria, polio), to frequent resistance to a specific infection (vivax malaria), as well as some other susceptibilities. **?** before the disease name is the equivalent of L (in limbo). The number in parentheses after the name of each disorder indicates whether the mutation was positioned by mapping the 'wildtype' gene (1), by mapping the disease phenotype itself (2), or by both approaches (3).

Disorder	Symbol	MIM #	Location
46,XY female (2)	ZFX	314980	Xp22.2-p21.2
Aarskog-Scott syndrome (2)	FGDY, AAS	305400	Xq13
?Abetalipoproteinemia (1)	APOB	107730	2p24
[Acanthocytosis, 1 form] (1)	EPB3, EMPB3	109270	17q21-q22
Acatalasemia (1)	CAT	115500	11p13
Acetyl-CoA carboxylase deficiency (1)	ACC	200350	17q21
Acid-maltase deficiency, adult (1)	GAA	232300	17q23
Acoustic neuroma (2)	NF2, ACN	101000	22q11.21-q13.1
?Acrokeratoelastoidosis (2)	AKE	101850	2p
ACTH deficiency (1)	POMC	176830	2p25
Acute alcohol intolerance (1)	ALDH2	100650	12q24.2
Acute lymphoblastic leukemia (2)	LALL	247640	9p22-p21
?Acyl-CoA dehydrogenase, long chain deficiency of (1)	HADH, ACADL, LCAD	143450	Chr.7
Acyl-CoA dehydrogenase, medium chain, deficiency of (1)	ACADM, MCAD	201450	1p31
Acyl-CoA dehydrogenase, short chain, deficiency of (1)	ACADS	201470	12q22-qter
Adenylosuccinase deficiency (1)	ADSL, ADS	103050	Chr.22
Adrenal hyperplasia, congenital, due to 11-beta-hydroxylase deficiency (1)	CYP11B1, P450C11	202010	8q21
Adrenal hyperplasia, congenital, due to 21-hydroxylase deficiency (3)	CYP21, CA21H, CAH1	201910	6p21.3
Adrenal hyperplasia II (1)	HSDB	201810	1p13
Adrenal hyperplasia V (1)	CYP17, P450C17	202110	Chr.10
Adrenal hypoplasia, primary (2)	AHC, AHX	300200	Xp21.3-p21.2
Adrenocortical carcinoma (2)	ADCR, ADCC	202300	11p15.5
Adrenoleukodystrophy (2)	ALD	300100	Xq28
AFP deficiency, congenital (1)	AFP	104150	4q11-q13
Agammaglobulinemia, type 2, X-linked (2)	AGMX2, XLA2, IMD6	300310	Xp22
Agammaglobulinemia, X-linked (2)	AGMX1, IMD1, XLA	300300	Xq21.3-q22
Aicardi syndrome (2)	AIC	304050	Xp22
Albinism (3)	TYR, ATN	203100	11q14-q21
Albinism-deafness syndrome (2)	ALDS, ADFN	300700	Xq26.3-q27.1
?Aldolase A deficiency (1)	ALDOA,ALDA	103850	16q22-q24
Alpha-1-antichymotrypsin deficiency (1)	AACT	107280	14q32.1
Alpha-NAGA deficiency (1)	NAGA	104170	22q11

Disorder	Symbol	MIM #	Location
Alport syndrome (2)	ATS, ASLN	301050	Xq22-q24
Alzheimer disease (2)	AD1	104300	21q11.2-q21
Amelogenesis imperfecta (1)	AMGS, AMG, ALGN, AIH1	301200	Xp22.3-p22.1
Amyloid neuropathy, familial, several allelic types (3)	PALB, TTR, TBPA	176300	18q11.2-q12.1
?Amyloidosis, cerebroarterial, Dutch type, 105160 (1)	APP, AAA, CVAP	104760	21q21.3-q22.05
Amyloidosis, Iowa form 105100 (1)	APOA1	107680	11q23-qter
(?Amyloidosis, secondary, susceptibility to) (2)	APCS, SAP	104770	1q12-q23
Anal canal carcinoma (2)	ANC	105580	11q22-qter
Analbuminemia (1)	ALB	103600	4q11-q13
Anemia, sideroblastic/hypochromic (3)	ALAS2, ASB, ANH1	301300	Xq13
Angelman syndrome (2)	ANCR, AGMS	234400	15q11-q13
Angioedema, hereditary (1)	C1NH, C1I, HANE	106100	11q11-q13
Anhidrotic ectodermal dysplasia (2)	EDA, HED	305100	Xq12.2-13.1
Aniridia of WAGR syndrome (2)	WAGR, WTCR1	194070	11p13
Aniridia-1 (2)	AN1	106200	2p25
Aniridia-2 (2)	AN2	106210	11p13
?ANLL-M2 (1)	MRS	159560	8q21.1-q23
Anterior segment mesenchymal dysgenesis (2)	ASMD	107250	4q28-q31
Antithrombin III deficiency (3)	AT3	107300	1q23.1-q23.9
ApoA-I and apoC-III deficiency, combined (1)	APOA1	107680	11q23-qter
Apolipoprotein B-100, defective (1)	APOB	107730	2p24
[Apolipoprotein H deficiency] (1)	APOH	138700	Chr.17
Argininemia (1)	ARG1	207800	6q23
Argininosuccinicaciduria (1)	ASL	207900	7cen-q11.2
Arteriohepatic dysplasia (2)	AGS, AHD	118450	20p11.2
Aspartylglucosaminuria (1)	AGA	208400	4q21-qter
Ataxia-telangiectasia (2)	AT1	208900	11q22-q23
Atopy (2)	APY, IGEL	147050	11q12-q13
Atransferrinemia (1)	TF	190000	3q21
Atrial septal defect, secundum type (2)	ASD2	108800	6p21.3
?Batten disease, 1 form, 204200 (1)	CTSH	116820	15q24-q25
Batten disease (2)	NCL, BD	204200	16q22
Becker muscular dystrophy (3)	DMD, BMD	310200	Xp21.2
Beckwith-Wiedemann syndrome (2)	BWCR, BWS, WBS	130650	11pter-p15.4
?Branchiootic syndrome (2)	BOS	113650	8q13.3
Breast cancer, ductal (2)	BRCD2	211420	1p36
Breast cancer, ductal (2)	BRCD1, DBC, BCDS1	211410	Chr.13
?Brody myopathy (1)	ATP2B	108740	Chr.12
Burkitt lymphoma (3)	MYC	190080	8q24.1
?C1q deficiency (1)	C1QA	120550	1p
?C1q deficiency (1)	C1QB	120570	1p
C1r/C1s deficiency, combined (1)	C1R	216950	12p13
C1r/C1s deficiency, combined (1)	C1S	120580	12p13
C2 deficiency (3)	C2	217000	6p21.3
C3 deficiency (1)	C3	120700	19p13.3-p13.2

Disorder	Gene symbol	MIM number	Location
C3b inactivator deficiency (1)	IF	217030	4q25
C4 deficiency (3)	C4A, C4S	120810	6p21.3
C4 deficiency (3)	C4B, C4F	120820	6p21.3
C5 deficiency (1)	C5	120900	9q34.1
C6 deficiency (1)	C6	217050	Chr.5
C7 deficiency (1)	C7	217070	Chr.5
C8 deficiency, type I (2)	C8A	120950	1p22
C8 deficiency, type II (2)	C8B	120960	1p22
C9 deficiency (1)	C9	120940	5p13
?Campomelic dysplasia with sex reversal (2)	CMD1	211970	5q33.1
?Campomelic dysplasia with sex reversal (2)	CMD1	211970	8q21.4
Carbamoylphosphate synthetase I deficiency (1)	CPS1	237300	2p
[Carbonic anhydrase I deficiency] (1)	CA1	114800	8q22
Cat eye syndrome (2)	CECR, CES	115470	22q11
?Cataract, anterior polar (2)	CAP	115650	14q24
?Cataract, anterior polar (2)	CAP	115650	2p25
Cataract, Coppock-like (3)	CRYG1	123660	2q33-q35
Cataract, Marner type (2)	CPM, CAM	116800	16q22.1
Cataract, zonular pulverulent (2)	CAE	116200	1q2
Cerebral amyloid angiopathy (1)	CST3	105150	Chr.22
CETP deficiency (1)	CETP	118470	16q21
Charcot-Marie-Tooth disease, slow nerve conduction type Ia (2)	CMT1A	118220	17p11.2-q23
Charcot-Marie-Tooth disease, slow nerve conduction type Ib (2)	CMT1B	118200	1p22-q23
Charcot-Marie-Tooth disease, X-linked (2)	CMTX, CMT2	302800	Xq13
Cholesterol ester storage disease (1)	LIPA	278000	10q24-q25
Chondrodysplasia punctata, X-linked dominant (2)	CDPX2, CPXD, CPX	302960	Xq28
Chondrodysplasia punctata, X-linked recessive (2)	CPXR	302950	Xpter-p22.32
Choroideremia (2)	TCD	303100	Xq21.2
Chronic granulomatous disease due to deficiency of NCF-1 (1)	NCF1	233700	Chr.7
Chronic granulomatous disease due to deficiency of NCF-2 (1)	NCF2	233710	1cen-q32
Citrullinemia (1)	ASS	215700	9q34
Cleft palate, X-linked (2)	CPX	303400	Xq21
CMO II deficiency (1)	CYP11B1, P450C11	202010	8q21
Coffin-Lowry syndrome (2)	CLS	303600	Xp22.2-p22.1
?Coloboma of iris (2)	COI	120200	2pter-p25.1
Colorblindness, blue-monochromatic (3)	CBBM, BCM	303700	Xq28
Colorblindness, deutan (2)	GCP, CBD	303800	Xq28
Colorblindness, protan (2)	RCP, CBP	303900	Xq28
Colorblindness, tritan (2)	BCP, CBT	190900	7q22-qter
Colorectal adenoma (1)	KRAS2, RASK2	190070	12p12.1
?Colorectal cancer (1)	KRAS2, RASK2	190070	12p12.1
Colorectal cancer (1)	CRC18	120470	18q23.3
Colorectal cancer, 114500 (2)	CRCR2, CRC17	120460	17p12
Colorectal carcinoma, 114500 (1)	TP53	191170	17p13.105-p12
Combined C6/C7 deficiency (1)	C6	217050	Chr.5
?Combined variable hypogammaglobulinemia (1)	IGH		14q32.33

Disorder	Symbol	MIM #	Location
Conductive deafness with stapes fixation (2)	DFN3	304400	Xq13-q21.1
Coproporphyria (1)	CPRO, CPO	121300	Chr.9
{Coronary artery disease, susceptibility to} (1)	LPA	152200	6q27
Cortisol resistance (1)	GRL	138040	5q31
CR1 deficiency (1)	CR1, C3BR	120620	1q32
Craniosynostosis (2)	CRS, CSO	123100	7p21.3-p21.2
[Creatine kinase, brain type, ectopic expression of] (2)	CKBE	123270	14q32
?Creutzfeld-Jacob disease, 123400 (2)	PRIP, PRNP	176640	20pter-p12
?Cryptorchidism (2)	GTD	306190	Xp21
[Cystathioninuria] (1)	CTH	219500	Chr.16
Cystic fibrosis (2)	CF	219700	7q31.3-q32
Dentinogenesis imperfecta-1 (2)	DGI1	125490	4q13-q21
Diabetes insipidus, nephrogenic (2)	DIR, DI1	304800	Xq28
?Diabetes insipidus, neurohypophyseal, 125700 (1)	ARVP, VP	192340	Chr.20
?Diabetes mellitus, insulin dependent (2)	IDDM	222100	6p21.3
Diabetes mellitus, insulin-resistant, with acanthosis nigricans (1)	INSR	147670	19p13.3-p13.2
Diabetes mellitus, rare form (1)	INS	176730	11p15.5
?Diaphragmatic hernia (2)	DH	222400	1q32.3-q42.3
?Diastrophic dysplasia (2)	DD	222600	Chr.18
DiGeorge syndrome (2)	DGCR, DGS	188400	22q11
{Diphtheria, susceptibility to} (1)	DTS	126150	5q23
?Dubin-Johnson syndrome (2)	DJS	237500	13q34
Duchenne muscular dystrophy (3)	DMD, BMD	310200	Xp21.2
[Dysalbuminemic hyperthyroxinemia] (1)	ALB	103600	4q11-q13
[Dysalbuminemic hyperzincemia] (1)	ALB	103600	4q11-q13
Dysfibrinogenemia, alpha types (1)	FGA	134820	4q26-q28
Dysfibrinogenemia, beta types (1)	FGB	134830	4q26-q28
Dysfibrinogenemia, gamma types (1)	FGG	134850	4q26-q28
Dyskeratosis congenita (2)	DKC	305000	Xq28
?Dyslexia-1 (2)	DLX1	127700	15q11
Dysplasia-gigantism syndrome, X-linked (2)	SDYS, DGSX, GDS	312870	Xq13-q21
Dysplasminogenemic thrombophilia (1)	PLG	173350	6q26-q27
Dysprothrombinemia (1)	F2	176930	11p11-q12
[Dystransthyretinemic hyperthyroxinemia](1)	PALB, TTR, TBPA	176300	18q11.2-q12.1
Ehlers-Danlos syndrome, type IV (3)	COL3A1	120180	2q31
Ehlers-Danlos syndrome, type VIIA1 (3)	COL1A1	120150	17q21.31-q22.05
Ehlers-Danlos syndrome, type VIIA2 (3)	COL1A2	120160	7q21.3-q22.1
?Ehlers-Danlos syndrome, type X (3)	FN1	135600	2q34-q36
Elliptocytosis-1 (3)	EL1	130500	1p36.2-p34
?Elliptocytosis-2 (2)	EL2	130600	1q2
Elliptocytosis-2 (2)	SPTA1	182860	1q21
Elliptocytosis-3 (2)	SPTB, SPH1	182870	14q22-q23.2
Emery-Dreifuss muscular dystrophy (2)	EMD	310300	Xq28
Emphysema-cirrhosis (1)	PI, AAT	107400	14q32.1
Enolase deficiency (1)	ENO1, PPH	172430	1pter-p36.13
?Eosinophilic myeloproliferative disorder (2)	MPE, EMP	131440	12p13

Disorder	Gene	MIM	Location
Epidermolysis bullosa dystrophica, recessive (3)	CLG, EBR1, CLGN	226600	11q11-q23
Epidermolysis bullosa, Ogna type (2)	EBS1	131950	8q24
Epidermolysis bullosa progressiva (2)	EBR3	226500	ULG
Epilepsy, juvenile myoclonic (2)	EJM, JME	254770	6q21
?Erythremia (1)	EPO	133170	7q21-q22
Erythremias, alpha- (1)	HBA1	141800	16pter-p13.3
Erythremias, beta- (1)	HBB	141900	11p15.5
Erythroblastosis fetalis (1)	RH		1p36.2-p34
Erythrokeratodermia variabilis (2)	EKV	133200	1p36.2-p34
[Euthyroidal hyper- and hypothyroxinemia] (1)	TBG	314200	Xq21-q22
Ewing sarcoma (2)	ES	133450	22q12
Exertional myoglobinuria due to deficiency of LDH-A (1)	LDHA	150000	11p15-p14
Fabry disease (3)	GLA	301500	Xq22
Factor V deficiency (1)	F5	227400	1q23
Factor VII deficiency (1)	F7	227500	13q34
Factor X deficiency (1)	F10	227600	13q34
Factor XI deficiency (1)	F11	264900	4q35
Factor XII deficiency (1)	F12, HAF	234000	5q33-qter
Factor XIII, A component deficiency (1)	F13A1	134570	6p25-p24
Familial aneurysm (2)	COL3A1	120180	2q31
?Familial colorectal cancer (2)	APC, GS, FPC	175100	5q22-q23
?Familial Mediterranean fever, 249100 (1)	ITIL, ITI, HCP	176870	9q32-q33
?Fanconi anemia (1)	PPOL, PARP	173870	1q41-q42
Favism (1)	G6PD1	305900	Xq28
?Fetal alcohol syndrome (1)	ALDH2	100650	12q24.2
?Fetal hydantoin syndrome (1)	EPHX, EPOX	132810	1p22-qter
Focal dermal hypoplasia (2)	DHOF, FODH	305600	Xp22.31
Friedreich ataxia (2)	FRDA, FAT	229300	9q13-q21.1
Fructose intolerance (1)	ALDOB	229600	9q22
?Fryns syndrome (2)	FRNS	229850	1q24-q31.2
Fucosidosis (1)	FUCA1,FUCA	230000	1p34
?Fumarase deficiency (1)	FH	136850	1q42.1
Fumarylacetoacetate deficiency (1)	FAH	276700	15q23-q25
G6PD deficiency (3)	G6PD1	305900	Xq28
Galactokinase deficiency (1)	GALK	230200	17q21-q22
Galactose epimerase deficiency (1)	GALE	230350	1pter-p32
Galactosemia (1)	GALT	230400	9p13
Galactosialidosis (1)	GSL, NGBE	256540	Chr.20
Gardner syndrome (2)	APC, GS, FPC	175100	5q22-q23
Gaucher disease (1)	GBA	230800	1q21
Gerstmann-Straussler disease, 137440 (2)	PRIP, PRNP	176640	20pter-p12
Glanzmann thrombasthenia (1)	GP3A	173470	17q21.1-q21.3
Glanzmann thrombasthenia (1)	GP2B	273800	17q21.32
Glaucoma, congenital (2)	GLAU1	231300	Chr.11
Glioblastoma multiforme	GBM	137800	10p12-q23.2
Glucose/galactose malabsorption (1)	SGLT1, NAGT	182380	22q11.2-qter

Disorder	Symbol	MIM #	Location
Glutaricaciduria, type II (1)	ETFA, GA2	231680	15q23-q25
Glutathioninuria (1)	GGT, GTG	231950	22q11.1-q11.2
Glycerol kinase deficiency (2)	GK	307030	Xp21.3-p21.2
Glycogen storage disease, type VII (1)	PFKM	232800	1cen-q32
Glycogen storage disease VIII (1)	PHKA	306000	Xq12-q13
[Glyoxalase II deficiency] (1)	HAGH,GLO2	138760	16p13
GM1-gangliosidosis (1)	GLB1	230500	3p21-p14.2
GM2-gangliosidosis, AB variant (1)	GM2A	272750	Chr.5
GM2-gangliosidosis, juvenile, adult (1)	HEXA, TSD	272800	15q22-q25.1
Goemime TKCR syndrome (2)	TKCR	314300	Xq28
?Goiter, adolescent multinodular, 138800 (1)	TG	188450	8q24.2-q24.3
?Goldenhar syndrome (2)	GHS	141400	7p
Gonadal dysgenesis, XY female type (2)	GDXY, TDFX	306100	Xp22-p21
Gonadoblastoma (2)	WAGR, WTCR1	194070	11p13
?Gonadotropin deficiency (2)	GTD	306190	Xp21
Granulomatous disease, chronic, X-linked (3)	CYBB, CGD	306400	Xp21.1
Greig craniopolysyndactyly syndrome (2)	GCPS	175700	7p13
?Growth hormone deficiency, X-linked (2)	GHDX	312000	Xq21.3-q22
?Gynecomastia, familial, due to increased aromatase activity (1)	CYP19, ARO	107910	15q21.1
Gyrate atrophy of choroid and retina (1)	OAT	258870	10q26
Harderoporphyria (1)	CPRO,CPO	121300	Chr.9
Hb H mental retardation syndrome (2)	HBHR	141750	16pter-p13.3
Heinz body anemias, alpha- (1)	HBA1	141800	16pter-p13.3
Heinz body anemias, beta- (1)	HBB	141900	11p15.5
Hemochromatosis (2)	HFE	235200	6p21.3
Hemodialysis-related amyloidosis (1)	B2M	109700	15q21-q22
Hemolytic anemia due to ADA excess (1)	ADA	102700	20q13.11
Hemolytic anemia due to adenylate kinase deficiency (1)	AK1	103000	9q34.1
Hemolytic anemia due to bisphosphoglycerate mutase deficiency (1)	BPGM	222800	7q22-q34
Hemolytic anemia due to G6PD deficiency (1)	G6PD1	305900	Xq28
Hemolytic anemia due to glucosephosphate isomerase deficiency (1)	GPI	172400	19cen-q12
Hemolytic anemia due to glutathione peroxidase deficiency (1)	GPX1	138320	3p13-q12
Hemolytic anemia due to glutathione reductase deficiency (1)	GSR	138300	8p21.1
Hemolytic anemia due to hexokinase deficiency (1)	HK1	142600	10p11.2
Hemolytic anemia due to PGK deficiency (1)	PGKA,PGK1	311800	Xq13
Hemolytic anemia due to phosphofructokinase deficiency (1)	PFKL	171860	21q22.3
Hemolytic anemia due to triosephosphate isomerase deficiency (1)	TPI1,TPI	190450	12p13
Hemophilia A (3)	HEMA, F8C	306700	Xq28
Hemophilia B (3)	HEMB, F9	306900	Xq27.1-q27.2
Hemorrhagic diathesis due to 'antithrombin' Pittsburgh (1)	PI, AAT	107400	14q32.1
Hemorrhagic diathesis due to PAI1 deficiency (1)	PLANH1, PAI1	173360	7q21.3-q22
?Hepatic lipase deficiency (1)	LIPC, LIPH, HL, HTGL	151670	15q21-q23
Hepatocellular carcinoma (3)	HVBS6, HCC2	142380	4q32.1
[Hereditary persistence of alpha-fetoprotein] (3)	HPAFP	104140	4q11-q13
?Hereditary persistence of fetal hemoglobin (3)	HBGR	142270	11p15.5
Hers disease, or glycogen storage disease VI (1)	PYGL, PPYL	232700	Chr.14

Disorder	Symbol	MIM	Location
Heterocellular hereditary persistence of fetal hemoglobin (2)	HPFH, FCP, HHPF	142470	11p15
?Heterocellular hereditary persistence of fetal hemoglobin (2)	FCPX	305430	Xq28
[Hex A pseudodeficiency] (1)	HEXA, TSD	272800	15q22-q25.1
?HHH syndrome (2)	HHHS	238970	13q34
[Histidinemia] (1)	HIS, HSTD	235800	12q22-q23
?Holoprosencephaly (2)	HPEC	236100	2p21
?Holt-Oram syndrome (2)	HOS	142900	14q23-q24.2
Homocystinuria, B6-responsive and nonresponsive types (1)	CBS	236200	21q22.3
HPFH, deletion type (1)	HBB	141900	11p15.5
HPFH, nondeletion type A (1)	HBG1	142200	11p15.5
HPFH, nondeletion type G (1)	HBG2	142250	11p15.5
HPRT-related gout (1)	HPRT	308000	Xq26-q27.2
Huntington disease (2)	HD	143100	4p16.3
Hurler syndrome (1)	IDUA, IDA	252800	22q11
Hurler-Scheie syndrome (1)	IDUA, IDA	252800	22q11
Hydrops fetalis (1)	GPI	172400	19cen-q12
Hyperbetalipoproteinemia (1)	APOB	107730	2p24
Hypercholesterolemia, familial (3)	LDLR,FHC	143890	19p13.2-p13.1
?Hyperglycinemia, isolated nonketotic, type I (2)	NKH1	238300	9p22
?Hypergonadotropic hypogonadism (1)	LHB	152780	19q13.32
?Hyperimmunoglobulin G1 syndrome (2)	IGHR	144120	14q32.33
?Hyperleucinemia-isoleucinemia or hypervalinemia (1)	BCT1	113520	12pter-q12
Hyperlipoproteinemia I (1)	LPL, LIPD	238600	8p22
Hyperlipoproteinemia, type Ib (1)	APOC2	207750	19q13.1
Hyperlipoproteinemia, type III (1)	APOE	207760	19q13.1
[Hyperphenylalaninemia, mild] (3)	PAH, PKU1	261600	12q24.1
[?Hyperproglucagonemia] (1)	GCG	138030	2q36-q37
Hyperproinsulinemia, familial (1)	INS	176730	11p15.5
Hypertriglyceridemia, 1 form (1)	APOA1	107680	11q23-qter
?Hypervalinemia or hyperleucine-isoleucinemia (1)	BCT2	113530	Chr.19
Hypoalphalipoproteinemia (1)	APOA1	107680	11q23-qter
Hypobetalipoproteinemia (1)	APOB	107730	2p24
[Hypoceruloplasminemia, hereditary] (1)	CP	117700	3q21-q24
Hypofibrinogenemia, gamma types (1)	FGG	134850	4q26-q28
?Hypogonadotropic hypogonadism due to GNRH deficiency , 227200 (1)	GNRH,LHRH	152760	8p21-q11.2
Hypomagnesemia, X-linked primary (2)	HOMG, HSH, HMGX	307600	Xp22
?Hypomelanosis of Ito (2)	ITO	146150	15q11-q13
?Hypomelanosis of Ito (2)	ITO	146150	9q33-qter
?Hypoparathyroidism, familial (1)	PTH	168450	11p15
Hypoparathyroidism, X-linked (2)	HPTX, HYPX	307700	Xq26-q27
?Hypophosphatasia, adult 146300 (1)	ALPL, HOPS	171760	1p36.2-p34
Hypophosphatasia, infantile 241500 (3)	ALPL, HOPS	171760	1p36.2-p34
Hypophosphatemia, hereditary (2)	HYP, HPDR1	307800	Xp22
?Hypophosphatemia with deafness (2)	GY	307810	Xp22
Hypoprothrombinemia (1)	F2	176930	11p11-q12
Hypothyroidism, hereditary congenital, 1 or more types (1)	TG	188450	8q24.2-q24.3

Disorder	Symbol	MIM #	Location
Hypothyroidism, nongoitrous (1)	TSHB	188540	1p22
Hypothyroidism, nongoitrous, due to TSH resistance (1)	TSHR	275200	22q11-q13
?Ichthyosis vulgaris, 146700 (1)	FLG	135940	1q21
Ichthyosis, X-linked (3)	STS,SSDD	308100	Xpter-p22.32
Immunodeficiency, X-linked, with hyper-IgM (2)	HIGM1, IMD3	308230	Xq24-q27
Incontinentia pigmenti (2)	IP1, IP	308300	Xp11.2
Incontinentia pigmenti, familial (2)	IP2	308310	Xq27-q28
Infertile male syndrome (1)	AR, DHTR, TFM	313700	Xcen-q13
[Inosine triphosphatase deficiency] (1)	ITPA	147520	20p
Interferon, alpha, deficiency (1)	IFNA, IFL,IFA	147660	9p21
Interferon, immune, deficiency (1)	IFNG, IFI, IFG	147570	12q24.1
?Isolated growth hormone deficiency due to defect in GHRF (1)	GHRF	139190	20p11.23-qter
Isolated growth hormone deficiency, Illig type with absent GH and Kowarski type with bioinactive GH (3)	GH1, GHN	139250	17q22-q24
Isovalericacidemia (1)	IVD	243500	15q14-q15
Kallmann syndrome (2)	KAL, KMS	308700	Xpter-p22.32
Kennedy disease (2)	SBMA, KD, SMAX1	313200	Xq21.3-q22
?Kniest dysplasia (1)	COL2A1	120140	12q13.1-q13.3
?Kostmann agranulocytosis (2)	NDF	202700	6p21.3
Krabbe disease (1)	GALC	245200	Chr.17
?Lactase deficiency, adult, 223100 (1)	LCT, LAC, LPH	223000	Chr.2
?Lactase deficiency, congenital (1)	LCT, LAC, LPH	223000	Chr.2
Langer-Giedion syndrome (2)	LGCR, LGS, TRPS2	150230	8q24.11-q24.13
Langer-Saldino achondrogenesis- hypochondrogenesis (1)	COL2A1	120140	12q13.1-q13.3
Laron dwarfism (1)	GHR, GHBP	262500	5p13-p12
?Laryngeal adductor paralysis (2)	LAP	150270	6p21.3-p21.2
[Lead poisoning, susceptibility to] (1)	ALAD	125270	9q34
?Leiomyomata, multiple hereditary cutaneous (2)	MCL	150800	18p11.32
Leprechaunism (1)	INSR	147670	19p13.3-p13.2
Lesch-Nyhan syndrome (3)	HPRT	308000	Xq26-q27.2
?Letterer-Siwe disease (2)	LSD	246400	13q14-q31
?Leukemia, acute lymphocytic, with 4/11 translocation (3)	IGCJ, JCH	147790	4q21
Leukemia, acute T-cell (2)	TCL2	151390	11p13
Leukemia, chronic myeloid (3)	BCR, CML, PHL	151410	22q11.21
Leukemia, chronic myeloid (3)	ABL	189980	9q34.1
Leukemia, T-cell acute lymphocytic (2)	TCL3	186770	10q24
Leukemia/lymphoma, B-cell, 1 (2)	BCL1	151400	11q13.3
Leukemia/lymphoma, B-cell, 2 (2)	BCL2, BCL3	151430	18q21.3
Leukemia/lymphoma, T-cell (2)	TCL1	186960	14q32.1
Leukemia/lymphoma, T-cell (3)	TCRA	186880	14q11.2
Leukocyte adhesion deficiency (2)	CD18, LCAMB, LAD	116920	21q22.1-qter
Lipoamide dehydrogenase deficiency (1)	DLD, LAD	246900	Chr.7
Lipoid adrenal hyperplasia, congenital (1)	CYP11A, P450SCC, P450C11A1	201710	Chr.15
Lipoma (2)	BABL, LIPO	151900	12q13-q14
Liver cell carcinoma (1)	HVBS1, HBVS1	114550	11p14-p13

Disorder	Symbol	MIM	Location
?Long QT syndrome (2)	LQT	192500	6p21.3
Lowe syndrome (2)	OCRL, LOCR	309000	Xq25
Lymphoproliferative syndrome, X-linked (2)	LYP, IMD5, XLP, XLPD	308240	Xq25-q26
?Lynch cancer family syndrome II (2)	LCFS2	114400	18q11-q12
?Lysosomal acid phosphatase deficiency (1)	ACP2	171650	11p12-p11
Macrocytic anemia of 5q- syndrome, refractory (2)	MAR	153550	5q12-q32
Macular dystrophy, atypical vitelliform (2)	VMD1	153840	8q24
Macular dystrophy, ?vitelline type (2)	VMD2	153700	6q25-qter
?Male infertility, familial (1)	FSHB	136530	11p13
?Male pseudohermaphroditism due to defective LH (1)	LHB	152780	19q13.32
Malignant hyperthermia (2)	MHS	145600	19q13.1-q13.3
Malignant melanoma, cutaneous (2)	CMM, HCMM	155600	1p36
?Manic-depressive illness (2)	MAFD1, MD1	125480	11p15.5
Manic-depressive illness, X-linked (2)	MAFD2, MDX	309200	Xq28
Mannosidosis (1)	MANB	248500	19p13.2-q12
Maple syrup urine disease (1)	BCKDHA, MSUD1	248600	Chr.19
Marfan syndrome, atypical (1)	COL1A2	120160	7q21.3-q22.1
?Marfan syndrome, atypical, 154700(1)	COL1A1	120150	17q21.31-q22.05
Maroteaux-Lamy syndrome (1)	ARSB	253200	5q11-q13
Martin-Bell syndrome (2)	FRAXA	309550	Xq27.3
MASA syndrome (2)	MASA	309250	Xq28
McArdle disease (1)	PYGM, MGP	232600	11q13
[McLeod phenotype] (2)	XK	314850	Xp21.2-p21.1
Medullary thyroid carcinoma (2)	MEN2A, MEN2	171400	10q21.1
?Megacolon (2)	MGC	249200	13q22.1-q32.1
?Megaloblastic anemia (1)	DHFR	126060	5q11.1-q13.2
Megalocornea, X-linked (2)	MGCN	309300	Xq21.3-q22
Meningioma (2)	MGCR, MGM	156100	22q12.3-qter
?Menkes disease (1)	EPA, TIMP	305370	Xp11.4-p11.23
Menkes disease (2)	MNK, MK	309400	Xq12-q13
Mental retardation of WAGR (2)	WAGR, WTCR1	194070	11p13
Mental retardation, X-linked nonspecific, I (2)	MRX1	309530	Xp22
Mental retardation, X-linked nonspecific, II (2)	MRX2	309540	Xq11-q12
Mental retardation-skeletal dysplasia (2)	MRSD, CHRS	309620	Xq28
Metachromatic leukodystrophy (1)	ARSA	250100	22q13.31-qter
Metachromatic leukodystrophy due to deficiency of SAP-1 (1)	SAP1, SAP2	249900	10q21-q22
Methemoglobinemia, enzymopathic (1)	DIA1	250800	22q13.31-qter
Methemoglobinemias, alpha- (1)	HBA1	141800	16pter-p13.3
Methemoglobinemias, beta- (1)	HBB	141900	11p15.5
Methylmalonicaciduria, mutase deficiency type (1)	MUT, MCM	251000	6p21.2-p12
?Microcephaly, true (2)	MCT	251200	1q31-q32.1
Miller-Dieker lissencephaly syndrome (2)	MDCR, MDLS, MDS	247200	17p13.3
MODY, one form, 125850 (3)	INS	176730	11p15.5
Mucolipidosis II (1)	GNPTA	252500	4q21-q23
Mucolipidosis III (1)	GNPTA	252500	4q21-q23

Disorder	Symbol	MIM #	Location
Mucopolysaccharidosis I (1)	IDUA, IDA	252800	22q11
Mucopolysaccharidosis II (2)	IDS, MPS2, SIDS	309900	Xq27.3
Mucopolysaccharidosis IVB (1)	GLB1	230500	3p21-p14.2
Mucopolysaccharidosis VII (1)	GUSB	253220	7q21.1-q22
Multiple endocrine neoplasia I (1)	MEN1	131100	11q13
Multiple endocrine neoplasia II (2)	MEN2A, MEN2	171400	10q21.1
Multiple endocrine neoplasia III(2)	MEN3, MEN2B	162300	10q21.1
?Multiple exostoses (2)	EXT	133700	8q23-q24.1
?Multiple lipomatosis (2)	BABL, LIPO	151900	12q13-q14
Myeloperoxidase deficiency (1)	MPO	254600	17q21.3-q23
Myopathy due to phosphoglycerate mutase deficiency (1)	PGAM2, PGAMM	261670	7p13-p12
Myotonic dystrophy (2)	DM	160900	19q13
Myotubular myopathy, X-linked (2)	MTM1, MTMX	310400	Xq28
Myxoid liposarcoma (2)	BABL, LIPO	151900	12q13-q14
Nail-patella syndrome (2)	NPS1	161200	9q34
Nance-Horan syndrome (2)	NHS	302350	Xp22.3-p21.1
Neuroblastoma (2)	NB, NBS	256700	1p32
Neurofibromatosis, von Recklinghausen (2)	NF1, VRNF	162200	17q11.2
?Nevoid basal cell carcinoma syndrome (2)	NBCCS, BCNS, NBCS	109400	1p
Niemann-Pick disease (1)	SMPD1, NPD	257200	Chr.17
Nightblindness, congenital stationary, type I (2)	CSNB1	310500	Xp11.3
Norrie disease (2)	NDP, ND	310600	Xp11.4
Norum disease (3)	LCAT	245900	16q22.1
Nucleoside phosphorylase deficiency, immunodeficiency due to (2)	NP, NP1	164050	14q13.1
Ocular albinism, Forsius-Eriksson type (2)	OA2	300600	Xp21.3-p21.1
Ocular albinism, Nettleship-Falls type (2)	OA1	300500	Xp22.3
?Optic atrophy, Kjer type (2)	OAK	165500	2p
Ornithine transcarbamylase deficiency (3)	OTC	311250	Xp21.1
Orofacial cleft (2)	OFC, CL	119530	6pter-p23
Oroticaciduria (1)	UMPS, OPRT	258900	3q13
Osteoarthrosis, precocious (3)	COL2A1	120140	12q13.1-q13.3
Osteogenesis imperfecta, 2 or more clinical forms (3)	COL1A1	120150	17q21.31-q22.05
Osteogenesis imperfecta, 2 or more clinical forms (3)	COL1A2	120160	7q21.3-q22.1
Osteosarcoma, retinoblastoma-related (2)	OSRC	259500	13q14.1
Ovarian failure, premature (2)	POF	311360	Xq26-q27
?Paget disease of bone (2)	PDB	167250	6p21.3
(?Parkinsonism, susceptibility to) (1)	CYP2D, P450C2D	124030	22q11.2-q12.2
Pelizaeus-Merzbacher disease (3)	PLP, PMD	312080	Xq22
?Pendred syndrome (2)	PDS	274600	8q24
Periodontitis, juvenile (2)	JPD, JP	170650	4q11-q13
Persistent Mullerian duct syndrome (1)	AMH, MIF	261550	19p13.3-p13.2
Phenylketonuria (3)	PAH, PKU1	261600	12q24.1
Phenylketonuria due to dihydropteridine reductase deficiency (1)	QDPR, DHPR	261630	4p15.3
Phosphoribosylpyrophosphate synthetase-related gout (1)	PRPS1	311850	Xq22-q26
?Phosphorylase kinase deficiency of liver and muscle, 261750 (2)	PHKB	172490	16q12-q13.1
?Piebaldism (2)	PBT	172800	4q12

Disorder	Gene Symbol	MIM No.	Map Location
PK deficiency hemolytic anemia (1)	PKLR, PK1, PKR	266200	1q21-q22
[Placental lactogen deficiency] (1)	CSA, PL, CSH1	150200	17q22-q24
Placental steroid sulfatase deficiency (3)	STS,SSDD	308100	Xpter-p22.32
Plasmin inhibitor deficiency (1)	PLI	262850	18p11.1-q11.2
Plasminogen activator deficiency (1)	PLAT, TPA	173370	8p12
Plasminogen deficiency, types I and II (1)	PLG	173350	6q26-q27
Plasminogen Tochigi disease (1)	PLG	173350	6q26-q27
[Polio, susceptibility to) (2)	PVS	173850	19q12-q13.2
Polycystic kidney disease (2)	PKD1, APKD	173900	16p13.31-p13.12
Polycystic ovarian disease (1)	EDHB17	264300	17q11-q12
Polyposis coli, familial (2)	APC, GS, FPC	175100	5q22-q23
Pompe disease (1)	GAA	232300	17q23
Porphyria, acute hepatic (1)	ALAD	125290	9q34
Porphyria, acute intermittent (1)	PBGD, UPS	176000	11q23.2-qter
Porphyria cutanea tarda (1)	UROD	176100	1p34
Porphyria, hepatoerythropoietic (1)	UROD	176100	1p34
Porphyria variegata (2)	VP, PPOX	176200	14q32
Postanesthetic apnea (1)	CHE1	177400	3q25.2
Prader-Willi syndrome (2)	PWCR, PWS	176270	15q11
Progressive cone dystrophy (2)	COD1, PCDX	304020	Xp21.1-p11.3
?Prolidase deficiency, 264130 (1)	PEPD	170100	19cen-q13.11
Properdin deficiency, X-linked (3)	PFC, PFD	312060	Xp11.4
Propionicacidemia, type I or pccA type (1)	PCCA	232000	Chr.13
Propionicacidemia, type II or pccB type (1)	PCCB	232050	3q13.3-q22
Protein C deficiency (1)	PROC	176860	2q13-q14
Protein S deficiency (1)	PSA, PROS	176880	3p11.1-q11.2
Pseudohermaphroditism, male, with gynecomastia (1)	EDHB17	264300	17q11-q12
Pseudohypoaldosteronism (1)	MLR, MCR, MR	264350	4q31.1
Pseudohypoparathyroidism, type Ia (1)	GNAS1, GNAS, GPSA	139320	Chr.20
Pseudo-Zellweger syndrome (1)	ACAA	261510	3p23-p22
?Pyridoxine dependency with seizures (1)	GAD	266100	Chr.2
Pyropoikilocytosis (1)	SPTA1	182860	1q21
Pyruvate carboxylase deficiency (1)	PC	266150	11q
Pyruvate dehydrogenase deficiency (1)	PDHA1, PHE1A	312170	Xp22.2-p22.1
?Rabson-Mendenhall syndrome (1)	INSR	147670	19p13.3-p13.2
?Ragweed sensitivity (2)	RWS	179450	6p21.3
Reifenstein syndrome (1)	AR, DHTR, TFM	313700	Xcen-q13
Renal cell carcinoma (2)	RCC1, RCC	144700	3p14.2
[Renal glucosuria] (2)	GLUR	233100	6p21.3
Renal tubular acidosis-osteopetrosis syndrome (1)	CA2	259730	8q22
?Retinal cone dystrophy-1 (2)	RCD1	180020	6q25-q26
?Retinal cone-rod dystrophy (2)	RCRD1	120970	18q21-q22.2
Retinitis pigmentosa 2 (2)	RP2	312600	Xp11.3
Retinitis pigmentosa 3 (2)	RP3	312610	Xp21
Retinitis pigmentosa-1 (2)	RP1	180100	3q21-q23
Retinoblastoma (2)	RB1	180200	13q14.1-q14.2

Disorder	Symbol	MIM #	Location
Retinol binding protein, deficiency of (1)	RBP4	180250	10q23-q24
Retinoschisis (2)	RS	312700	Xp22
Rhabdomyosarcoma (2)	RMS, RMSCR	268210	11pter-p15.5
Rhabdomyosarcoma, alveolar (2)	RMSA	268220	2q37
Rh-null disease (1)	MER6, RHN	268150	3cen-q22
?Rh-null hemolytic anemia (1)	RH		1p36.2-p34
Rieger syndrome (2)	RGS	180500	4q23-q27
Salivary gland pleomorphic adenoma (2)	SGPA, PSA	181030	8q12
Sandhoff disease (1)	HEXB	268800	5q13
Sanfilippo syndrome D (1)	GNS, G6S	252940	12q14
Sarcoma, synovial (2)	SSRC	312820	Xp11.2
Scheie syndrome (1)	IDUA, IDA	252800	22q11
Schizophrenia (2)	SCZD1	181510	5q11.2-q13.3
SCID, X-linked (2)	SCIDX1, SCIDX, IMD4	300400	Xq13.1-q21.1
Scleroylosis (2)	TYS	181600	4q28-q31
Seizures, benign neonatal (2)	EBN, BNS	121200	Chr.20
Severe combined immunodeficiency due to ADA deficiency (1)	ADA	102700	20q13.11
Severe combined immunodeficiency (SCID), HLA class II-negative type (1)	RFX	209920	19p13
?Sialidosis (1)	NEU, NEUG	256550	Chr.10
?Sialidosis (2)	NEU, NEU1	162050, 256550	6p21.3
Sickle cell anemia (1)	HBB	141900	11p15.5
?SLE (1)	CR1, C3BR	120620	1q32
Small-cell cancer of lung (2)	SCLC1, SCCL	182280	3p23-p21
?Smith-Lemli-Opitz syndrome (2)	SLO	270400	7q34-qter
Spastic paraplegia, X-linked, uncomplicated (2)	SPG2, SPPX2	312920	Xq21-q22
Spherocytosis, recessive (1)	SPTA1	182860	1q21
Spherocytosis-1 (3)	SPTB, SPH1	182870	14q22-q23.2
Spherocytosis-2 (2)	ANK, SPH2	182900	8p11
Spinocerebellar ataxia-1 (2)	SCA1	164400	6p21.3-p21.2
Spondyloepiphyseal dysplasia congenita (3)	COL2A1	120140	12q13.1-q13.3
Spondyloepiphyseal dysplasia tarda (2)	SEDL, SEDT	313400	Xp22
Stickler syndrome (3)	COL2A1	120140	12q13.1-q13.3
Sucrose intolerance (1)	SI	222900	3q25-q26
?Susceptibility to amyloid in FMF, 249100 (1)	SAA	104750	11pter-p12
Tay-Sachs disease (1)	HEXA, TSD	272800	15q22-q25.1
Testicular feminization (1)	AR, DHTR, TFM	313700	Xcen-q13
Thalassemias, alpha- (1)	HBA1	141800	16pter-p13.3
Thalassemias, beta- (1)	HBB	141900	11p15.5
Thrombophilia due to elevated HRG (2)	HRG	142640	Chr.3
?Thrombophilia due to excessive plasminogen activator inhibitor (1)	PLANH1, PAII	173360	7q21.3-q22
Thrombophilia due to heparin cofactor II deficiency (1)	HCF2, HC2	142360	Chr.22
Thyroid hormone resistance, 274300, 188570 (3)	THRB, THR1, ERBA2	190160	3p24.3
Thyroid iodine peroxidase deficiency (1)	TPO, TPX	274500	2pter-p12
Thyroid papillary carcinoma (1)	TST1, PTC, TPC	188550	10q11-q12
Torsion dystonia (2)	DYT1	128100	9q32-q34
?Tourette syndrome (2)	GTS	137580	18q22.1

Disorder	Gene	MIM No.	Location
Transcobalamin II deficiency (1)	TCN2, TC2	275350	22q11.2-qter
?Treacher Collins mandibulofacial dysostosis (2)	MFD1	154500	5q11
Trichorhinophalangeal syndrome, type I (2)	TRPS1	190350	8q24.12
Trypsinogen deficiency (1)	TRY1, TRP1	276000	7q22-qter
Tuberous sclerosis-1 (2)	TSC1, TSC, TS	191100	9q33-q34
Tuberous sclerosis-2 (2)	TSC2	191090	11q23
Tyrosinemia, type II (1)	TAT	276600	16q22.1-q22.3
Urolithiasis, 2,8-dihydroxyadenine (1)	APRT	102600	16q24
Usher syndrome, type 2 (2)	US2	276900	1q32
van der Woude syndrome (2)	LPS, PIT, VDWS	119300	1q32
Vitamin D dependency, type I (2)	VDD1	264700	12q14
{Vivax malaria, susceptibility to} (1)	FY	110700	1q21-q22
von Hippel-Lindau syndrome (2)	VHL	193300	3p25-p24
von Willebrand disease (1)	F8VWF,VWF	193400	12pter-p12
Waardenburg syndrome, type I (2)	WS1	193500	2q37.3
?Watson syndrome (2)	WSS	193520	17q11.2
Wieacker-Wolff syndrome (2)	WWS	314580	Xq13-q21
Wilms tumor (2)	WAGR, WTCR1	194070	11p13
Wilms tumor, type 2 (2)	WT2, WTCR2	194090	11p15.5
Wilson disease (2)	WND, WD	277900	13q14-q21
Wiskott-Aldrich syndrome (2)	WAS, IMD2	301000	Xp11.3-p11
Wolf-Hirschom syndrome (3)	HOX7	142983	4p16.1
Wolman disease (1)	LIPA	278000	10q24-q25
?Xeroderma pigmentosum (1)	PPOL, PARP	173870	1q41-q42
?Xeroderma pigmentosum, 1 form (1)	ERCC1, UV20	126380	19q13.2-q13.3
?Xeroderma pigmentosum A (1)	XPAC, XPA	278700	1q42-qter
Xeroderma pigmentosum, group B, 278710 (1)	ERCC3, XPB	133510	2p23-qter
Xeroderma pigmentosum, group F (2)	XPF	278760	Chr.15
?Xeroderma pigmentosum, one type (1)	UVDR,ERCM2	192060	Chr.13
Zellweger syndrome (2)	ZWS, ZS	214100	7q11.12-q11.23

APPENDIX 3   SUMMARY TABLE

							Expression	
Name of disease	Chap. no.	Frequency	Mode of inheritance	Mutant gene product	Chromosomal location	Altered DNA structure	Disturbed protein function	Disrupted cell and organ function
Part 2: Chromosomes								
Down syndrome (Trisomy 21)	7	1:1000 live births (mean); increases with maternal age; higher rates in fetuses	Sporadic in most cases; translocation forms (<5% of total) may sometimes be inherited	Increased amounts of numerous normal gene products	Genes in 21q22 are implicated in dysmorphic features and heart disease; genes in other regions may be involved in mental retardation and other manifestations	Trisomy of chromosome 21 or duplication of part of chromosome 21	50% increase in synthesis and concentration of many gene products	Aberrant morphogenesis, short stature, fewer cortical neurons, mental retardation, hypotonia, immune deficiency, increased risk of leukemia, male infertility, reduced life span.
Fragile X syndrome	8	1–2:2600 males 1–2:4100 females	X-linked but with significant deviation	Unknown	Xq27	Unknown	Unknown	Primary: unknown. Secondary: mental retardation, mild facial dysmorphism, macroorchidism.
Retinoblastoma	9	1:14,000	Autosomal dominant	*RB1*	13q14.1	Deletion	Deficient	Retinal differentiation, retinal tumors, osteogenic tumors.
Wilms tumor	9	1:10,000	Autosomal dominant	*WT1* (locus, gene not yet isolated)	11p13	Unknown	Unknown	Unknown.
Beckwith-Wiedemann syndrome	9	1:100,000	Autosomal dominant	Unknown	11p15	Unknown	Unknown	Unknown.
Part 3: Carbohydrates								
Diabetes mellitus, type 1 (insulin-dependent diabetes mellitus)	10	1:400 whites and blacks Less in Hispanics, Indians	Unknown	*DQ* locus product?	6p21.3 HLA-DQ	Unknown	Substitution of residue 57	Immune-mediated destruction of pancreatic β cell resulting in insulin deficiency/glucagon excess. Major complications probably due to hyperglycemia-induced sorbitol accumulation in tissues.
Diabetes mellitus, type 2 (non-insulin-dependent diabetes mellitus)	10	1:133 whites and blacks Higher in Hispanics and Indians	Unknown except in maturity-onset diabetes of youth (MODY), which is Mendelian dominant	Unknown	Unknown	Unknown	Unknown	Impaired insulin release in response to glucose coupled with insulin resistance. Relative insulin deficiency/glucagon excess. Major complications probably due to hyperglycemia-induced sorbitol accumulation in tissues.

SUMMARY TABLE (continued)

Part 3: Carbohydrates (continued)

Name of disease	Chap. no.	Frequency	Mode of inheritance	Mutant gene product	Chromosomal location	Altered DNA structure	Disturbed protein function	Disrupted cell and organ function
Essential fructosuria hepatic fructokinase deficiency	11	~1:130,000; more common in Jews	Autosomal recessive	Fructokinase	Unknown	Unknown	Deficient enzyme activity	Decreased phosphorylation of fructose to fructose 1-phosphate leads to alimentary hyperfructosemia and fructosuria. No clinical symptoms.
Hereditary fructose intolerance	11	1:20,000 in Switzerland	Autosomal recessive	Fructose 1,6-biphosphate aldolase B	9q13-q32	Unknown	Deficient enzyme activity	Ingestion of fructose causes the accumulation of fructose 1-phosphate and hence multiple dysfunctions in small intestine, liver, and kidneys.
Hereditary fructose 1,6-diphosphatase deficiency	11	85 cases	Autosomal recessive	Fructose 1,6-biphosphatase	Unknown	Unknown	Deficient enzyme activity	Gluconeogenesis is impaired, which during fasting leads to hypoglycemia, ketosis, lactic acidosis, and hyperalaninemia.
D-Glyceric aciduria	11	4 cases	Unknown	Unknown	Unknown	Unknown	Unknown	Metabolic acidosis.
Erythrocyte aldolase deficiency with nonspherocytic hemolytic anemia (aldolase A deficiency)	11	3 cases	? Autosomal recessive	Fructose 1,6-biphosphate aldolase A	Unknown	Point mutation	Deficient enzyme deficiency	Elevated fructose 1,6-biphosphate inhibits glucose-6-phosphate dehydrogenase and hence hexose monophosphate shunt activity in red cells.
Fructose malabsorption	11	Unknown (prevalence may be high)	Unknown	Unknown	Unknown	Unknown	Unknown	Oral fructose is incompletely absorbed causing abdominal symptoms and diarrhea.
Glycogen storage disease type Ia (von Gierke disease)	12	~1:100,000	Autosomal recessive	Glucose 6-phosphatase	Unknown	Unknown	Absent or deficient enzyme activity	Impaired gluconeogenesis, hypoglycemia, hyperlactic acidemia. Glycogen accumulation in liver & kidney.
Glycogen storage disease type Ib	12	~1:200,000	Autosomal recessive	Glucose 6-phosphate translocase	Unknown	Unknown	Deficient transport of glucose 6-phosphate across the membrane of endoplasmic reticulum	Same as type Ia plus leukocyte defect.
Glycogen storage disease type II	12	~1:175,000	Autosomal recessive	Lysosomal α-glucosidase	17q23	Unknown	Absent or deficient enzyme activity	Glycogen accumulates within lysosomes in all cells. Muscle weakness and heart failure are the main signs. Existence of infantile (Pompe disease), late infantile, and adult variants.

Disease		Frequency	Inheritance	Gene product	Chromosome	Mutation	Enzyme activity	Clinical features
Glycogen storage disease type III	12	~1:125,000	Autosomal recessive	Amylo-1, 6-glucosidase (debrancher enzyme)	Unknown	Unknown	Absent or deficient enzyme activity	Generalized accumulation of a glycogen with shorter outer chains (limit-dextrin). Moderate hypoglycemia and lacticacidemia. Muscle weakness mostly in adults.
Glycogen storage disease type IV (Andersen disease)	12	~1:million	Autosomal recessive	Amylo-1, 4:1,6-glucantransferase (Brancher enzyme)	Unknown	Unknown	Deficient enzyme activity	Generalized accumulation of a poorly branched glycogen (amylopectin-like). Rapidly fatal cirrhosis.
Glycogen storage disease type V (McArdle disease)	12	~1:million	Autosomal recessive	Muscle glycogen phosphorylase	11q13-qter (provisional)	Unknown	Absent or deficient enzyme activity	Accumulation of glycogen in striated muscle. Abnormal fatigue and cramps on exercise; sometimes myoglobinuria.
Glycogen storage disease X-linked phosphorylase kinase deficiency	12	1:125,000	X-linked recessive	Phosphorylase b-kinase	X	Unknown	Deficient or absent enzyme activity function	Accumulation of glycogen in liver causes hepatomegaly.
Glycogen storage disease autosomal phosphorylase kinase deficiency	12	~1:175,000	Autosomal recessive	Phosphorylase b-kinase	Unknown	Unknown	Deficient enzyme activity	Accumulation of glycogen in liver and muscle. Relatively benign.
Glycogen storage disease liver phosphorylase deficiency	12	~1:million	Autosomal recessive	Liver phosphorylase	Unknown	Unknown	Deficient enzyme activity	Accumulation of glycogen in liver causes hepatomegaly.
Glycogen storage disease type VII (Tarui disease)	12	~1:million	Autosomal recessive	Muscle phosphofructokinase 1	1cen-q32	Unknown	Deficient enzyme activity	Accumulation of glycogen in muscle. Exercise intolerance, hemolysis, hyperuricemia.
Liver glycogen synthase deficiency	12	?2 cases	Autosomal recessive	Liver glycogen synthase	Unknown	Unknown	Unknown	Fasting hypoglycemia.
Phosphoglycerate kinase deficiency	12	<1:million	Autosomal recessive X-linked	Phosphoglycerate kinase	Xq13	Unknown	Deficient enzyme	Impaired glycolysis in most cells leading to hemolytic anemia and muscle exercise intolerance without glycogenosis.
Phosphoglycerate mutase deficiency	12	<1:million	Autosomal recessive	Phosphoglycerate mutase	10q25.3 (provisional)	Unknown	Deficient enzyme	Intolerance for strenuous exercise, cramps, myoglobinuria.
Muscle lactate dehydrogenase deficiency	12	<1:million	Autosomal recessive	Muscle-specific subunit of lactate dehydrogenase (LDH)	11 (provisional)	Unknown	Absence of M subunit of LDH. Muscle LDH is a tetramer of the heart-specific subunit.	Myoglobinuria after intense exercise.
Glucose phosphate isomerase deficiency	12	?(1 case)	? Autosomal recessive	Glucose phosphate isomerase	19cen-q13.2	Unknown	Unknown	Liver glycogenosis, muscular fatigue, hemolytic disorder, and mental retardation.
Transferase deficiency galactosemia	13	1:35,000–60,000	Autosomal recessive	Galactose 1-phosphate uridyltransferase	9p13	Probable missense mutation(s)	Deficient enzyme activity	Accumulation of galactitol, galactose 1-phosphate, and galactonate causes cataracts, mental retardation, and liver and kidney dysfunction.

SUMMARY TABLE (continued)

Name of disease	Chap. no.	Frequency	Mode of inheritance	Mutant gene product	Chromosomal location	Altered DNA structure	Expression	
							Disturbed protein function	Disrupted cell and organ function
Part 3: Carbohydrates (continued)								
Galactokinase deficiency galactosemia	13	1:40,000	Autosomal recessive	Galactokinase	17q21-q25	Unknown	Deficient enzyme activity	Accumulation of galactitol in lens results in cataracts.
Epimerase deficiency galactosemia	13	Unknown, rare	Autosomal recessive	Uridine diphosphate galactose-4-epimerase	1pter-p32	Unknown	Deficient enzyme action in blood cells only (benign) or more rarely, in all tissues (generalized)	In the benign form, galactose 1-phosphate accumulates in red cells without clinical significance. In the generalized form the clinical and biochemical abnormalities resemble transferase-deficient galactosemia.
Pentosuria	14	1:2500 Ashkenazi Jews	Autosomal recessive	L-Xylulose reductase	Unknown	Unknown	Deficient enzyme activity	Accumulation of substrate (L-xylulose) leads to its continuous excretion in the urine without apparent clinical dysfunction.
Part 4: Amino acids								
Phenylketonuria (PKU)	15	~1:10,000 births (considerable regional variation)	Autosomal recessive (homozygous or compound)	Phenylalanine hydroxylase (PAH)	12q22-q24.1	6 different mutations known so far: splicing defect, missense mutations, and partial deletion. Known associations between RFLP haplotypes and PKU alleles	Deficient or absent PAH activity (<1% normal)	Hepatic enzyme deficiency causes hyperphenylalaninemia; plasma values persistently above 1.3 mM cause impaired cognitive development.
Non-PKU hyperphenylalaninemia	15	<1:20,000 in most populations	Autosomal recessive (homozygous or compound)	Phenylalanine hydroxylase (PAH)	12q22-q24.1	Unknown. Associated with RFLP haplotypes 1 & 4 in northern Europeans	Deficient PAH activity (>1% normal)	Benign phenotype for proband. Risk of maternal hyperphenylalaninemia effect on fetus carried by female proband.
"Malignant" hyperphenylalaninemia: DHPR-deficient form	15	~1:million (~1% of hyperphenylalaninemia cases)	Autosomal recessive (homozygous or compound)	Dihydropteridine reductase (DHPR)	4p15.3	Unknown; informative RFLP markers available	Deficient or absent DHPR activity	Impaired regeneration of tetrahydrobiopterin (BH$_4$) from qBH$_2$; inhibits hydroxylation of phenylalanine tyrosine and tryptophan; associated neurotransmitter deficiencies affect brain function.

Disorder	Chromosome	Incidence	Inheritance	Enzyme	Map location			Defect	Comments
"Malignant" hyperphenylalaninemia: GTP-CH–deficient form	15	~1:million (<1% of hyperphenylalaninemia cases)	Autosomal recessive	Guanosine triphosphate cyclohydrolase (GTP-CH)	Unknown	Unknown	Unknown	Deficient enzyme activity	Impairs tetrahydrobiopterin (BH_4) synthesis. BH_4 deficiency affects hydroxylation of phenylalanine, tyrosine, and tryptophan.
"Malignant" hyperphenylalaninemia: 6-PTS–deficient form	15	~1:million (~1% of hyperphenylalaninemia cases)	Autosomal recessive	6-Pyruvoyl tetrahydropterin synthase (6-PTS)	Unknown	Unknown	Unknown	Deficient enzyme activity	Impairs tetrahydrobiopterin (BH_4) synthesis. BH_4 deficiency affects hydroxylation of phenylalanine, tyrosine, and tryptophan. "Complete" form affects brain, liver, etc. "Peripheral" form spares brain.
Tyrosinemia IA (fumarylacetoacetate hydrolase deficiency)	16	1:20,000 with significant ethnic/regional variation	Autosomal recessive	Fumarylacetoacetate hydrolase	Unknown	Unknown	Unknown	Deficient enzyme activity; greater deficiency in acute than in chronic form	Increased succinylacetone, which inhibits renal tubular transport and hepatic enzymes.
Tyrosinemia IB (tentative) (maleylacetoacetate isomerase deficiency)	16	1 case	Autosomal recessive (provisional)	Maleylacetoacetate isomerase	Unknown	Unknown	Unknown	Deficient enzyme activity	No increase in succinylacetone; otherwise chemical and clinical findings are like type IA.
Tyrosinemia II (Tyrosine aminotransferase deficiency)	16	<100 cases	Autosomal recessive	Tyrosine aminotransferase (TAT)	16q22-q24	Unknown	Unknown	Deficient enzyme activity	Tyrosine crystals in cornea, inflammation in palm and sole skin and in cornea.
Urocanic aciduria	17	? (perhaps 1:200,000)	Unknown	Urocanase	Unknown	Unknown	Unknown	Absent urocanase activity	Increased substrate (urocanic acid); reduced products (imidazolonepropionate and FIGLU).
Histidinemia	17	1:10,000 general population	Autosomal recessive	Histidase (L-histidine ammonialyase)	Unknown	Unknown	Unknown	Absent or markedly reduced enzyme activity	Increased substrate; reduced products (urocanic acid and FIGLU).
Hyperprolinemia types I and II	18	1:200,000	Autosomal recessive	Type I, proline oxidase Type II, Δ-pyrroline-5-carboxylate dehydrogenase	Unknown; two loci	Unknown	Unknown	Deficient activity in types I and II	No apparent dysfunction; may have predisposition for neurological manifestations.
Hyperhydroxyprolinemia	18	Rare (<1:600,000)	Autosomal recessive	4-Hydroxy-L-proline oxidase	Unknown	Unknown	Unknown	Deficient activity	No apparent dysfunction (benign).
Prolidase deficiency (hyperimidodipeptiduria) and prolidase polymorphisms	18	1:50,000 (rare phenotypes, 28 cases) >1:100 (polymorphisms)	Autosomal recessive for rare alleles, codominant for polymorphisms	Peptidase D (prolidase)	19p13-cen	Unknown	Unknown	"Activity" mutations = prolidase deficiency "Structural" mutations = polymorphisms	Impaired imidodipeptide (X-Pro, X-Hypro) cleavage, (altered collagen metabolism?), imidodipeptiduria, skin changes, impaired development, and other problems.

SUMMARY TABLE (continued)

| | | | | | | | Expression | |
Name of disease	Chap. no.	Frequency	Mode of inheritance	Mutant gene product	Chromosomal location	Altered DNA structure	Disturbed protein function	Disrupted cell and organ function
Part 4: Amino acids (continued)								
Gyrate atrophy of the choroid and retina	19	~150 cases; ~1:50,000 in Finland	Autosomal recessive	Ornithine-δ-aminotransferase	10q26	Several point mutations and at least one deletion	Absent or deficient enzyme activity	Accumulation of substrate (ornithine) and reduced synthesis of creatine due to inhibition by ornithine of glycine transaminidinase. Mechanism of chorioretinal degeneration and cataract formation not known.
Hyperornithinemia-hyperammonemia-homocitrullinuria syndrome	19	15 cases	Autosomal recessive	Unknown	Unknown	Unknown	Impaired ornithine transport into mitochondria	Decreased availability of ornithine within mitochondria leads to decreased citrulline synthesis and impaired ammonia detoxification, causing hyperammonemia.
Carbamyl phosphate synthetase deficiency	20	1:70,000–100,000	Autosomal recessive	Carbamyl phosphate synthetase I	2p	Unknown	Absent of deficient enzyme activity	Impaired urea formation leads to ammonia intoxication.
Ornithine transcarbamylase deficiency	20	1:70,000–100,000	X-linked	Ornithine transcarbamylase	Xp21.1	Deletions, missense & nonsense mutations	Absent or reduced enzyme activity	Impaired urea formation leads to ammonia intoxication.
Argininosuccinic acid synthetase deficiency	20	1:70,000–100,000	Autosomal recessive	Argininosuccinic acid synthetase	9q34	Abnormal intron splicing?	Deficient enzyme activity	Accumulation of citrulline in blood, urine, and CSF leads to neurologic dysfunction.
Argininosuccinase deficiency	20	1:70,000–100,000	Autosomal recessive	Argininosuccinate lyase	7p21-cen	Unknown	Deficient enzyme activity	Accumulation of argininosuccinate in blood, urine, & CSF leads to neurologic problems.
Arginase deficiency	20	<1:100,000	Autosomal recessive	Liver arginase	6q23	Unknown	Deficient enzyme activity	Accumulation of arginine in blood and CSF leads to neurologic dysfunction.
Familial hyperlysinemia (variant: saccharopinuria)	21	Unknown (rare)	Autosomal recessive	α-Aminoadipic semialdehyde synthase (bifunctional enzyme: lysine-ketoglutarate reductase and saccharopine dehydrogenase activities)	Unknown	Unknown	Deficient enzyme activity	Severe hyperlysinemia. Saccharopinuria is less constant and less severe. No recognizable disruption of function.
Maple syrup urine disease or branched chain ketoacidemia	22	1:100,000 with ethnic/ regional variation	Autosomal recessive	Multiple loci and subunits	Unknown	Unknown	Impaired dehydrogenase activity, absent E₂ and E₁β subunits in rare variants	Enzyme deficiency causes accumulation of organic acids and amino acids; acute and chronic neurologic dysfunction occurs.

Cystathionine β-synthase deficiency	23	1:335,000	Autosomal recessive	Cystathionine β-synthase	21q21-q22.1	Unknown	Deficient enzyme activity	Vitamin B$_6$-responsive and -unresponsive forms. Vascular thrombosis, dislocation of ocular lens, and abnormal development.
α-Cystathionase deficiency	23	1:68,000–333,000	Autosomal recessive	α-Cystathionase	16	Unknown	Deficient enzyme activity	Benign.
Hepatic methionine adenosyltransferase deficiency	23	Unknown	? Autosomal recessive	Isoenzyme of methionine adenosyltransferase	Unknown	Unknown	Deficient enzyme activity	Benign.
Sarcosinemia	24	1:350,000	Autosomal recessive	Sarcosine dehydrogenase ?	Unknown	Unknown	Deficient enzyme activity	Believed to be a benign condition without clinical symptoms.
Nonketotic hyperglycinemia	25	1:250,000 (U.S.) 1:12,000 (northern Finland)	Autosomal recessive	1 of several proteins of glycine cleavage system	Unknown	Unknown	Deficient enzyme activity	Substrate (glycine) accumulates in body fluids including CSF. Severe retardation may be related to glycine role as a neurotransmitter.
Hyperuracil thyminuria	26	5 cases	Autosomal recessive	Dihydropyrimidine dehydrogenase	Unknown	Unknown	Deficient enzyme activity	Impaired CNS function; impaired disposal of fluorouracil.
Hyper-β-alaninemia	26	1 case	Autosomal recessive	β-Alanine-pyruvate transaminase (putative)	Unknown	Unknown	Deficient enzyme activity (or coenzyme binding)	Impaired CNS function.
Hyper-β-aminoisobutyric aciduria	26	5–95% of population	Autosomal (incompletely recessive)	R-β-aminoisobutyrate-pyruvate transaminase	Unknown	Unknown	Deficient enzyme activity (liver)	Benign metabolic polymorphism.
Pyridoxine dependency with seizures	26	uncommon	Autosomal recessive	Brain (type 1) glutamic acid decarboxylase (putative)	Unknown	Unknown	Deficient coenzyme binding? (brain)	Seizures controlled only by pharmacologic doses of vitamin B$_6$.
GABA aminotransferase deficiency	26	3 cases	Autosomal recessive	GABA-α-ketoglutarate transaminase (form not specified)	Unknown	Unknown	Deficient enzyme activity	Impaired CNS function, accelerated somatic growth, elevated plasma growth hormone levels.
4-Hydroxybutyricaciduria	26	6 cases	Autosomal recessive	Succinic semialdehyde dehydrogenase	Unknown	Unknown	Deficient enzyme activity	Cerebellar signs, hypotonia, and mental retardation.
Serum carnosinase deficiency (and homocarnosinosis)	26	20 cases	Autosomal recessive	Serum carnosinase	Unknown	Unknown	Deficient enzyme activity	Probably benign.

Part 5: Organic acids

Alcaptonuria	27	1:100,000–million	Autosomal recessive	Homogentisic acid oxidase	Unknown	Unknown	Absent or deficient enzyme activity	Homogentisic acid accumulates in the tissues and is excreted in the urine. Abnormal pigmentation of connective tissues (ochronosis) and arthritis commonly found in older alcaptonurics.

Name of disease	Chap. no.	Frequency	Mode of inheritance	Mutant gene product	Chromosomal location	Altered DNA structure	Expression	Disrupted cell and organ function
							Disturbed protein function	
Part 5: Organic acids (continued)								
Isovaleric acidemia	28	>45 cases	Autosomal recessive	Isovaleryl-CoA dehydrogenase	15q14-q15	Unknown	Deficient enzyme activity	Accumulation of isovaleryl-CoA causes episodes of severe metabolic acidosis and ketosis, often with neutropenia and thrombocytopenia, precipitated by infections or high protein intake.
Isolated 3-methylcrotonyl-CoA carboxylase deficiency	28	4 cases	Autosomal recessive	3-Methylcrotonyl-CoA carboxylase	Unknown	Unknown	Deficient enzyme activity	Accumulation of 3-methyl-crotonyl-CoA causes episodes of severe metabolic acidosis and hypoglycemia.
3-Methylglutaconic aciduria	28	2 mild cases 7 severe cases	Mild form: autosomal or X-linked Severe form: autosomal recessive	Mild form: 3-methylglutaconyl-CoA hydratase Severe form: unknown	Unknown	Unknown	Mild form: deficient enzyme activity Severe form: unknown	Mild form: Delayed speech development. Severe form: Progressive neurologic degeneration, optic atrophy.
3-Hydroxy-3-methylglutaryl-CoA lyase deficiency	28	19 cases	Autosomal recessive	3-Hydroxy-3-methylglutaryl-CoA lyase	Unknown	Unknown	Deficient enzyme activity	Accumulated 3-hydroxy-3-methylglutaryl-CoA causes episodes of severe metabolic acidosis without ketosis. Deficiency of enzyme blocks ketogenic pathway, leading to hypoglycemia on fasting.
Mevalonic aciduria	28	4 cases	Autosomal recessive	Mevalonate kinase	Unknown	Unknown	Deficient enzyme activity	Deficiency of enzyme in cholesterol and isoprenoid biosynthesis causes failure to thrive, anemia, lack of development.
2-Methylacetoacetyl-CoA thiolase deficiency	28	14 cases	Autosomal recessive	2-Methylacetoacetyl-CoA thiolase	Unknown	Unknown	Deficient enzyme activity	Accumulation of 2-methylacetoacetyl-CoA causes episodes of severe metabolic acidosis and ketosis.
3-Hydroxyisobutyryl-CoA deacylase deficiency	28	1 case	Autosomal recessive	3-Hydroxyisobutyryl-CoA deacylase	Unknown	Unknown	Deficient enzyme activity	Causes congenital malformations of vertebra and heart, lack of neurologic development.
Propionic acidemia (2 nonallelic disorders designated *pccA* and *pccBC*)	29	Rare	Autosomal recessive	Propionyl-CoA carboxylase (PCC)	α subunit: 13 β subunit: 3q13.3-q22	Unknown	Deficient enzyme activity (nonallelic variants reflect mutations in nonidentical subunits of PCC)	Accumulation of propionate and alternate pathway metabolites (methylcitrate, hydroxypropionate, and propionylglycine) leads to ketoacidosis and developmental retardation.

Disorder	References	Frequency	Inheritance	Enzyme or protein	Chromosome		Defect	Comments
Methylmalonic acidemia (two allelic variants designated *mut⁰* and *mut⁻*)	29	1:20,000	Autosomal recessive	Methylmalonyl-CoA mutase (MUT) apoenzyme	6p12-p21.2	Unknown	Absent MUT activity in *mut⁰*, deficient MUT activity due to reduced affinity for cofactor (adenosylcobalamin) in *mut⁻*	Accumulation of methylmalonate leading to metabolic ketoacidosis and developmental retardation.
Methylmalonic acidemia (two nonallelic variants designated *cb1A* and *cb1B*)	29, 82	1:20,000	Autosomal recessive	*cb1A* form: unknown *cb1B* form: ATP: cobalamin' adenosyltransferase	Unknown	Unknown	Unknown in *cb1A*; absent or deficient enzyme activity in *cb1B*	Impaired adenosylcobalamin synthesis leads to deficient methylmalonyl-CoA mutase (MUT) activity; clinical and chemical findings resemble those in apoprotein MUT deficiency.
Methylmalonic acidemia and homocystinuria (two nonallelic forms designated *cb1C* and *cb1D*)	29, 82	Rare	Autosomal recessive	Unknown	Unknown	Unknown	Unknown	Impaired synthesis of adenosylcobalamin and methylcobalamin leads to deficient activities of two cobalamin-dependent enzymes, N^5-methyltetrahydrofolate: homocysteine methyltransferase and methylmalonyl-CoA mutase. Hematologic and neurologic abnormalities predominate.
Methylmalonic acidemia (variant designated *cb1F*)	29, 82	Rare	? Autosomal recessive	Unknown	Unknown	Unknown	Impaired efflux of cobalamin from lysosomes into the cell	Impaired synthesis of both cobalamin coenzymes leads to deficient activities of methylmalonyl-CoA mutase and N^5-methyltransferase in vitro. In the one case described, homocystinuria was not present in vivo.
Glutaric acidemia type I	30, 34	~50 patients 1:30,000 in Sweden	Autosomal recessive	Glutaryl-CoA dehydrogenase	Unknown	Unknown	Deficient enzyme activity	Accumulation of compounds (glutaric acid, 3-hydroxyglutaric acid, glutaconic acid) related to enzyme substrate. Relation between enzyme defect and neurologic dysfunction is not understood.
2-Ketoadipic acidemia	30	Unknown	Autosomal recessive	Probably 2-ketoadipic dehydrogenase E_1 or E_2	Unknown	Unknown	Deficient enzyme activity	Substrate accumulation possibly of no pathologic significance.

SUMMARY TABLE (continued)

Name of disease	Chap. no.	Frequency	Mode of inheritance	Mutant gene product	Chromosomal location	Altered DNA structure	Disturbed protein function	Disrupted cell and organ function
Part 5: Organic acids (continued)							*Expression*	
Glutathione synthetase deficiency	31	Rare	Autosomal recessive	Glutathione synthetase	Unknown	Unknown	Decreased enzyme activity. Two forms: A, severe, generalized deficiency of enzyme activity; B, a mild form, possibly due to an unstable enzyme, with deficient function manifested only in red cells	Both forms have decreased erythrocyte glutathione and increased rate of hemolysis. In the generalized form there is 5-oxoproline overproduction, metabolic acidosis, and progressive brain dysfunction.
5-Oxoprolinase deficiency	31	Rare	Autosomal recessive	5-Oxoprolinase	Unknown	Unknown	Decreased enzyme activity	Increased urinary excretion of 5-oxoproline.
γ-Glutamylcysteine synthetase deficiency	31	Rare	Unknown	γ-Glutamylcysteine synthetase	Unknown	Unknown	Decreased enzyme activity	Decreased cellular levels of glutathione. Two patients described have had hemolytic anemia, spinocerebellar degeneration, peripheral neuropathy, myopathy, and aminoaciduria.
δ-Glutamyl transpeptidase deficiency	31	Rare	Autosomal recessive	δ-Glutamyl transpeptidase	Unknown	Unknown	Decreased enzyme activity	Increased extracellular levels and urinary excretion of glutathione. All patients have had central nervous system involvement.
Cytochrome oxidase deficiency	32	Unknown	Autosomal recessive	Cytochrome oxidase polypeptides	Unknown	Unknown	Decreased activity of the cytochrome oxidase complex	Neuronal loss in brain leading to psychomotor retardation and neurodegenerative disease.
Fumarase deficiency/fumaric acidemia	32	5 cases	? Autosomal recessive	Fumarase	1q	Unknown	Decreased enzyme activity	Mental retardation.
Pyruvate dehydrogenase complex deficiency—E₁ decarboxylase component	32	<1:250,000	Autosomal recessive	Pyruvate decarboxylase, either E₁α or E₁β	Unknown	Unknown	Decreased enzyme activity	Neuronal loss in brain leading to psychomotor retardation. Muscular hypotonia.
Combined α-ketoacid dehydrogenase deficiency/lipoamide dehydrogenase deficiency	22, 32	6 cases	Autosomal recessive	Lipoamide dehydrogenase	Unknown	Unknown	Decreased enzyme activity	Neuronal loss in brain leads to psychomotor retardation.
NADH-CoQ reductase deficiency	32	Unknown	? Autosomal recessive	Any of the nuclear genes encoding the 25 complex I polypeptides of mitochondria	Unknown	Unknown	Decreased activity of the overall complex I	Overwhelming acidosis due to lactic acid production from many types especially those of the brain.

Disorder	Ref.	Frequency	Inheritance	Enzyme/protein affected	Chromosome	Molecular defect	Enzyme defect	Clinical features
Pyruvate carboxylase deficiency	32	<1:250,000; higher in certain Amerindian groups	Autosomal recessive	Pyruvate carboxylase	11q	Unknown	Absent enzyme activity; seven cases absent enzyme, protein and mRNA	Neuronal loss in cerebral cortex leading to mental retardation.
Long-chain acyl-CoA dehydrogenase deficiency	33	Rare	Autosomal recessive	Long-chain acyl-CoA dehydrogenase	Unknown	Unknown	Deficient enzyme activity	Impaired β oxidation of long-chain fatty acids with recurrent episodes of coma, hypoglycemia, and inadequate ketogenesis. Hypotonia and cardiomyopathy occur.
Medium-chain acyl-CoA dehydrogenase deficiency	33	~1:10,000–25,000 (U.K.)	Autosomal recessive	Medium-chain acyl-CoA dehydrogenase	1p31	Unknown	Deficient enzyme activity	Impaired β oxidation of medium-chain fatty acids with recurrent episodes of coma, hypoglycemia, and inadequate ketogenesis.
Short-chain acyl-CoA dehydrogenase deficiency	33	Rare	Autosomal recessive	Short-chain acyl-CoA dehydrogenase	Unknown	Unknown	Deficient enzyme activity	Variable with some presenting in infancy with vomiting and lethargy; another case exhibited a proximal myopathy in otherwise asymptomatic adult.
Glutaric acidemia type I (See Chap. 30)	30, 34							
Glutaric acidemia type II	34	Unknown	Autosomal recessive	In some patients: electron transfer flavoprotein (ETF); in some patients: ETF: ubiquinone oxidoreductase	Unknown	Unknown	In some cases, no enzyme antigen; in others, no enzyme activity	Inability to oxidize fatty acids leads to lipid accumulation, hypoglycemia (nonketotic), myopathy, and cardiomyopathy. Cause of congenital anomalies is not known.
Primary hyperoxaluria type I	35	Unknown, rare	Autosomal recessive	Alanine: glyoxylate aminotransferase	Unknown	Unknown	Alteration of reaction rate	Glyoxylate leaves the peroxisome and is oxidized to oxalate.
Primary hyperoxaluria type II	35	Unknown, rare	Autosomal recessive	D-Glycerate dehydrogenase	Unknown	Unknown	Alteration of reaction rate	Glyoxylate leaves the peroxisome and is oxidized to oxalate.
Glycerol kinase deficiency (Gkd)	36	~30 cases	X-linked	Glycerol kinase and in microdeletion cases the products of linked loci, including *AHC*, *DMD*, and/or *OTC*	Xp21	Microdeletions in patients with complex phenotype. Less extensive mutations presumed in individuals with isolated Gkd	The microdeletion involves not only *GK* but also the other deleted loci: *AHC*, *DMD*, *OTC*, and other linked loci.	Disruption of adrenal, muscle, and/or liver and brain function as consequence of microdeletions in *AHC*, *DMD*, and/or *OTC* in patients with complex phenotypes. Not clear that isolated Gkd has any detrimental effect.

SUMMARY TABLE (continued)

Name of disease	Chap. no.	Frequency	Mode of inheritance	Mutant gene product	Chromosomal location	Altered DNA structure	Disturbed protein function	Disrupted cell and organ function
							Expression	
Part 6: Purines and pyrimidines								
Primary gout: idiopathic	37	1:500 in Western populations 1:50 in American males by age 60 1:10 males and 1:25 females in some Polynesian groups	Multifactorial	Unknown	Unknown	Unknown	Unknown	Mixed pathogenesis: increased biosynthesis and reduced renal clearance in most affected individuals.
Primary gout: superactive variant of phosphoribosyl-pyrophosphate (PP-ribose-P) synthetase	37	~20 families	X-linked recessive	PP-ribose-P synthetase	Xq	Unknown	Enhanced enzyme activity	Increased production of PP-ribose-P leads to increased purine synthesis de novo, causing gout.
Primary gout: partial deficiency of hypoxanthine-guanine phosphoribosyltransferase (HPRT)	37, 38	1:100,000 males	X-linked recessive	Hypoxanthine-guanine phosphoribosyltransferase (HPRT)	Xq26-q27	$Arg_{50} \rightarrow Gly$ $Ser_{109} \rightarrow Leu$ $Ser_{103} \rightarrow Arg$	Absent or deficient enzyme activity	Accumulation of substrate (phosphoribosylpyrophosphate) leads to enhanced purine biosynthesis de novo, causing gout.
Lesch Nyhan: deficiency of hypoxanthine-guanine phosphoribosyltransferase (HPRT)	38	1:10,000 males	X-linked recessive	Hypoxanthine-guanine phosphoribosyltransferase (HPRT)	Xq26-q27	$Arg_{193} \rightarrow Asn$ point mutations, deletions, insertions	Deficient enzyme activity	Increased PP-ribose-P leads to gout. Mechanism of neurologic dysfunction in Lesch-Nyhan unknown.
2,8-Dihydroxyadenine lithiasis (adenine phosphoribosyltransferase deficiency)	39	Type I: 32 cases Type II: 31 cases	Autosomal recessive	Adenine phosphoribosyltransferase	16q	Unknown	Type I: Absent enzyme activity Type II: Reduced affinity for PP-ribose-P	Adenine is metabolized through an alternative pathway leading to the formation of 2,8-dihydroxy-adenine, a product that is insoluble in the kidney or urinary tract. Urolithiasis frequently results.
Adenosine deaminase deficiency with severe combined immunodeficiency disease	40	100 families	Autosomal recessive	Adenosine deaminase	20q13.11	Multiple missense mutations and exon deletions	Absent or greatly diminished enzyme activity	Accumulation of substrates (adenosine and deoxyadenosine) which are toxic to lymphoid cells leads to immunodeficiency.
Purine nucleoside phosphorylase deficiency with cellular immunodeficiency	40	21 cases	Autosomal recessive	Purine nucleoside phosphorylase	14q13	$Glu_{89} \rightarrow Lys$	Absent or greatly diminished enzyme activity	Accumulation of substrates (primarily deoxyguanosine) toxic to T lymphocytes causes cellular immunodeficiency.
Myoadenylate deaminase deficiency	41	1–2% of all muscle biopsies submitted for pathological evaluation	? Autosomal recessive	Myoadenylate deaminase	Unknown	Unknown	No enzyme activity; no immunoreactive protein	Only skeletal muscle is affected; all other tissues are normal.

Disorder		Frequency	Inheritance	Protein	Chromosome		Absent enzyme activity	Consequences
Xanthinuria	42	1:45,000	Autosomal recessive	Xanthine dehydrogenase (xanthine oxidase)	Unknown	Unknown	Absent enzyme activity	Accumulated substrate (xanthine) crystallizes in urinary tract and muscle, causing nephrolithiasis and myopathy.
Hereditary orotic aciduria	43	13 cases	Autosomal recessive	UMP synthase	3q13	Unknown	Deficient enzyme activity (probably unstable protein)	Block in UMP biosynthesis leads to overproduction of orotic acid, megaloblastic anemia, failure to thrive, possible malformations.
Pyrimidine 5'-nucleotidase deficiency	43	~100 cases	Autosomal recessive	Pyrimidine 5'-nucleotidase	Unknown	Unknown	Absent or unstable enzyme	Accumulation of pyrimidine nucleotides leads to hemolytic anemia.
Dihydropyrimidine dehydrogenase deficiency	43	1 case	Autosomal recessive	Dihydropyrimidine dehydrogenase	Unknown	Unknown	Absent or unstable enzyme	Accumulation of uracil and thymine in blood and elevated urine excretion. Physiological consequences unclear.

Part 7: Lipoproteins and lipids

Disorder		Frequency	Inheritance	Protein	Chromosome		Absent enzyme activity	Consequences
Chylomicron retention disease	44B	~10 cases	? Autosomal recessive	Unknown	Unknown	Unknown	Apo B-48 retained in intestine and absent from plasma	Abnormality of release of apo B-48 from intestine associated with fat malabsorption.
Familial combined hyperlipidemia	44B	~1:100	Autosomal dominant	Unknown	Unknown	Unknown	Increased apo B in plasma	Increased LDL or VLDL or both. Increased risk of myocardial infarction.
Lp(a) hyperlipoproteinemia	44B	? major gene frequency of 0.10	? Autosomal dominant or polygenic	Unknown, ? Lp(a) protein	Unknown	Unknown	Increased Lp(a) in plasma	Increased LP(a) associated with increased risk of coronary disease by unknown mechanism.
Abetalipoproteinemia	44B	~50 cases	Autosomal recessive	Unknown, ? apo B in some	2p24 for apo B	Unknown, increased apo B mRNA in some	Apo B not detectable in some	Lack of synthesis and/or secretion of apoprotein B prevents formation of chylomicrons, VLDL, and LDL. This leads to decreased vitamin E transport, which in turn causes neurologic and retinal abnormalities. Heterozygotes have normal plasma levels of apoprotein B.
Familial hypobetalipoproteinemia	44B	~10 cases	Autosomal recessive	? Apo B in some	2p24 for apo B	Unknown, decreased mRNA for apo B in some	Decreased apo B in some	Homozygotes have syndrome similar to abetalipoproteinemia. Heterozygotes have one-half of the normal levels of apoprotein B in plasma and are asymptomatic.
Normotriglyceridemic abetalipoproteinemia	44B	1 case	? Autosomal recessive	Probably apo B	2p24	Unknown	Absent apo B-100, apo B-48 present	Absent LDL able to absorb fat and form chylomicrons.
Hypobetalipoproteinemia with apo B-37	44B	1 family	? Autosomal recessive	Apo B	2p24	Unknown	Truncated apo B-37 formed	Very low LDL, mild fat malabsorption, mild phenotype.

SUMMARY TABLE (continued)

Part 7: Lipoproteins and lipids (continued)

Name of disease	Chap. no.	Frequency	Mode of inheritance	Mutant gene product	Expression			
					Chromosomal location	Altered DNA structure	Disturbed protein function	Disrupted cell and organ function
Familial lipoprotein lipase deficiency	45	~100 cases, 1:million	Autosomal recessive	Lipoprotein lipase	Unknown	Unknown	Nonfunctional protein in some, nondectable enzyme activity and protein in others	Accumulation of substrate (chylomicrons and VLDL) in plasma as triglyceride, associated with pancreatitis and eruptive xanthomas of skin.
Apolipoprotein C-II deficiency	45	~30 cases	Autosomal recessive	Apo C-II (activator of lipoprotein lipase)	19	Unknown	Decreased lipoprotein lipase activity due to absence of normal apo C-II	Same as familial lipoprotein lipase deficiency. Apo C-II activates lipoprotein lipase.
Familial lipoprotein lipase inhibitor	45	3 cases in one family	Autosomal dominant	Unknown	Unknown	Unknown	Decreased lipoprotein lipase activity	Same as familial lipoprotein lipase deficiency.
Familial chylomicronemia syndrome	45	~1:10,000	Complex, multiple loci	Unknown	Unknown	Unknown	Unknown	Same as familial lipoprotein lipase deficiency.
Familial lecithin: cholesterol acyltransferase deficiency	46	~50 cases	Autosomal recessive	Lecithin: cholesterol acyltransferase	16q	Unknown	Absent enzyme protein or deficient enzyme activity	Accumulation of unesterified cholesterol in plasma and tissues leads to anemia, dyslipoproteinemia, proteinuria, and renal failure and corneal opacities.
Familial type III hyperlipoproteinemia (dysbetalipoproteinemia)	47	1:1000–5000	Autosomal recessive (with modifiers)	Apolipoprotein E	19	Point mutation leading to single amino acid substitution in apolipoprotein E	Decreased binding to lipoprotein receptors	Accumulation in plasma of chylomicron and very low density lipoprotein remnants (collectively, β-very low density lipoproteins), leading to hyperlipidemia and atherosclerosis.
Familial hypercholesterolemia, multiple allelic types	48	1:500 in most populations; more frequent in Lebanese and Afrikaaners	Autosomal dominant	LDL receptor	19 p13.1-p13.3	13 different mutations characterized at DNA level; include deletion insertion, nonsense, frameshift, and missense mutations	Absent or deficient receptor activity (homozygotes); half normal receptor activity (heterozygotes)	Absent or deficient receptor-mediated endocytosis of LDL causes LDL to accumulate in plasma. Hypercholesterolemia and artherosclerosis results.
Hepatic triglyceride lipase (HGTL) deficiency	49	Rare; 3 families	Autosomal recessive	Unknown	Unknown	Unknown	Quantitative deficiency of HGTL	Hypercholesterolemia, hypertriglyceridemia, and increased susceptibility to arteriosclerosis.

Apolipoprotein A-I deficiency: Type I (apo A-I/apo C-III deficiency) Type II (apo A-I deficiency without xanthoma) Type III (apo A-I deficiency with xanthoma)	49	All rare	Autosomal recessive	Only known for type I; apo A-I and apo C-III both affected	11q23	5.5-kb inversion in 4th exon of apo A-I gene producing gene fusion of apo A-I and C-III genes	Deficiency of apo A-I and apo C-III	Low apo A-I level leads to low HDL levels, and accumulation of cholesteryl containing deposits in the cornea, the blood vessels. Xanthoma occurs in types I and III. Coronary insufficiency is the most serious disability.
Fish eye disease	49	2 families	Unknown	Unknown	Unknown	Unknown	Quantitative deficiency of lecithin-cholesterol acyltransferase, which esterifies free cholesterol in HDL	Low HDL cholesterol, corneal opacities.
Cholesteryl ester transport protein (CETP) deficiency	49	2 families from Japan	Unknown	Unknown	Unknown	Unknown	Quantitative deficiency of enzyme which transfers cholesteryl ester from HDL to VLDL and LDL	Hypercholesterolemia, hypertriglyceridemia, elevated HDL cholesterol levels. No arteriosclerotic heart disease or xanthoma.
Lipoprotein lipase deficiency	49	Covered in Chap. 45						
Tangier disease	50	Rare mutant	Autosomal codominant	Unknown	Unknown	Unknown	HDL-deficiency due to hypercatabolism of apo A-I-containing lipoproteins	Cholesteryl ester storage in histiocytes, Schwann cells, nevus cells, and others. Splenomegaly and hyperplastic orange-yellow tonsils.
Cerebrotendinous xanthomatosis	51	More than 100 but less than 150 cases	Autosomal recessive	Hepatic mitochondrial 26-hydroxylase involved in bile acid biosynthesis	Unknown	Unknown	Markedly reduced enzyme activity	Accumulation of cholesterol and intermediates in bile acid biosynthesis. Reduced biosynthesis of normal bile acids. Excretion of huge amounts of bile alcohols in feces and urine.
Phytosterolemia (sitosterolemia)	51	22 cases	? Autosomal recessive	Unknown	Unknown	Unknown	Unknown	Hyperabsorption of phytosterols and shellfish sterols leading to tendon and tuberous xanthoma and a strong predisposition for premature coronary atherosclerosis.
Part 8: Porphyrins and heme								
δ-Aminolevulinic acid dehydratase porphyria	52	3 cases	Autosomal recessive	δ-Aminolevulinic acid dehydratase	Unknown	Unknown	Minimal enzyme activity	Overproduction of δ-aminolevulinic acid, leading to neurologic disturbances.
Acute intermittent porphyria	52	1:10,000–20,000 (U.S.A.)	Autosomal dominant	Porphobilinogen deaminase	11q23-qter	Unknown	Decreased enzyme activity (~50%)	Overproduction of porphyrin precursors, leading to neurologic disturbances.

SUMMARY TABLE (continued)

Name of disease	Chap. no.	Frequency	Mode of inheritance	Mutant gene product	Chromosomal location	Expression		
						Altered DNA structure	Disturbed protein function	Disrupted cell and organ function
Part 8: Porphyrins and heme (continued)								
Congenital erythropoietic porphyria	52	<200 cases	Autosomal recessive	Uroporphyrinogen III cosynthase	Unknown	Unknown	Decreased enzyme activity	Overproduction of type I porphyrin isomers, leading to photosensitivity and hemolytic anemia.
Porphyria cutanea tarda (familial form)	52	Unknown	Autosomal dominant	Uroporphyrinogen decarboxylase	1pter-p21	Unknown	Decreased enzyme activity ($\sim$50%)	Excessive hepatic production of 8- and 7-carboxylate porphyrins, leading to photosensitivity.
Hepatoerythropoietic porphyria	52	16 cases	Autosomal recessive	Uroporphyrinogen decarboxylase	1pter-p21	$Gly_{281}\rightarrow Glu$ mutation (in one case)	Minimal enzyme activity	Excessive hepatic production of 8- and 7-carboxylate porphyrins, leading to photosensitivity.
Hereditary coproporphyria	52	1:500,000 (Denmark)	Autosomal dominant	Coproporphyrinogen oxidase	Unknown	Unknown	Decreased enzyme activity ($\sim$50%)	Overproduction of porphyrin precursors and coproporphyrin leading to neurologic disturbances $\pm$ photosensitivity.
Variegate porphyria	52	1:75,000 (Finland)	Autosomal dominant	Protoporphyrinogen oxidase	Unknown	Unknown	Decreased enzyme activity	Overproduction of porphyrin precursors and protoporphyrin, leading to neurologic disturbances $\pm$ photosensitivity.
Erythropoietic protoporphyria	52	300 cases (1961–1976)	Autosomal dominant	Ferrochelatase	Unknown	Unknown	Decreased enzyme activity	Overproduction of protoporphyrin leading to mild to moderate photosensitivity.
Crigler-Najjar syndrome type I	53	Over 70 cases	Autosomal recessive	Hepatic bilirubin UDPglucuronyl transferase	Unknown	Unknown	Absent enzyme activity	Substrate (unconjugated bilirubin) accumulates in brain, resulting in kernicterus.
Crigler-Najjar syndrome type II	53	Uncommon	? Autosomal recessive	Hepatic bilirubin UDPglucuronyl transferase	Unknown	Unknown	Reduced enzyme activity	Partial ability to conjugate bilirubin leads to mild unconjugated hyperbilirubinemia with increased proportion of bilirubin monoglucuronide in bile. Usually benign disorder.

Disorder	No.	Frequency	Inheritance		Location			Clinical features
Gilbert syndrome	53	~1:30	? Autosomal dominant	Unknown	Unknown	Unknown	Unknown	Impaired hepatic uptake of bilirubin and reduced activity of hepatic bilirubin uridine diphosphoglucuronyl transferase lead to mild unconjugated hyperbilirubinemia and increased proportion of bilirubin monoglucuronide in bile. Benign disorder.
Dubin-Johnson syndrome	53	Rare worldwide; 1:1300 in Persian Jews	Autosomal recessive	Unknown	Unknown	Unknown	Unknown	Failure of biliary excretion of conjugated bilirubin produces mild conjugated hyperbilirubinemia.
Rotor syndrome	53	Rare	Autosomal recessive	Unknown	Unknown	Unknown	Unknown	Partial failure of biliary excretion of conjugated bilirubin causes mild hyperbilirubinemia.

Part 9: Metals

Disorder	No.	Frequency	Inheritance		Location			Clinical features
Menkes disease	54	1:100,000	X-linked recessive	Unknown	? Xq13	Unknown	Unknown	Defective intracellular transport of copper leads to deficiency of copper-containing enzymes and causes arterial and brain degeneration.
Occipital horn syndrome	54	Rare	X-linked recessive	Unknown	Unknown—? allelic to Menkes disease	Unknown	Unknown	Defective biliary excretion of copper leads to deficiency of lysyl oxidase and causes skin and joint laxity, hernias, and urinary tract diverticula.
Wilson disease	54	1:50,000	Autosomal recessive	Unknown	13q14	Unknown	Unknown	Defective biliary excretion of copper leads to accumulation in liver (cirrhosis), cornea (Kayser-Fleischer rings), and basal ganglia (movement disorder).
Hereditary (idiopathic) hemochromatosis	55	~1:200–500 of European populations (males and females) are homozygous for hereditary hemochromatosis. A majority of cases are clinically unexpressed.	Autosomal	Unknown recessive	6p21.3	Unknown	Unknown	A greater proportion of the dietary iron taken up by the mucosal cells of the intestinal tract is absorbed into the body. When the body iron content reaches massive proportions (usually 15 g), many organs are severely damaged, including the liver, heart, and pancreas.

SUMMARY TABLE (continued)

Name of disease	Chap. no.	Frequency	Mode of inheritance	Mutant gene product	Chromosomal location	Altered DNA structure	Disturbed protein function	Disrupted cell and organ function
							Expression	
Part 9: Metals (*continued*)								
Molybdenum cofactor deficiency	56	15 cases	Autosomal recessive	Enzyme required for molybdenum cofactor biosynthesis	Unknown	Unknown	Absent or deficient activities of sulfite oxidase, xanthine dehydrogenase, and aldehyde oxidase	Sulfite, thiosulfate, S-sulfocysteine, hypoxanthine, and xanthine levels are elevated. Mental retardation, neurologic disturbances (seizures), and dislocated ocular lenses occur.
Part 10: Peroxisomes								
Peroxisome biogenesis, disorders of: Zellweger syndrome Neonatal adrenoleukodystrophy Infantile Refsum disease Hyperpipecolic acidemia	57	Combined incidence estimated at 1:25,000–50,000	Autosomal recessive for all	Unknown	Unknown	Unknown	Unknown for all	Failure of peroxisome assembly and deficiency of multiple peroxisomal enzymes in Zellweger syndrome. Impaired peroxisomal function, by any cause, results in accumulation of very long chain fatty acids, pipecolic acid, and phytanic acid and reduced synthesis of plasmalogens and bile acids. Biochemical alterations result in pathologic changes in brain, liver, kidney, eye, adrenal, bone, and other organs.
Adrenoleukodystrophy	58	1:100,000 minimum	X-linked	Unknown	Xq28	Unknown	Unknown	Accumulation of unbranched saturated very long chain fatty acids ($C_{24.0}$–$C_{26.0}$) occurs. How this relates to the clinical phenotype of progressive dementia, visual impairment, seizures, and adrenal insufficiency is not known.
Adrenomyeloneuropathy	58	1:50,000 minimum	X-linked	Unknown	Xq28	Unknown	Unknown	A milder phenotype of adrenoleukodystrophy which may occur in the same kindred. There is also accumulation of very long chain fatty acids, but the clinical phenotype is paraparesis and sphincter

Disorder		Frequency	Inheritance	Enzyme/protein	Chromosome		Enzyme activity	Comment
Adrenomyeloneuropathy (continued)								disturbance progressing over several decades and adrenal insufficiency. From 10 to 15% female heterozygotes develop a phenotype resembling adrenomyeloneuropathy.
Refsum disease	59	~100 cases	Autosomal recessive	Phytanic acid α-hydroxylase	Unknown	Unknown	Deficient enzyme activity	Accumulation of substrate (phytanic acid) is associated with the development of retinitis pigmentosa, ataxia, and peripheral neuropathy in young adults.
Acatalasemia	60	1:25,000–250,000 (worldwide)	Autosomal recessive	Catalase (mutations probably multiple, all uncharacterized)	11p13	Unknown	Unstable enzyme or decreased enzyme synthesis	Deficiency most marked in red cells. Associated gum disease in some patients. Otherwise, affected subjects are normal.

Part 11: Lysosomal enzymes

Disorder		Frequency	Inheritance	Enzyme/protein	Chromosome		Enzyme activity	Comment
Mucopolysaccharidosis I & V (Hurler, Scheie, and Hurler-Scheie syndromes)	61	~1:100,000 for Hurler syndrome 1:600,000 for Scheie syndrome	Autosomal recessive; disorders are allelic.	α-L-iduronidase	22pter-q11	Unknown	Absent enzyme activity	Defective lysosomal degradation of dermatan sulfate and heparan sulfate leads to storage of the incompletely degraded glycosaminoglycans. Nearly all cells and organs are affected.
Mucopolysaccharidosis II (Hunter syndrome)	61	1:70,000 in Israel; rarer in British and British Columbian surveys	X-linked recessive	Iduronate sulfatase	Xq26-q28	Unknown	Absent enzyme activity	Defective lysosomal degradation of dermatan sulfate and heparan sulfate leads to storage of the incompletely degraded glycosaminoglycans. Nearly all cells and organs are affected.
Mucopolysaccharidosis III (Sanfilippo syndrome) types A–D	61	1:24,000 (all types combined) in the Netherlands IIIA and IIIB most common; A > B in northern Europe, B > A in southern Europe	Autosomal recessive Four types nonallelic	IIIA: heparan-N-sulfatase IIIB: α-N-acetylglucosaminidase IIIC: acetyl-CoA: α-glucosaminide acetyltransferase IIID: N-acetylglucosamine-6-sulfatase	Unknown	Unknown	Absent enzyme activity	Defective lysosomal degradation of heparan sulfate leads to lysosomal storage of the partially degraded glycosaminoglycan. Cellular function is disrupted primarily in the central nervous system.
Mucopolysaccharidosis IV (Morquio syndrome) types A and B	61	1:300,000	Autosomal recessive Two types nonallelic	IVA: galactose-6-sulfatase IVB: β-galactosidase	IVA: unknown IVB: 3p21-cen	Unknown	IVA: absent enzyme activity IVB: defective enzyme activity	Defective lysosomal degradation of keratan sulfate leads to lysosomal storage of the glycosaminoglycan. Cellular function is disrupted primarily in cornea, skeletal, and cardiovascular systems.

SUMMARY TABLE (continued)

Part 11: Lysosomal enzymes (continued)

Name of disease	Chap. no.	Frequency	Mode of inheritance	Mutant gene product	Chromosomal location	Altered DNA structure	Expression	
							Disturbed protein function	Disrupted cell and organ function
Mucopolysaccharidosis VI (Maroteaux-Lamy syndrome)	61	Rare	Autosomal recessive	N-acetylgalactosamine-4-sulfatase (arylsulfatase B)	5p11-q13	Unknown	Absent enzyme activity	Defective lysosomal degradation of dermatan sulfate leads to lysosomal storage of the partially degraded glycosaminoglycan. Cellular function is disrupted in most tissues.
Mucopolysaccharidosis VII (Sly syndrome)	61	Very rare	Autosomal recessive	β-Glucuronidase	7q11.2-q22	Unknown	Absent or deficient enzyme activity	Defective lysosomal degradation of dermatan sulfate, heparan sulfate, and chondroitin sulfates leads to lysosomal storage of the partially degraded glycosaminoglycans. Cellular function is disrupted in most tissues.
I-cell disease (ML-II)	62	Rare (less rare in Japan?)	Autosomal recessive	UDP-N-acetylglucosamine: lysosomal enzyme N-acetylglucosaminyl-1-phosphotransferase	Unknown	Unknown	Phosphorylation of many lysosomal enzymes	Impaired lysosomal function in mesenchymal cells, especially fibroblasts.
Pseudo-Hurler polydystrophy (ML III)	62	Rare	Autosomal recessive	UDP-N-acetylglucosamine: lysosomal enzyme N-acetylglucosaminyl-1-phosphotransferase	Unknown	Unknown	Phosphorylation of many lysosomal enzymes	Impaired lysosomal function in mesenchymal cells, especially fibroblasts.
Mannosidosis	63	50-100 cases	Autosomal recessive	Lysosomal α-D-mannosidase	19p13-q13	Unknown	Deficient or unstable enzyme activity	Accumulation of oligosaccharides causes tissue damage.
Sialidosis	63	50-100 cases	Autosomal recessive	Lysosomal α-neuraminidase (glycoprotein substrate)	10pter-q23	Unknown	Deficient enzyme activity	Accumulation of oligosaccharides causes tissue damage.
Aspartylglycosaminuria	63	70-100 cases in Finland; extremely rare elsewhere	Autosomal recessive	Lysosomal aspartylglycosaminidase	4q	Unknown	Deficient enzyme activity	Accumulation of glycopeptides causes tissue damage.
Fucosidosis	63	30-60 cases	Autosomal recessive	Lysosomal α-L-fucosidase	1p34	Unknown	Deficient enzyme activity	Accumulation of glycolipid, glycopeptides, and oligosaccharides causes tissue damage.

#	Disease	Frequency	Inheritance	Deficient enzyme	Chromosome	Mutation	Deficient enzyme activity	Consequences
64	Wolman disease and cholesteryl ester storage disease	Wolman disease; 45 cases. Cholesteryl ester storage disease; 25 cases	Autosomal recessive	Acid lipase	10q	Unknown	Deficient enzyme activity	Cholesteryl esters and triglycerides accumulate in lysosomes of body cells producing hepatic, intestinal, and adrenal dysfunction. Death in infancy in Wolman disease. Hyperlipidemia and atherosclerosis with survival to early adulthood in cholesteryl ester storage disease.
65	Ceramidase deficiency (Farber lipogranulomatosis)	Rare; 40 cases	Autosomal recessive	Lysosomal acid ceramidase	Unknown	Unknown	Deficient enzyme activity	Accumulation of substrate (ceramide) leads to granulomatous reaction in joints, subcutaneous tissues, larynx, and other tissues. Accumulation of ceramides and gangliosides in lysosomes of neurons leads to spinal cord and brain dysfunction.
66	Niemann-Pick disease type I (primary sphingomyelin storage)	Rare (regional variations)	Autosomal recessive	Type I: sphingomyelinase	Unknown	Unknown	Type I: deficient sphingomyelinase activity	Type I: Accumulation of sphingomyelin and cholesterol in cells leads to dysfunction.
66	Niemann-Pick disease type II (secondary sphingomyelin storage)	Rare	Autosomal recessive	Type II: unknown	Unknown	Unknown	Type II: unknown	Type II: Accumulation of cholesterol, glycolipid, bis (monoacylglycero) phosphate, and some sphingomyelin.
67	Gaucher disease type 1 (nonneurologic)	1:600 among Ashkenazi Jews; rare in the general population	Autosomal recessive	Glucocerebrosidase	1q21	Probably many $Asn_{370} \rightarrow Ser$	Decreased catalytic activity and some instability of enzyme protein	Accumulation of glucosylceramide in lysosomes of macrophages leads to injury of it and surrounding cells (not including neurons).
67	Gaucher disease type 2 (infantile neurologic)	Rare; no ethnic predilection	Autosomal recessive	Glucocerebrosidase	1q21	Probably many $Leu_{444} \rightarrow Pro$	Small decrease in catalytic activity but major decrease in enzyme protein stability which results in little or no lysosomal glucocerebrosidase	Accumulation of glucosylceramide in lysosomes of macrophages which leads to injury of cell and surrounding cells (including neurons).
67	Gaucher disease type 3 (juvenile neurologic)	Rare; genetic isolate in Boden, Sweden	Autosomal recessive	Glucocerebrosidase	1q21	Unknown	Small decrease in catalytic activity and unstable enzyme protein result in significant decreased lysosomal glucocerebrosidase	Accumulation of glucosylceramide in lysosomes of macrophages which leads to injury of cell and surrounding cells (including neurons).

155

SUMMARY TABLE (continued)

Part 11: Lysosomal enzymes (continued)

Name of disease	Chap. no.	Frequency	Mode of inheritance	Mutant gene product	Chromosomal location	Altered DNA structure	Expression	
							Disturbed protein function	Disrupted cell and organ function
Globoid-cell leukodystrophy (Krabbe disease)	68	1:50,0000 in Sweden, much lower elsewhere 1:170 in unusual inbred Druze population in Israel	Autosomal recessive	Lysosomal galactosylceramidase (galactocerebroside β-galactosidase)	Unknown	Unknown	Absent enzyme activity	Accumulation of a toxic natural substrate (galactosylsphingosine-psychosine) leads to disappearance of oligodendroglia and cessation of myelination, resulting in destruction of CNS white matter and peripheral neuropathy.
Multiple sulfatase deficiency	69	40 cases	Autosomal recessive	6 lysosomal sulfatases and steroid sulfatase	Unknown	Unknown	Unstable enzyme proteins	Failure to hydrolyze sulfatides and sulfated mucopolysaccharides leads to their accumulation in neural and extraneural tissues causing progressive CNS deterioration, facial and skeletal dysmorphism, hepatosplenomegaly, sulfatiduria, and mucopolysacchariduria.
Metachromatic leukodystrophy	69	1:100,000	Autosomal recessive	Arylsulfatase A	22q13	Unknown	Deficient enzyme activity	Failure to hydrolyze sulfatides leads to their accumulation in the nervous system, kidney, gallbladder, and other organs, causing demyelination, progressive CNS deterioration, and sulfatiduria.
Fabry disease	70	1:40,000: panethnic	X-linked	α-Galactosidase A	Xq22	Partial deletions, partial duplications, missense mutations	Nonfunctional or unstable enzyme protein	Accumulation of substrates with terminal galactosyl moieties (globotriaosylceramide, galabiaosylceramide, blood group B substances) particularly in vascular endothelial lysosomes, leading to ischemia and infarction.

Disorder	Page	Frequency	Inheritance	Enzyme/protein	Chromosomal location	Probable point mutations	Deficient activity	Comments
Schindler disease (α-N-acetylgalactosaminidase deficiency)	70	Unknown, very rare	Autosomal recessive	α-N-acetylgalactos-aminidase	22q13-qter		Deficient activity of α-N-acetylgalactosaminidase	Accumulation of glycoprotein, glycopeptide, glycosphingolipid, and mucopolysaccharide substrates with α-N-galactosaminyl residues. Major pathologic substrate deposition is the terminal axons primarily in gray matter.
G_{M1} gangliosidosis	71	Unknown	Autosomal recessive	Acid β-galactosidase (GLB1)	3p21-cen	Unknown	Deficient enzyme activity	Lysosomal storage of ganglioside G_{M1} and galactosyl oligosaccharides.
Galactosialidosis	71	Uncommon but not rare in Japan; rare elsewhere	Autosomal recessive	20	Unknown	Unknown	Reduced to absent 32-kDa lysosomal protective protein which is required for realizing or stabilizing activities of β-galactosidase and oligosaccharide neuraminidase	Lysosomal accumulation of glycolipids and oligosaccharides producing dysostosis multiplex, some Hurler-like features, and CNS abnormalities including dementia.
G_{M2} gangliosidosis: hexosaminidase α-subunit deficiency (variant B, Tay-Sachs disease)	72	1:300,000; 100 times higher in Ashkenazi Jews	Autosomal recessive	α subunit of β-hexosaminidase	15q22-q25.1	Multiple alleles: deletion (French-Canadian) and nondeletion	Absent or defective hexosaminidase A (αβ) activity	Accumulation of ganglioside G_{M2} in lysosomes causes neuronal dysfunction.
G_{M2} gangliosidosis: hexosaminidase β-subunit deficiency (variant O, Sandhoff disease)	72	1:300,000	Autosomal recessive	β subunit of β-hexosaminidase	5q13	Multiple alleles: deletion and nondeletion	Absent hexosaminidase A (αβ) and B (ββ) activity	Accumulation of ganglioside G_{M2} and water-soluble substrates causes neuronal dysfunction and organomegaly.
G_{M2} gangliosidosis: G_{M2} activator deficiency	72	Very rare	Autosomal recessive	G_{M2} activator protein	5	Unknown	Absent or defective G_{M2} activator	Accumulation of ganglioside G_{M2} in lysosomes causes neuronal dysfunction.

Part 12: Hormones: synthesis and action

Disorder	Page	Frequency	Inheritance	Enzyme/protein	Chromosomal location	Probable point mutations	Deficient activity	Comments
Pendred syndrome	73	~1:15,000	Autosomal recessive	Unknown	Unknown	Unknown	Unknown	Defect of H_2O_2-generating system, hypothyroidism and goiter, deaf-mutism.
Hereditary hyperthyroidism	73	Very rare	Autosomal dominant	Unknown	Unknown	Unknown	Unknown	Constitutive stimulation of the thyrocytes with autonomy and hyperthyroidism, goiter.
Thyrotropin resistance, *see also* Pseudohypoparathyroidism Ia	73	Rare	Autosomal recessive	Unknown	Unknown	Unknown	Unknown	Unresponsiveness of thyrocytes to thyrotropin and consequent hypothyroidism.
Iodide transport defect	73	Rare	? Autosomal recessive	Unknown	Unknown	Unknown	Unknown	Absence of iodide transport; hypothyroidism and goiter.
Iodotyrosine deiodinase defect	73	Rare	Autosomal recessive	Unknown	Unknown	Unknown	Defect in iodotyrosine deiodinase	Loss of iodotyrosines, and consequently of iodine, from the thyroid and in the urine; hypothyroidism and goiter.

SUMMARY TABLE (continued)

Part 12: Hormones: synthesis and action (continued)

Name of disease	Chap. no.	Frequency	Mode of inheritance	Mutant gene product	Chromosomal location	Altered DNA structure	Expression	
							Disturbed protein function	Disrupted cell and organ function
Thyroxine-binding globulin deficiency	73	~1:4000	X-linked	Unknown	Xq	Unknown	Absence of serum thyroxine-binding globulin	None, benign.
Thyroglobulin defect	73	Rare	Autosomal recessive with one exception	? Thyroglobulin in some	8q24 for thyroglobulin	Unknown	Possibly abnormal thyroglobulin, proven in cattle	Reduced or dysfunctional thyroglobulin leading to hypothyroidism.
Classic steroid 21-hydroxylase deficiency salt-wasting type	74	1:19,000	Autosomal recessive	Steroid 21-hydroxylase	6p23 (HLA complex)	Deletions, gene conversions, and nonsense mutations	Absent or truncated enzyme with no activity	Nearly absent synthesis of cortisol and aldosterone in zona fasciculata of adrenal cortex. Deficiency of these hormones leads to impaired salt and water homeostasis.
Classic steroid 21-hydroxylase deficiency simple virilizing type	74	1:58,000	Autosomal recessive	Steroid 21-hydroxylase	6p23 (HLA complex)	Multiple point mutations	Decreased enzyme activity	Markedly decreased synthesis of cortisol in zona fasciculata of adrenal cortex. Compensatory overproduction of cortisol precursors and adrenal androgens leads to virilization.
Nonclassic steroid 21-hydroxylase deficiency	74	1:100 in some ethnic groups	Autosomal recessive	Steroid 21-hydroxylase	6p23 (HLA complex)	Associated with duplicated CYP21A pseudogene; point mutations	Decreased enzyme activity	Decreased cortisol synthesis in zona fasciculata of adrenal cortex.
Disorders of the androgen receptor (complete testicular feminization, incomplete testicular feminization, Reifenstein syndrome, infertile male syndrome)	75	1:64,000 with 46XY (complete testicular feminization)	X-linked recessive	Androgen receptor protein	Xq	Unknown	Absent, unstable, or deficient protein	Abnormality of the androgen receptor complex in androgen target cells leads to defective androgen action in utero and in postembryonic life.
Steroid 5α-reductase deficiency	75	Rare	Autosomal recessive	Steroid 5α-reductase	Unknown	Unknown	Absent or unstable enzyme activity	Deficiency of product (dihydrotestosterone) leads to a form of male pseudohermaphroditism in which genetic males have male genitalia, but female external genitalia.

Disorder	Page	Frequency	Inheritance	Gene product	Chromosome	Molecular defect	Biochemical/hormonal defect	Comments
Steroid sulfatase deficiency (X-linked ichthyosis)	76	1:2000–6000 males	X-linked recessive	3 β-hydroxysteroid sulfatase	Xp22.3-pter	Gene deletion in 90% of cases	Absent immunoreactive and enzymatically active protein (both deletion and nondeletion patients)	Accumulation of cholesterol sulfate in stratum corneum is responsible for abnormal desquamation. Some patients have other abnormalities due to deletion of contiguous genes.
Isolated human chorionic somatomammotropin deficiency	77	Rare	Autosomal recessive	Chorionic somatomammotropin	17q22-q24	Gene deletion of both functional loci (type 1A) or of one locus (type 1B)	Absent (type 1A) or deficient (type 1B)	Absent or deficient chorionic somatomammotropin during pregnancy. Affected children have normal intrauterine and postnatal growth.
Rieger syndrome	77	Rare	Autosomal dominant	Unknown	Unknown	Unknown	Deficient human growth hormone and other anterior pituitary hormones (ACTH, FSH, LH, and TSH)	Deficiency of pituitary hormones causes dwarfism, adrenal insufficiency, hypothyroidism, and delayed sexual development.
Pituitary aplasia	77	Rare	Autosomal recessive or sporadic	Unknown	Unknown	Unknown	Absent or deficient human growth hormone and other anterior pituitary hormones (ACTH, FSH, LH, and TSH)	Aplasia of pituitary results in panhypopituitarism, dwarfism, and adrenal insufficiency.
Holoprosencephaly	77	Unknown	Autosomal dominant or recessive, associated with chromosomal defects, or sporadic	Unknown	Unknown	Unknown	Absent or deficient ACTH, FSH, LH, and TSH	Developmental defect associated with median cleft lip and palate. Associated anomalies of the hypothalamus can cause anterior pituitary hormone deficiencies.
Ectrodactyly-ectodermal dysplasia-clefting (EEC) syndrome	77	Unknown	Autosomal recessive	Unknown	Unknown	Unknown	Deficiency of growth hormone and other anterior pituitary hormone deficiency in associated with CNS malformations that occur in some of these patients	Defects of hands and feet; ectodermal dysplasia causes fair skin, anodontia, and cleft palate. Patients with dwarfism due to human growth hormone deficiency usually respond to human growth hormone.
Panhypopituitary dwarfism type II	77	Rare	X-linked	Unknown	X	Unknown	Deficient human growth hormone, ACTH, FSH, LH, and TSH	Deficiency of human growth hormone causes dwarfism. Associated endocrine deficiencies cause delayed sexual development, hypothyroidism, and adrenal insufficiency.
Panhypopituitary dwarfism type I	77	Rare	Autosomal recessive	Unknown	Unknown	Unknown GH1 locus does not cosegregate with disorder	Deficient human growth hormone, ACTH, FSH, LH, and TSH	Panhypopituitinism results in dwarfism, delayed sexual development, hypothyroidism, and adrenal insufficiency.

SUMMARY TABLE (continued)

Name of disease	Chap. no.	Frequency	Mode of inheritance	Mutant gene product	Chromosomal location	Altered DNA structure	Disturbed protein function	Disrupted cell and organ function
							Expression	
Part 12: Hormones: synthesis and action (continued)								
Laron dwarfism	77	Unknown	Autosomal recessive	Unknown	Unknown	Unknown	Deficient growth hormone receptor function?	Normal amounts of normal growth hormone are produced, but insulinlike growth factor 1 levels are low and do not respond to exogenous growth hormone. This defect in the mediator of growth hormone function results in dwarfism.
Isolated growth hormone deficiency type IA (IGHD1A)	77	25 cases	Autosomal recessive	Growth hormone	17q22-q24	Gene deletion	Growth hormone absent	Absence of human growth hormone results in severe dwarfism. Patients often produce anti-growth hormone antibodies when given growth hormone.
Isolated growth hormone deficiency type IB (IGHD1B)	77	Unknown	Autosomal recessive	Unknown	Unknown	Unknown	Growth hormone deficiency	Deficiency of human growth hormone results in dwarfism. Patients usually respond to exogenous growth hormone.
Isolated growth hormone deficiency type II	77	Unknown	Autosomal dominant	Unknown	Unknown	Unknown	Growth hormone deficiency	Deficiency of growth hormone results in dwarfism. Patients usually respond to exogenous growth hormone.
Isolated growth hormone deficiency type III	77	Rare	X-linked	Unknown	X	Unknown	Growth hormone deficiency	Deficiency of growth hormone results in dwarfism. Patients usually respond to exogenous growth hormone. Hypogammaglobulinemia (deficient IgG, IgA, IgM, and IgE) also occurs.
Nephrogenic diabetes insipidus	78	Uncommon but not rare	X-linked with mild and variable manifestations in females	Unknown	Xq28	Unknown	Unknown	Renal tubular cells fail to accumulate cyclic AMP in response to vasopressin. The resulting vasopressin unresponsiveness leads to polyuria, hyposthenuria, and polydipsia.

Disorder		Number of cases	Inheritance	Gene product			Protein defect	Comments
Pseudohypoparathyroidism type Ia	79	Unknown; over 100 cases	? Autosomal dominant	α Subunit of stimulatory guanine nucleotide–binding protein associated with adenylate cyclase (?)	Unknown	Unknown	Reduced synthesis of protein	Deficiency of protein leads to generalized hormone resistance with hypoparathyroidism, hypothyroidism, and hypogonadism most prominent clinically. Other abnormalities include: obesity, short stature, mental retardation, and bony anomalies collectively termed *Albright osteodystrophy*.
Pseudohypoparathyroidism type Ib	79	Unknown; over 50 cases	Unknown	Unknown	Unknown	Unknown	Unknown	Isolated resistance to parathyroid hormone due to defect in receptor-adenylate cyclase complex leads to parathyroidism.
Hereditary simple and selective deficiency of 1,25(OH)$_2$D (pseudo-vitamin D deficiency type I, vitamin D dependency type I)	80	Unknown	Autosomal recessive	25(OH)D$_3$-1 α-hydroxylase (so far confirmed only in similar disease in pigs)	Unknown	Unknown	Deficient enzyme activity (putative and by analogy with pig model)	Deficient product [1,25(OH)$_2$D] causes features of vitamin D deficiency.
Hereditary generalized resistance to 1,25(OH)$_2$D (pseudo-vitamin D deficiency type II, vitamin D dependency type II)	80	Unknown	Autosomal recessive	Receptor for 1,25(OH)$_2$D	Unknown	Unknown several alleles, (at one or more loci ?)	1. Hormone binding negative 2. Decreased maximal capacity of hormone binding 3. Decreased affinity of hormone binding 4. Normal hormone binding but undetectable nuclear localization 5. Nuclear localization positive	Disrupted cell and organ Decreased or absent 1,25(OH)$_2$D action in all cells causes features of vitamin D deficiency. The most severely affected cases show alopecia.
Idiopathic hypercalcemia with supravalvular aortic stenosis (Williams-Beuren syndrome)	80	Unknown	Unknown	Unknown	Unknown	Unknown	Unknown	Hypercalcemia, supravalvular aortic stenosis, characteristic "elfin" facies.

Part 13: Vitamins

Disorder		Number of cases	Inheritance	Gene product			Protein defect	Comments
Methylenetetrahydrofolate reductase deficiency	81	>25 cases	Autosomal recessive	Methylenetetrahydrofolate reductase	Unknown	Unknown	Absent or deficient enzyme activity	Lack of formation of methyltetrahydrofolate results in elevated levels of homocysteine and decreased levels of methionine. Considerable phenotypic heterogeneity, but most patients have severe neurologic disturbances.

Part 13: Vitamins (continued)

Name of disease	Chap. no.	Frequency	Mode of inheritance	Mutant gene product	Chromosomal location	Expression		
						Altered DNA structure	Disturbed protein function	Disrupted cell and organ function
cblG (functional methionine synthase deficiency)	81	3 cases	Autosomal recessive	Unknown	Unknown	Unknown	Decreased activity of vitamin B_{12}–dependent methionine synthase	Elevated homocysteine and low methionine levels; failure to regenerate tetrahydrofolate. Patients have megaloblastic anemia and neurologic abnormalities.
cblE (functional methionine synthase deficiency)	81	4 cases	? Autosomal recessive; all cases male	Unknown	Unknown	Unknown	Decreased activity of a reducing system associated with B_{12}-dependent methionine synthase	Impaired methylcobalamin formation results in elevated homocysteine levels, decreased methionine levels, and failure to regenerate tetrahydrofolate. Patients have megaloblastic anemia and neurologic abnormalities.
Glutamate formininotransferase deficiency	81	Rare; 13 cases	Autosomal recessive	Glutamate forminotransferase	Unknown	Unknown	Low levels of enzyme reported in liver and erythrocytes	Elevated levels of forminoglutamic acid. Some patients have neurologic abnormalities; significance not clear.
Hereditary folate malabsorption	81	12 cases	? Autosomal recessive, excess of females	Unknown	Unknown	Unknown	Defective transport system for folates in intestine and choroid plexus	Deficiency of folate derivatives leading to megaloblastic anemia and neurologic abnormalities.
Homocystinuria (cobalamin-dependent) (two nonallelic forms designated *cblE* and *cblG*)	82	Rare (6 cases)	Unknown	Unknown	Unknown	Unknown	Unknown	Impaired cytoplasmic utilization of cobalamin results in decreased activity of N^5-methyltetrahydro-folate-homocysteine methyltransferase and deficient synthesis of methylcobalamin and methionine. Clinical findings include developmental delay and megaloblastic anemia.
Transcobalamin II deficiency	82	Rare	Autosomal recessive	Transcobalamin II (TC II)	22q	Unknown	Absent TC II protein; decreased binding of TC II–cobalamin to cellular receptors	Defective function of TC II leads to abnormal transport of cobalamin into cells and to functional cellular cobalamin deficiency. Megaloblastic anemia and eventual neurologic and immunologic dysfunction are important findings.

Disorder	Page	Frequency	Inheritance	Protein/gene product	Chromosome	Mutation	Biochemical defect	Consequence
Enterocyte cobalamin malabsorption (Imerslünd-Grasbeck syndrome) (possibly multiple nonallelic forms)	82	Rare (more common in Finns and North African Jews)	? Autosomal recessive; others unknown	Enterocyte intrinsic factor receptor	Unknown	Unknown	Failure of specific enterocyte receptor to bind intrinsic factor–cobalamin complex; failure of transfer of cobalamin from intrinsic factor to transcobalamin II	Impaired transintestinal transport of cobalamin leads to functional cobalamin deficiency. Hematologic and neurologic abnormalities are major clinical findings.
Intrinsic factor deficiency	82	Rare	Autosomal recessive	Intrinsic factor (IF)	Unknown	Unknown	Absent IF protein; increased lability of IF; decreased binding of cobalamin to IF; decreased binding of IF to specific enterocyte receptors	Defective IF function leads to reduced intestinal cobalamin transport and functional cobalamin deficiency. Hematologic abnormalities, particularly megaloblastic anemia, and neurologic dysfunction are prominent.
Holocarboxylase synthetase deficiency	83	Rare	Autosomal recessive	Holocarboxylase synthetase ?	Unknown	Unknown	Deficient holocarboxylase synthetase activity	Failure to biotinylate enzymes causes secondary deficiency of four carboxylases causing organic acidemia.
Biotinidase deficiency	83	1:50,000–70,000 whites by newborn screening	Autosomal recessive	Biotinidase	Unknown	Unknown	Deficient biotinidase activity	Failure to absorb and recycle biotin causes secondary deficiency of four carboxylases causing organic acidemia.

Part 14: Blood and blood forming tissues

Disorder	Page	Frequency	Inheritance	Protein/gene product	Chromosome	Mutation	Biochemical defect	Consequence
Protein C deficiency	84	Rare ?	Autosomal dominant	Protein C	2	Missense and nonsense known	Decreased anticoagulant activity	Impaired regulation of blood coagulation.
Prothrombin deficiency	84	<50 cases	Autosomal recessive	Prothrombin	11p11-q12	Several, Barcelona $Arg_{271} \rightarrow Cys$; Tokushima $Arg_{98} \rightarrow Trp$	Barcelona prevents cleavage by factor Xa. Tokushima has 21% clotting activity.	Impaired blood coagulation.
Factor VII deficiency	84	Estimated 1:500,000	Autosomal recessive	Factor VII	13q34-qter	Not established	Decreased factor VII coagulant activity	Impaired blood coagulation.
Factor IX deficiency (hemophilia B)	84	1:70,000	X-linked	Factor IX	Xq26-q27	Deletions, splicing abnormalities, and missense	Absence of protein, protein with reduced coagulant activity or abnormal susceptibility to cleavage for activation	Impaired blood coagulation.
Factor X deficiency	84	About 50 families	Autosomal recessive	Factor X	13q34-qter	Not established	Decreased coagulation activity	Impaired blood coagulation.
Afibrinogenemia	85	150 cases	Autosomal recessive	Fibrinogen	4q23-q32	Unknown	Absence of fibrinogen	Absence of fibrinogen leads to defective platelet aggregation.

SUMMARY TABLE (continued)

Part 14: Blood and blood forming tissues (continued)

Name of disease	Chap. no.	Frequency	Mode of inheritance	Mutant gene product	Chromosomal location	Expression		
						Altered DNA structure	Disturbed protein function	Disrupted cell and organ function
Dysfibrinogenemia	85	130 cases	Autosomal recessive (in several cases autosomal codominant)	Fibrinogen	4q23-q32	Point mutations	Defective fibrinogen	Dysfunction of fibrinogen can lead to hemorrhage, spontaneous abortion, or thromboembolism.
Factor XIII deficiency	85	1:5 million in U.K. and Japan	Autosomal recessive	The A subunit of factor XIII	6p24-p21	Not determined	Absent or deficient enzyme activity	Deficiency of factor XIII leads to delayed bleeding and wound healing and to habitual abortion.
Factor VIII deficiency (hemophilia A, classic hemophilia)	86	1:10,000 males	X-linked recessive	Factor VIII	Xq28	Missense, nonsense, deletion	Factor VIII deficiency or dysfunction	Factor VIII fails to function as a cofactor for activation of factor X and impairs clotting cascade.
Factor V deficiency (parahemophilia)	86	Extremely rare (<1:million)	Autosomal recessive	Factor V	1q21-q25	Unknown	Factor V deficiency	Factor V fails to function as a cofactor for activation of prothrombin and impairs clotting cascade.
von Willebrand disease	87	1:125 but only 1:8000 clinically significant	Variable mostly autosomal dominant	von Willebrand factor	12p12-pter	Unknown, very heterogeneous	Quantitative or qualitative binding protein deficiency	Abnormal platelet adhesion and mildly reduced factor VIII levels cause bleeding.
von Willebrand disease type III (severe)	87	1:200,000–2 million higher in Arabs	Autosomal recessive	von Willebrand factor	12p12-pter	Gene deletions in some; unknown and heterogenous in most	Total binding protein deficiency	Abnormal platelet adhesion and markedly reduced factor VIII levels cause severe bleeding.
Factor XI deficiency	88	~1:1000 in Ashkenazi Jews of Israel	Autosomal recessive	Factor XI	Unknown	Unknown	Decreased levels of factor XI	Deficiency of protein leads to impaired contact activation and mild bleeding tendency.
Antithrombin deficiency	89	~1:5000	Autosomal dominant	Antithrombin	1q23-q25	Deletions point mutations	Deficient or dysfunctional antithrombin	Impaired inhibition of coagulation factors IIa, IXa, and Xa in plasma causes recurrent venous thrombosis.
Glanzmann thrombasthenia	90	Uncommon, but not rare	Autosomal recessive	Platelet membrane glycoprotein IIb-IIIa complex	The genes for glycoproteins IIb and IIIa are both on chromosome 17	Unknown	Quantitative or qualitative defects in glycoprotein IIb-IIIa (receptor for fibrinogen, fibronectin, and von Willebrand factor)	Failure of activated platelets to interact with extracellular adhesive proteins and intracellular contractile proteins results in defective platelet aggregation, platelet spreading, and clot retraction, causing moderate bleeding.

Disorder	Frequency	Inheritance	Protein	Chromosome	Mutations	Defect	Description
Bernard-Soulier disease 90	<50 cases	Autosomal recessive	Platelet membrane glycoprotein Ib-IX-(V)	Unknown	Unknown	Absent or decreased platelet membrane glycoproteins Ib, IX, and V (receptor for von Willebrand factor)	Failure of platelets to bind plasma von Willebrand factor results in defective platelet adhesion to blood vessel subendothelium, causing moderate bleeding.
Glucose-6-phosphate dehydrogenase deficiency (favism; primaquine sensitivity) 91	Very variable; up to 30% in parts of Africa and Asia; about 13% in U.S. black males	X-linked	Glucose-6-phosphate dehydrogenase (G6PD)	Xq28	Point mutations (missense), about 300 different variants known	Some variants unstable; some with altered enzyme kinetics; some with both	Red cells tend to hemolyze because of inadequate NADPH production; very rarely, impaired granulocyte function.
Hereditary methemoglobinemia, secondary to cytochrome b_5 reductase deficiency, types I, II, and III 92	~300 cases	Autosomal recessive	Cytochrome b_5 reductase	22	Unknown	Deficient enzyme activity in erythrocyte cytosol only (type I), in all tissues (type II), and in all hematopoetic cells (type III)	Failure to reduce substrate cytochrome b_5 leads to accumulation of methemoglobin in erythrocytes and cyanosis (types I, II, and III). Patients with type II also have severe progressive neurologic dysfunction.
Hereditary methyemoglobinemia secondary to cytochrome b_5 deficiency 92	1 case	Unknown	Cytochrome b_5	Unknown	Unknown	Deficiency of this electron transferring protein	Defective transfer of electrons to methemoglobin results in methemoglobin accumulation and cyanosis.
Hemoglobinopathies (selected entries): α-Thalassemia, multiple allelic disorders 93	High frequency in Mediterranean, African, and Asian populations	Autosomal recessive	α-Globin	16p13	Deletion of both loci (α° thalassemia); deletion of one α locus (α^+ thalassemia); single nucleotide mutation of termination codon (HB Constant Spring); nondeletion defects due to (1) mutation within intervening sequence and (2) unknown mutations	Deficiency of α-globin	Decreased α-globin synthesis leads to uncombined β-globin chains, which disrupts erythroid cell maturation and function, causing microcytosis, ineffective erythropoiesis, and hemolysis.
β-Thalassemia, multiple allelic disorders 93	High frequency in Mediterranean and Asian populations	Autosomal recessive	β-Globin	11p15.5	Gene deletion; nonsense mutation; frame shift mutation; mutation in intervening sequence causing abnormal processing	Decreased or absent β-globin	Decreased β-globin leads to uncombined α-globin chains, which disrupts erythroid cell maturation and function, causing microcytosis, ineffective erythrocytosis, and hemolysis.

Name of disease	Chap. no.	Frequency	Mode of inheritance	Mutant gene product	Chromosomal location	Altered DNA structure	Disturbed protein function	Disrupted cell and organ function
							Expression	
Part 14: Blood and blood forming tissues (continued)								
Sickle-cell anemia	93	High frequency in African, Mediterranean, and Middle Eastern populations	Autosomal recessive	β-Globin	11p15.5 single nucleotide change	(A→T) in 6th codon	Glu→Val substitution at 6th residue of β chain	Phenotype liable to tactoid formation and sickle deformation of RBC under reduced O_2 pressure with effect on microcirculation.
Pyruvate kinase deficiency hemolytic anemia	94	1:20,000 Caucasians	Autosomal recessive	Pyruvate kinase	Unknown	Unknown	Deficient enzyme activity	Deficiency of product (ATP) leads to hemolysis.
Hexokinase deficiency hemolytic anemia	94	~14 cases	Autosomal recessive	Hexokinase	10 for type I	Unknown	Deficient enzyme activity	Impaired glycolysis. Hemolysis.
Glucose phosphate isomerase deficiency hemolytic anemia	94	>40 severely deficient cases	Autosomal recessive	Glucosephosphate isomerase	19q12-q13.2	Unknown	Deficient enzyme activity	Hemolytic anemia. Rarely hydrops fetalis.
Phosphofructokinase hemolytic anemia	94	>20 kindreds	Autosomal recessive	Usually of M (muscle) subunit	1cen-q32	Unknown	Partial enzyme activity deficiency	Hemolytic anemia. Myopathy.
Aldolase deficiency hemolytic anemia	94	Very rare; two kindreds	Autosomal recessive	Aldolase	Unknown	Unknown	Enzyme activity deficiency	Hemolytic anemia? Other tissue disorders.
Triose-phosphate isomerase deficiency hemolytic anemia	94	25 cases	Autosomal recessive	Triosephosphate isomerase	12p13	Glu_{104}→Asp	Enzyme activity deficient in all tissues	Hemolytic anemia, severe neurologic deficits, multisystem disease.
Phosphoglycerate kinase deficiency hemolytic anemia	94	About 12 deficiency variants documented	X-linked	Phosphoglycerate kinase	Xq13	Four missense	Deficient enzyme activity in hemizygotes	Hemolytic anemia. Often neurologic abnormalities.
2,3-Diphosphoglyceromutase and phosphatase deficiency	94	One kindred unequivocally documented	Autosomal recessive	2,3-Diphosphoglyceromutase and phosphatase (one protein)	Unknown	Uncertain	Enzyme activity deficient	Mild erythrocytosis. Nearly absent 2,3-DPG in red cells.
Lactate dehydrogenase deficiency	94	2 kindreds	Autosomal recessive	1. H subunit 2. M subunit	H subunit 12q12.1-p12.2 M subunit 11p14-p15	Unknown	Enzyme activity deficiency	1. No manifestations. 2. Myopathy.
6-Phosphogluconate dehydrogenase deficiency	94	Unknown; severe deficiency detected in surveys	Autosomal recessive	6-Phosphogluconate dehydrogenase	Unknown	Unknown	Enzyme activity deficiency	None known.
Glutathione peroxidase deficiency	94	Uncertain; very rare	Autosomal recessive	Glutathione peroxidase	3q13-q12	Unknown	Diminished enzyme activity	Uncertain? Hemolytic syndrome under some circumstances.
Glutathione reductase deficiency	94	1 kindred with unequivocal apoenzyme deficiency	Autosomal recessive	Glutathione reductase	8p21.1	Unknown	Enzyme activity deficiency	Hemolysis with oxidant stress such as fava bean ingestion.
Glutathione synthetase deficiency hemolytic anemia	94	Rare; several kindreds	Autosomal recessive	Glutathione synthetase	Unknown	Unknown	Enzyme activity deficiency	Hemolysis. Pyroglutamic aciduria. Variable neurologic deficits.
γ-Glutamylcysteine deficiency hemolytic anemia	94	1 kindred	Autosomal recessive	γ-Glutamylcysteine synthetase	Unknown	Unknown	Enzyme activity deficiency	1. Hemolytic anemia exacerbated by oxidant stress. 2. Spinocerebellar ataxia.

Disorder		Frequency	Inheritance	Protein	Chromosome		Molecular defect	Consequence
Adenosine deaminase hyperactivity hemolytic anemia	94	3 families	Autosomal dominant	Adenosine deaminase	20q13-qter	Unknown	Overproduction of structurally normal enzyme protein mediated at mRNA translation level	Decreased erythrocyte ATP salvage via adenosine kinase.
Pyrimidine nucleotidase deficiency hemolytic anemia	94	Rare	Autosomal recessive	Pyrimidine nucleotidase	Unknown	Unknown	Deficient enzyme activity	Accumulation of pyrimidine degradation products of RNA normally cleared during reticulocyte maturation.
Hereditary spherocytosis	95	~1:5000 Caucasians	Autosomal dominant	1. Unknown 2. β-Spectrin 3. ? Ankyrin	1. Unknown 2. 14 3. 8 (?8q11.1)	1. Unknown 2. Unknown 3. ? Deletion	Common denominator: Spectrin deficiency (primary or secondary) 1. Unknown primary defect 2. Decreased binding of protein 4.1 by defective β-spectrin weakened spectrin-actin interaction 3. ? Ankyrin deficiency decreased spectrin binding	All forms: Membrane loss causes spherocytosis, splenic sequestration, and hemolytic anemia.
Hereditary spherocytosis	95	~1:20,000	? Autosomal recessive	Spectrin, probably α subunit	1q22-q25	Unknown	Spectrin deficiency	Membrane loss causes spherocytosis, splenic sequestration, and hemolytic anemia.
Hereditary elliptocytosis	95	~1:2500 (all forms)	Autosomal dominant	1. α-Spectrin 2. β-Spectrin 3. Protein 4.1 4. Glycophorin C	1. 1 2. 14 3. 1p34-p36 4. 2q14-q21	Unknown (all forms)	1 & 2: Defective spectrin self-association 3. Decreased protein 4.1 4. Decreased glycophorin C (and decreased Gerbich antigen)	All forms: Membrane cytoskeletal weakness and elliptocytosis (? mechanism). Severe forms only: Red cell fragmentation and hemolysis.
Hereditary pyropoikilocytosis	95	Unknown	Autosomal recessive	α-Spectrin	1q22-q25	Unknown	Defective spectrin self-association	Membrane weakness leads to red cell fragmentation and hemolytic anemia.

SUMMARY TABLE (continued)

Name of disease	Chap. no.	Frequency	Mode of inheritance	Mutant gene product	Chromosomal location	Altered DNA structure	Disturbed protein function	Disrupted cell and organ function
Part 14: Blood and blood forming tissues (continued)								
α_1-Antitrypsin deficiency (Z variant)	96	1:7000 northern Europeans 1:3000 Scandinavians	Autosomal recessive	α_1-Antitrypsin	14q32.1	Missense mutations	Z, (Glu$_{342}$ → Lys); S, (Glu$_{264}$ → Val). Aggregated, nonsecreted protein PI$_Z$. Other phenotypes unknown	Liver storage of polypeptide; plasma deficiency of enzyme.
Hereditary amyloidosis	97	1:100,000–million	Autosomal dominant	Prealbumin (Transthyretin) Several allelic disorders	18q11.2-q12.1	Seven missense identified	Abnormal prealbumin	Abnormal prealbumin is deposited extracellularly as amyloid; causes peripheral neuropathy, cardiomyopathy, and nephropathy.
Part 15: Membrane transport systems								
Renal glycosuria	98	? <5% of the glycosuria in children	Type A: autosomal dominant (autosomal recessive mode not excluded)	Unknown	6 ?	Unknown several alleles	Defect in glucose carrier in nephron	Glucosuria—no clinical significance.
Congenital selective glucose and galactose intestinal malabsorption	98	<50 cases	Autosomal recessive	Unknown	Unknown	Unknown	Defect in intestinal carrier shared by glucose and galactose	Unabsorbed substrates (glucose and galactose) accumulate in intestinal lumen and exert an osmotic effect. This in turn leads to abdominal fullness, cramping abdominal pain, and diarrhea. Failure to thrive.
Cystinuria (3 allelic types)	99	1:7000	Autosomal recessive	Unknown	Unknown	Unknown	Defect in shared transport system for cystine and diabasic amino acids (ornithine, arginine, lysine) in renal tubule and intestinal mucosa	Elevated urinary excretion of cystine causes urinary tract calculi. Intestinal transport defect causes no clinical dysfunction.

	Number	Frequency	Inheritance				Defect	Clinical Features
Lysinuric protein intolerance	100	~80 cases worldwide; 1:60,000 (Finland)	Autosomal recessive	Unknown	Unknown	Unknown	Deficient function of the dibasic amino acid transporter in the basolateral membranes of epithelial cells and the plasma membrane of parenchymal cells	Impaired gastrointestinal absorption and increased renal losses of lysine, arginine, and ornithine leads to growth failure, osteoporosis, and reduced function of the urea cycle with protein intolerance and hyperammonemia.
Hyperdibasic aminoaciduria	100	Rare	Autosomal recessive	Unknown	Unknown	Unknown	Deficient function of a dibasic amino acid transporter whose cellular distribution is not yet well delineated	Reduced gastrointestinal absorption and increased renal clearance of the dibasic amino acids, without protein intolerance of hyperammonemia. Heterozygotes have milder but demonstrable absorption defects.
Hartnup disorder	101	1:24,000	Autosomal recessive	Unknown	Unknown	Unknown; more than one allele	Defect in neutral amino acid transport in kidney and intestine	Increased neutral amino acid loss in urine and feces. Pellagralike episodes or delayed development in some probands.
Familial renal iminoglycinuria	102	1:15,000	Autosomal recessive homozygotes and compounds; completely and incompletely recessive heterozygous phenotypes	Unknown; several alleles	Unknown	Unknown; several alleles	Defect in shared transport system for imino acids and glycine in renal tubule and intestine (brush-border membrane)	Aminoaciduria without clinical significance.
Distal renal tubular acidosis type I	103	Not rare	Autosomal dominant	Unknown	Unknown	Unknown	Defect in acidification in collecting tubule of nephron as a result of impaired H^+ secretion (H^+-ATPase) or abnormally high permeability of luminal membrane	Chronic hyperchloremic metabolic acidosis associated with inability to acidify urine below pH 5.5 Often associated with hypokalemia, hypercalciuria, hypocitriuria, and nephrolithiasis.

SUMMARY TABLE (continued)

Name of disease	Chap. no.	Frequency	Mode of inheritance	Mutant gene product	Chromosomal location	Altered DNA structure	Expression	
							Disturbed protein function	Disrupted cell and organ function
Part 15: Membrane transport systems (continued)								
Idiopathic Fanconi syndrome	104	Not rare	Autosomal recessive and dominant	Unknown	Unknown	Unknown	Unknown	Impaired renal tubular reabsorption of multiple solutes and ions and water. Primary Mendelian disorders that cause FS (e.g., cystinosis, hereditary fructose intolerance, galactosemia, hereditary tyrosinemia 1, Wilson disease, hereditary and vitamin D deficiency) have associated primary dysfunctions.
Oculocerebrorenal syndrome (Lowe syndrome)	104	Rare	X-linked	Unknown	Xq25	Unknown, most cases; deletion (contiguous gene syndrome) rare	Unknown	Fanconi-like tubular dysfunction plus ocular manifestations (cataracts, glaucoma) and mental retardation.
Familial hypophosphatemic rickets (vitamin D–resistant rickets, X-linked hypophosphatemia)	105	1:20,000	X-linked dominant	Unknown	Xp22	Unknown	Unknown	Defect in renal tubular phosphate reabsorption and in regulation of renal vitamin D metabolism.
Hereditary hypophosphatemic rickets with hypercalciuria	105	Rare	Autosomal dominant (probably) with variable expressivity	Unknown	Unknown	Unknown	Unknown	Defect in renal tubular phosphate reabsorption.
Hereditary renal hypouricemia	106	21 families	Autosomal recessive	Unknown	Unknown	Unknown	Unknown	Increased fractional clearance of urate (FC_{ur}) due to defective reabsorption of urate in the renal proximal tubule, manifested in hypouricemia.
Cystinosis	107	1:100,000	Autosomal recessive	Unknown	Unknown	Unknown	Transport of cystine across lysosomal membranes	Lysosomal cystine storage.
Salla disease	107	1:7000 (northern Finland)	Autosomal recessive	Unknown	Unknown	Unknown	Transport of free sialic acid across lysosomal membranes	Lysosomal storage of free sialic acid.

Disorder		Frequency	Inheritance	Gene product	Chromosome	Molecular defect	Laboratory findings	Clinical features
Cystic fibrosis	108	1:2000–3000 Caucasians; rare in other ethnic groups	Autosomal recessive	Cloned transmembrane protein	7q31	Deletion of Phe 508 in 70–75%.	Impaired chloride transport: apical membrane of epithelium; exact function of gene product unknown	Dysfunction of exocrine cells leads to pulmonary infections, exocrine pancreatic insufficiency, meconium ileus, and atrophy of the vas deferens.

Part 16: Defense and immune mechanisms

Disorder		Frequency	Inheritance	Gene product	Chromosome	Molecular defect	Laboratory findings	Clinical features
X-linked agammaglobulinemia	109	Not rare	X-linked recessive	Unknown	Xq	Unknown	Unknown	Inadequate antibody synthesis due to an absence of mature B cells. Pre-B cell numbers are normal, indicating a developmental arrest in B cell maturation. Recurrent pyogenic infections occur.
X-linked agammaglobulinemia with growth hormone deficiency	109	Multiple members of a single family	X-linked	Unknown	X	Unknown	Unknown	Hypogammaglobulinemia and reduced numbers of B cells. Growth hormone levels reduced in response to provocative testing. Short stature, delayed puberty, and recurrent infections.
Common variable immunodeficiency	109	Not rare	Autosomal recessive in some families; no definite Mendelian pattern in most	Unknown	Unknown	Unknown	Unknown	Abnormal B-cell development; recurrent infections beginning at any age.
Selective IgA deficiency	109	~1:600	Unclear; patterns consistent with autosomal recessive and autosomal dominant observed in a few families	Probably several; all unknown	Unknown	Unknown	Markedly reduced or absent IgA	Immature IgA-bearing B cells. Most affected individuals asymptomatic; some with recurrent respiratory infections and/or gastrointestinal disease. Frequency of autoimmune disease increased.
IgG subclass deficiency	109	Rare	Unclear	Unknown	Unknown	Unknown	Reduced levels of one or more IgG subclasses	Defective heavy chain genes or an abnormality in the regulation of immunoglobulin isotype switching. Recurrent infections.
Immunodeficiency with elevated IgM	109	Uncommon	X-linked and autosomal recessive	Unknown	X in some families; in others unknown	Unknown	Unknown	Reduced IgG- and IgA-bearing B cells. Recurrent pyogenic infection.
Severe combined immunodeficiency	109	Uncommon	X-linked or autosomal recessive in some families	Adenosine deaminase and nucleoside phosphorylase are two so far identified	Variable	Unknown	Deficient enzyme activity in some	Impaired humoral and cellular immunity; survival beyond 1 year unusual without treatment.

SUMMARY TABLE *(continued)*

Name of disease	Chap. no.	Frequency	Mode of inheritance	Mutant gene product	Chromosomal location	Expression: Altered DNA structure	Expression: Disturbed protein function	Expression: Disrupted cell and organ function
Part 16: Defense and immune mechanisms (continued)								
Ataxia-telangiectasia	110	1:40,000	Autosomal recessive	Unknown	Unknown	Unknown	Unknown	Variable defects in humoral and cellular immunity associated with cerebellar dysfunction and telangiectasias. Endocrine abnormalities, malignancies, and infections occur with increased frequency. Chromosomal breakage following irradiation of cultured cells is increased and has been used to define multiple complementation groups.
Wiskott-Aldrich syndrome	110	~1:500,000	X-linked recessive	Unknown	Unknown	Unknown	Unknown	Selective defects in humoral and cellular immunity with thrombocytopenia and eczema. Autoimmune disease and malignancies occur with increased frequency. Heterozygous females are clinically normal but show a nonrandom pattern of X inactivation in their T and B lymphocytes, monocytes, and granulocytes.
Severe combined immunodeficiency (*see also* Adenosine Deaminase Deficiency)	110	Rare	Heterogeneous; best delineated subtypes listed below and in Chap. 40	Variable	Variable	Unknown	Unknown	Profound dual system immunodeficiency, usually fatal.
Severe combined immunodeficiency and with MHC class I and/or class II antigen deficiency ("bare lymphocyte syndrome")	110	Rare	Autosomal recessive	Unknown	Unknown	Unknown	Abnormal expression of major histocompatibility class I and/or class II antigens	Profound dual system immunodeficiency, usually fatal.
X-linked severe combined immunodeficiency	110	Rare	X-linked	Unknown	X	Unknown	Unknown	Profound dual system immunodeficiency usually fatal. Heterozygous females are asymptomatic but exhibit a nonrandom pattern of X inactivation in their T and B lymphocytes.

Disorder		Frequency	Inheritance	Gene/protein	Chromosome	Molecular defect	Protein defect	Functional consequence
C1q deficiency/dysfunction	111	Rare	Autosomal recessive	Complement component C1q, B chain	1p	Unknown	Absence of C1q in some kindreds and presence of dysfunctional C1q in others	Markedly reduced activation of the classic pathway.
C1r/C1s deficiency	111	Rare	Autosomal recessive	Unknown	12p13	Unknown	Absent C1r and reduced C1s	Markedly reduced activation of the classic pathway.
C2 deficiency	111	~1:10,000	Autosomal recessive	Complement component 2	6p21.3	Unknown but no mRNA expressed	Absent C2	Markedly reduced activation of the classic pathway.
C3 deficiency	111	Rare	Autosomal recessive	Complement component 3	19q13	Unknown	Absent C3	Markedly reduced C3-dependent opsonization and reduced C3-dependent activation of C5–C9.
C4 deficiency	111	Rare	Autosomal recessive	Complement component 4	6q21.3	Some due to gene deletion; others unknown	Absent C4	Markedly reduced activation of the classic pathway.
C5 deficiency	111	Rare	Autosomal recessive	Complement component 5	9q22-q34	Unknown	Absent C5	Markedly reduced C5-dependent chemotaxis and reduced C5-dependent activation of C6–C9.
C6 deficiency	111	Rare	Autosomal recessive	Complement component 6	Unknown	Unknown	Absent C6	Markedly reduced C6-dependent serum bactericidal activity.
C7 deficiency	111	Rare	Autosomal recessive	Complement component 7	Unknown	Unknown	Absent C7	Markedly reduced C7-dependent serum bactericidal activity.
C8 deficiency	111	Rare	Autosomal recessive	Complement component 8	1q36-p22	Unknown	One form has absent α-γ subunit and the other absent β subunit	Markedly reduced C8-dependent serum bactericidal activity.
C9 deficiency	111	Rare	Autosomal	Complement component 9	Unknown	Unknown	Absent C9	Moderately reduced C9-dependent serum bactericidal activity.
Factor H deficiency	111	Rare	Autosomal recessive	Complement factor H	1q32	Unknown	Absent factor H	Lack of inhibition of the alternative pathway leading to continuous activation and consumption of C3.
Factor I deficiency	111	Rare	Autosomal recessive	Complement factor I	4q23-q25	Unknown	Absent factor I	Lack of inhibition of the alternative pathway leading to continuous activation and consumption of native C3.
C1 esterase inhibitor deficiency	111	Unknown	Autosomal dominant	C1 esterase inhibitor	11q12-q13	Genetic heterogeneity	Absence of C1 inhibitor in some kindreds and presence of dysfunctional C1 inhibitor in others	Lack of inhibition of C1r and C1s leading to uncontrolled activation of the classic pathway and edema.
Properdin deficiency	111	Rare	X-linked recessive	Properdin, complement factor B	Xp21-cen	Unknown	Absent properdin	Lack of stabilization of the alternative pathway C3-cleaving enzyme.

SUMMARY TABLE (continued)

Name of disease	Chap. no.	Frequency	Mode of inheritance	Mutant gene product	Chromosomal location	Altered DNA structure	Disturbed protein function	Disrupted cell and organ function
							Expression	

Part 16: Defense and immune mechanisms (continued)

Name of disease	Chap. no.	Frequency	Mode of inheritance	Mutant gene product	Chromosomal location	Altered DNA structure	Disturbed protein function	Disrupted cell and organ function
Immotile cilia syndrome (Kartagener syndrome)	112	~1:40,000	Autosomal recessive	Unknown	Unknown	Unknown	Absence of structural and enzymatic proteins of cilia (dynein arms or other structures)	Ciliary immotility or dyskinesis causes abnormalities of the respiratory tract (bronchiectasis) and spermatozoa (male sterility).
Leukocyte adhesion deficiency	113	50 cases	Autosomal recessive	β Subunit of CD18 adherence complex	21	Abnormal or absent mRNA in some	Deficient or defective β subunit of CD18 complex with secondary absence of α subunits	Abnormal leukocyte adherence complex disturbs leukocyte chemotaxis with bacterial infections; fatal in severe forms.
Myeloperoxidase deficiency	114	1:2000	Autosomal recessive	Myeloperoxidase	17q22-q23	Unknown	Absent or deficient enzyme activity	Deficiency of product (OCl⁻, a potent antimicrobial oxidant) by neutrophils and monocytes leads to impaired bacterial killing.
Chronic granulomatous disease	114	Uncommon, but not rare	X-linked recessive Autosomal recessive	β Subunit of cytochrome b (X-linked) Autosomal recessive form, product unknown	Xp21.1 (X-linked form)	One partial deletion, one abnormal mRNA	Absent or deficient activity or enzyme responsible for respiratory burst	Deficiency of product (O_2^-) prevents neutrophils, macrophages, and monocytes from expressing respiratory burst. This in turn leads to impaired bacterial killing and chronic infections.
Leukocyte glucose 6-phosphate dehydrogenase (G6PD) deficiency	114	Rare	X-linked recessive	G6PD	Xq28	Unknown	Absent enzyme activity in neutrophils	Deficiency of product (NADPH) prevents neutrophils from expressing respiratory burst. Impaired bacterial killing promotes infections.

Part 17: Connective tissues

Name of disease	Chap. no.	Frequency	Mode of inheritance	Mutant gene product	Chromosomal location	Altered DNA structure	Disturbed protein function	Disrupted cell and organ function
Osteogenesis imperfecta type I	115	1:20,000–40,000	Autosomal dominant	COL1A1, COL1A2	COL1A1 at 17q21.3-q22 COL1A2 at 7q21.3-q22.1	1. Frame shift in COL1A1 2. Splice mutations in COL1A1	Synthesis of half normal amount of type I	Bone fragility.
Osteogenesis imperfecta type II	115	1:20,000–40,000	Autosomal dominant (new mutations) (Autosomal recessive— rare)	COL1A1, COL1A2	COL1A1 at 17q21-q22 COL1A2 at 7q21.3-q22.1	COL1A1: Missense for glycine; deletion in triple helix; insertion in triple helix COL1A2: Deletion in triple helix; small deletion on background of null allele	Decreased secretion and thermal stability of type I procollagen	Bone fragility.

Osteogenesis imperfecta type III	115	Rare (? 1:60,000)	Autosomal dominant (frequent new mutations) Autosomal recessive—rare in most populations	COL1A1, COL1A2 Unknown	COL1A1 at 17q21.3-q22, COL1A2 at 7q21.3-q22.1	COL1A1: Missense for glycine in triple helix	Poor secretion, decreased thermal stability Failure to incorporate pro 2(I) chains into type I procollagen	Bone fragility and deformity.
Osteogenesis imperfecta type IV	115	1:20,000–50,000	Autosomal dominant	COL1A1, COL1A2	COL1A1 at 17q21.3-q22 COL1A2 at 7q21.3-q22.1	COL1A1: Missense near end of triple-helical domain COL1A2: Missense for glycine; small deletions	Decreased secretion and thermal stability. Free sulfhydryl (due to unpaired cysteine in 1(I) or 2(I) chains).	Bone fragility.
Ehlers-Danlos syndrome type I	115	1:20,000–40,000	Autosomal dominant	Unknown	Unknown	Unknown	Unknown	Altered morphology of collagen in skin. Altered mechanical properties of skin.
Ehlers-Danlos syndrome type II	115	1:20,000–40,000	Autosomal dominant	Unknown	Unknown	Unknown	Unknown	Altered morphology of collagen in skin. Altered mechanical properties of skin.
Ehlers-Danlos syndrome type III	115	1:5000–10,000	Autosomal dominant	Unknown	Unknown	Unknown	Unknown	Altered morphology of collagen in skin. Altered mechanical properties of skin.
Ehlers-Danlos syndrome type IV	115	1:100,000	Autosomal dominant (possibly rare autosomal recessive)	COL3A1	2q31-q32.3	Point mutations, deletions, insertions	Type III procollagen, unstable, poor secretion, abnormal structure	Tissues rich in type III collagen—skin, vessels, GI tract, uterus.
Ehlers-Danlos syndrome type V	115	Very rare	X-linked recessive	Unknown	Unknown	Unknown	Unknown	Altered morphology of collagen in skin. Altered mechanical properties of skin.
Ehlers-Danlos syndrome type VI	115	Rare	Autosomal recessive	Lysyl hydroxylase	Unknown	Unknown	Lysyl hydroxylase enzyme deficiency	Lax ligaments, vessel and globe fragility.
Ehlers-Danlos syndrome type VII	115	Rare	Autosomal dominant	COL1A1, COL1A2	COL1A1 at 17q21.3-q22, COL1A2 at 7q21.3-q22.1	COL1A1, COL1A2: deletion of exon 6 by splice junction mutation	Failure to convert procollagen to collagen	Marked joint instability.
Ehlers-Danlos syndrome type VIII	115	Rare	Autosomal dominant	Unknown	Unknown	Unknown	Unknown	Abnormal collagen structure in dermis and severe periodontal disease.
Ehlers-Danlos syndrome type IX	115	Rare	X-linked recessive	Unknown	Unknown	Unknown	Intracellular copper accumulation and defective function of some copper enzymes	Bladder diverticula, skeletal dysplasia.
Ehlers-Danlos syndrome type X	115	Rare	? Autosomal recessive	Fibronectin	2q	Unknown	Defective platelet binding	Joint laxity, bruising.
Marfan syndrome	115	1:10,000	Autosomal dominant	Unknown (COL1A2, very rare)	(7q-COL1A2)	Small insertion in COL1A2	Insertion in pro 2(I) chains	Aortic dissection.

SUMMARY TABLE (continued)

Name of disease	Chap. no.	Frequency	Mode of inheritance	Mutant gene product	Chromosomal location	Expression		
						Altered DNA structure	Disturbed protein function	Disrupted cell and organ function
Part 17: Connective tissues (continued)								
Stickler syndrome	115	1:20,000	Autosomal dominant	COL1A2	7q21.3-q22.1	Unknown	Unknown	Early degenerative joint disease. Vitreal degeneration.
Achondrogenesis type II	115	Rare	New dominant mutation	COL2A1	12q14.3	Unknown (probably point mutations)	Thermal instability of type II collagen	Poor secretion of abnormal molecules.
Epidermolysis bullosa, recessive dystrophic form	115	1:50,000	Autosomal recessive	Collagenase	Unknown	Unknown	Increased activity	Blistering with scar formation.
Hypophosphatasia	116	1 in 100,000 live births for severe forms; mild forms more common	Autosomal recessive (severe forms) Autosomal dominant (mild forms)	Probably alkaline phosphatase (bone, liver, kidney isozyme)	1p (provisional)	Unknown; allelic variation likely	Deficient activity of the tissue nonspecific alkaline phosphatase isoenzyme	Decreased hydrolysis of phosphoethanolamine, inorganic pyrophosphate, and pyridoxal 5'-phosphate in extracellular fluid. Accumulation of inorganic pyrophosphate. Defective skeletal mineralization.
Carbonic anhydrase II deficiency syndrome (osteopetrosis with renal tubular acidosis)	117	Unknown; rare except in the Middle East	Autosomal recessive	Unknown	Unknown	Unknown	Quantitative deficiency of carbonic anhydrase II	Defect in bone resorption produces osteopetrosis, defect in urinary acidification produces metabolic acidosis; cerebral calcification is late consequence. Growth failure and mental retardation common.
Part 18: Muscle								
Duchenne-Becker muscular dystrophy	118	~1:3500-4000 male births	X-linked	Cloned; total length c. 2×10^6 base pairs, with around 60 exons	Xp21	Gene deletions of varying length account for at least half of all cases; duplication and disruption by translocation also recorded	Specific protein 'dystrophin' characterized by reverse genetics techniques. Absent in most classic Duchenne cases. Reduced in some milder cases with "Becker" phenotype	Skeletal and cardiac muscle primarily involved; to a lesser extent smooth muscle and CNS. Dystrophin is localized in sarcolemmal membrane (and perhaps in triad regions of myofibrils).

Emery-Dreifuss muscular dystrophy	118	Unknown	X-linked	Unknown (not allelic to DMD)	Xq28	Unknown	Unknown	Muscle involvement, in particular cardiac and skeletal.
Myotonic dystrophy	118	5–15:100,000	Autosomal dominant	Unknown	19q	Unknown	Unknown	No primary defect identified. Widespread involvement of many organ systems, in particular muscle (skeletal, cardiac, smooth) CNS, endocrine organs.
Facioscapulohumeral muscular dystrophy	118	Unknown	Autosomal dominant	Unknown	Unknown	Unknown	Unknown	Skeletal muscle principally involved.

Part 19: Skin

Albinism, oculocutaneous, autosomal dominant type	119	Rare: 2 kindreds	Autosomal dominant	Unknown	Unknown	Unknown	Unknown	Decreased melanin. Secondary: decreased visual acuity. Susceptibility to solar-induced skin changes.
Albinism, ocular with deafness	119	Rare: 2 kindreds	X-linked recessive	Unknown	X	Unknown	Unknown	Decreased melanin in eye. Secondary: decreased visual acuity. Ear: sensorineural hearing loss.
Albinism, oculocutaneous, rufous type	119	? Caucasians; has been observed in U.S. Caucasians and blacks. Prevalent in New Guinea natives and African blacks	Autosomal recessive	Unknown	Unknown	Unknown	Unknown	Reduced eumelanin, increase in pheomelanin. Secondary reduced visual acuity.
Albinism, ocular, X-linked type	119	1:180,000 Caucasians occurs in U.S. blacks	X-linked recessive	Unknown	Xq22.1	Unknown	Unknown	Reduction of melanin in eye with abnormal melanin bodies in eye and skin. Secondary decreased visual acuity; decussation defects in optic neuronal tracts.
Albinism, oculocutaneous, tyrosinase-negative type	119	1:39,000 U.S. Caucasians 1:28,000 U.S. blacks 1:15,000 Irish	Autosomal recessive	Tyrosinase	Unknown	Unknown	Absent enzyme activity	Absence of melanin. Secondary decreased visual acuity. Decussation defects of optic and otic neuronal tracts. Susceptibility to squamous-cell carcinoma of skin.
Albinism, oculocutaneous, tyrosinase-positive type	119	1:36,000 U.S. Caucasians 1:15,000 U.S. blacks 1:3000–4000 African blacks 1:140–240 in S.W. Amerindians	Autosomal recessive	Unknown	Unknown	Unknown	Unknown	Reduced melanin formation. Secondary decreased visual acuity. Decussation defects in optic and otic neuronal tracts. Susceptibility to squamous-cell carcinoma of skin.

SUMMARY TABLE (continued)

Name of disease	Chap. no.	Frequency	Mode of inheritance	Mutant gene product	Chromosomal location	Altered DNA structure	Expression	
							Disturbed protein function	Disrupted cell and organ function
Part 19: Skin (continued)								
Chédiak-Higashi syndrome	119	? Reported in all major races	Autosomal recessive	Unknown	Unknown	Unknown	Unknown	Defect in lysosomes and lysosomal-like organelles including melanosomes. Secondary: susceptibility to infections and lymphoreticular malignancy. Decreased melanin and visual acuity. Abnormal decussation of optic and otic neuronal tracts.
Albinism, ocular with lentigines and deafness	119	Rare: 1 family	Autosomal dominant	Unknown	Unknown	Unknown	Unknown	Decreased melanin. Eye: decreased visual acuity. Ear: sensorineuronal deafness.
Albinism, ocular, autosomal recessive type	119	1:180,000 U.S. Caucasians	Autosomal recessive	Unknown	Unknown	Unknown	Unknown	Reduced melanin in eye. Secondary decreased visual acuity. Decussation defect in optic neuronal tracts.
Albinism, oculocutaneous, Hermansky-Pudlak syndrome	119	Unknown U.S. 1:2000 Puerto Ricans Prevalent in Indians from Madras, Dutch, and Swiss	Autosomal recessive	Unknown	Unknown	Unknown	Unknown	Reduced melanin, accumulation of ceroid in lysosomes with restrictive lung disease, granulomatous colitis, kidney failure, cardiomyopathy, and storage pool–deficient platelets. Secondary reduced visual acuity. Decussation defects in optic and otic neuronal tracts. Susceptibility to squamous-cell carcinoma.
Albinism, oculocutaneous, platinum type	119	1:200,000 U.S. Caucasians	Autosomal recessive	Tyrosinase	Unknown	Unknown	Reduced enzyme activity	Reduction of melanin. Secondary decreased visual acuity; decussation defects of optic and otic neuronal tracts. Susceptibility to squamous-cell carcinoma of skin.
Albinism, oculocutaneous, brown type	119	Occurs in Afro-Americans. 1:10,000 Ibos of Nigeria	Autosomal recessive	Unknown	Unknown	Unknown	Unknown	Moderate reduction in melanin. Secondary reduced visual acuity; decussation defect in optic neuronal tract.

Disorder	Page	Frequency / Epidemiology	Inheritance	Protein	Chromosomal location		Defect	Description
Albinism, oculocutaneous, yellow mutant type	119	1:180,000 U.S. Caucasians Higher in Amish	Autosomal recessive	Tyrosinase	Unknown	Unknown	Reduced enzyme activity	Reduced eumelanin formation. Secondary decreased visual acuity; decussation defects in optic and otic neuronal tracts; susceptibility to solar skin damage.
Albinism, oculocutaneous, minimal pigment type	119	? 6 Caucasian families in U.S.	Autosomal recessive	Probably tyrosinase	Unknown	Unknown	Reduced tyrosinase activity	Decreased melanin formation. Secondary decreased visual acuity; decussation defects in optic and otic neuronal tracts. Susceptibility to solar skin damage.
Xeroderma pigmentosum	120	1:250,000	Autosomal recessive	Unknown	Unknown	Unknown	Unknown	Defective repair of ultraviolet and chemical carcinogen damage to DNA leading to actinic carcinogenesis and neurologic dysfunction.
Part 20: Intestine								
Congenital sucrase-isomaltase deficiency	121	~200 cases ~2% frequency of heterozygotes in white Americans 4–10% frequency of homozygotes in Greenland and among Canadian Eskimos and Indians	Autosomal recessive	Unknown	3q25-q26	Unknown	Absent or deficient sucrase and isomaltase activities; defective homing of pro-sucrase-isomaltase from the endoplasmic reticulum to the brush borders (polymorphism possible)	Deficient intestinal digestion of sucrose, of linear oligo-1,4-α-glucanes and of α-limit dextrins.
Congenital lactase deficiency	121	Not more than 40 cases	Autosomal recessive (?)	Lactase	Chromosome 2	Unknown	Absent or deficient enzyme activity	Deficient intestinal digestion of lactose. Severe manifestations.
Congenital (?) trehalase deficiency	121	10–15% among Greenland Eskimos; one or two families elsewhere	Autosomal recessive	Trehalase	Unknown	Unknown	Absent or deficient enzyme activity	Deficient intestinal digestion of trehalose.
Lactase persistence (LAC*P) and restriction (LAC*R) polymorphic phenotypes	122	5–90% for LAC*R depending on ethnic group	LAC*P autosomal dominant; LAC*R recessive	Lactase (or regulator of activity) LAC*P is the variant in *H. sapiens*; LAC*R is the variant in Caucasians.	Unknown (chromosome 2?)	Unknown	Decreased lactase activity in LAC*R	Deficient intestinal digestion of lactose, after weaning.